CURRENT TRENDS IN TREATMENT IN PSYCHIATRY

CURRENT TRENDS IN TREATMENT IN PSYCHIATRY

Edited by

T G Tennent DM FRCPsych
Medical Director
St Andrew's Hospital
Northampton

PITMAN MEDICAL

First Published 1980

Catalogue Number 21-3593-81

Pitman Medical Limited
57 High Street, Tunbridge Wells, Kent

Associated Companies:

Pitman Publishing Pty Ltd, Melbourne
Pitman Publishing New Zealand Ltd, Wellington

British Library Cataloguing in Publication Data

Current trends in treatment in psychiatry.
   1. Psychiatry — Congresses
   I. Tennent, T G
   616.8'91   RC475

ISBN 0-272-79596-8

Printed and bound in Great Britain
at The Pitman Press, Bath

PREFACE

Postgraduate education in psychiatry is a sadly neglected area. Opportunities for even the most conscientious consultant to keep up with the change in opinions, drugs and treatment techniques that have occurred in psychiatry are few and far between and too many of the symposia and meetings that consultants are invited to attend are specifically promotional venues for drug companies or the presentation of original papers that ignore the different viewpoints against which the paper is set.

This book reports the proceedings of a conference held at St Andrew's Hospital, Northampton, which was organised with the intention of providing consultant psychiatrists both with information regarding the current trends in treatment in various fields of psychiatry and the opportunity of discussing them with acknowledged experts. The format of the conference was somewhat unusual both in that the drug companies who kindly sponsored several of the meetings were able to do so outside the sphere of their own special drug interests but, more particularly, in that the main review papers were circulated to participants four weeks prior to the conference to be read before the meeting.

In order to provoke discussion and to avoid the prevalence of too idiosyncratic a viewpoint, two commentary papers illustrating and expanding each main paper were presented at the meeting. These papers were followed by a reply from the principal speaker and the session was then thrown open to general discussion. Unfortunately in one of the sessions (that of Psychotherapy) the principal speaker did not produce a paper and so the intended discussant speakers had to alter their papers into more free communications which unfortunately, although providing for interesting discussion at the meeting, read less well in book form.

This book then presents the main and commentary papers together with the principal speakers' summation and, as such, provides a short up-to-date review of the literature in a form which could be useful to all consultants and senior registrars looking for a recent conspectus on their acquired knowledge.

In putting together these conference papers and trying to present them in a consistent literary form, I am most grateful to my secretary Mrs A H Gee and to Dr J G Westerman for their assistance. My thanks also to Mr K N Coates who checked all the references.

Gavin Tennent

LIST OF CONTRIBUTORS

A P Bedford
Principal Clinical Psychologist, St Andrew's Hospital, Billing Road, Northampton NN1 5DG, UK

D H Bennett
Consultant Psychiatrist, The Maudsley Hospital, Denmark Hill, London SE5 8AZ, UK

P K Bridges
Consultant Psychiatrist, Guy's Hospital Medical School, London Bridge, London SE1 9RT, UK

A W Clare
Senior Lecturer in Psychiatry, Institute of Psychiatry, De Crespigny Park, Denmark Hill, London SE5 8AF, UK

D Curson
Consultant Psychiatrist, St Andrew's Hospital, Billing Road, Northampton NN1 5DG, UK

P G Eames
Consultant Neuropsychiatrist, St Andrew's Hospital, Billing Road, Northampton NN1 5DG, UK

H C Ferguson
Consultant Psychiatrist, St Andrew's Hospital, Billing Road, Northampton NN1 5DG, UK

F Fransella
Reader in Clinical Psychology, Royal Free Hospital School of Medicine, University of London, 8 Hunter Street, Brunswick Square, London WC1N 1BP, UK

D G Grahame-Smith
Professor of Clinical Pharmacology, MRC Unit of Clinical Pharmacology, Radcliffe Infirmary, Woodstock Road, Oxford OX2 6HE, UK

D E Hawton
Consultant Psychiatrist and Clinical Tutor in Psychiatry, Department of Psychiatry, Oxford University, The Medical School, Oxford, UK

S R Hirsch
Professor of Psychiatry, Charing Cross Hospital Medical School, The Reynolds Building, St Dunstan's Road, London W6 8RP, UK

R McAuley
Consultant Child Psychiatrist, The Royal Belfast Hospital for Sick Children, 180 Falls Road, Belfast BT12 6BE, UK

I M Marks

Professor of Experimental Psychopathology, Institute of Psychiatry, De Crespigny Park, Denmark Hill, London SE5 8AF, UK

A Mathews

Professor of Psychology, St George's Hospital Medical School, Cranmer Terrace, London SW17 0RE, UK

K L K Trick

Consultant Psychiatrist, St Andrew's Hospital, Billing Road, Northampton NN1 5DG, UK

C R M Wilson

Consultant Psychiatrist, St Andrew's Hospital, Billing Road, Northampton NN1 5DG, UK

K J T Wright

Senior Lecturer in Psychotherapy, Middlesex Hospital, Mortimer Street, London W1N 8AA, UK

M Yaffe

Senior Clinical Psychologist, York Clinic, Guy's Hospital, St Thomas Street, London SE1 9RT, UK

CONTENTS

CURRENT TRENDS IN BEHAVIOUR THERAPY

Isaac Marks

Behavioural psychotherapy is a form of treatment of increasing importance for the relief of a wide variety of problems in adults and in children. This psychotherapeutic approach tends to deal directly with clinical problems rather than to solve postulated underlying conflicts. It has been claimed that behavioural methods are based on learning theory, though this is debatable as many of the major clinical advances in the field have been on a pragmatic basis. There is no need to have extensive psychological training to have excellent results with behavioural treatment, as is testified by the good outcomes obtained by psychiatrists and by nurses who form an increasing number of behavioural practitioners (Marks et al, 1977; Marks, Bird and Lindley, 1978).

The roots of behavioural treatment reach back over the centuries. John Locke three hundred years ago initiated the same principle of exposure which is the essence of behavioural treatment today for reducing fears and rituals. That behavioural principles have been known so widely for so long indicates they are rooted in commonsense which is as old as the human species. What is new is that these commonsense principles have been welded together in the past 20 years into a potent therapeutic technology which can relieve several formerly untreatable conditions and holds promise for further advances.

Commonsense is of course not always correct, but it often points to universal processes of human behaviour. Commonsense principles seem disarmingly simple, but they can be notoriously difficult to apply, and it is in this area that behavioural approaches have made major advances. We all know that exercise is healthy, but few of us take exercise. Yet if a dog needs to be taken for regular walks we might walk the soles off our shoes for it. Many people are terribly lonely only yards away from others who long for company, but cannot push themselves to make a first approach. Yet provide an apartment house with a communal room with washing machines and they meet and gradually develop friendships. We know we should go for walks or arrange social contacts, but we

1

don't often act on commonsense until a suitable framework is provided. Behavioural treatment is a framework for applying commonsense to behavioural problems. Anxiety can be overcome more effectively within such a framework than by a simple command to 'pull yourself together' or 'use your willpower'. In some ways behavioural treatment can be regarded as a scientific approach to willpower. It can do for the reduction of anxiety what the dog does for exercise and the communal laundry does for socialising.

Like all treatments, behavioural psychotherapy has indications and contraindications. At present it is probably the treatment of choice in about 25% of all adult neurotic patients presenting at psychiatric hospitals, which means about 12% of all adult patients. The area of applicability is slowly widening, though it is clear that the behavioural approach is not a panacea for all treatments and takes its place alongside other forms of psychiatric management. For successful behavioural treatment appropriate selection is essential. The first question is whether the patient has a problem suitable for behavioural treatment. Behavioural psychotherapy is the treatment of choice for phobic disorders of all kinds including social anxiety (Marks, 1978a).

Compulsive rituals generally respond well to behavioural treatment, as does sexual dysfunction (the various forms of impotence and frigidity), sexual deviations (for example exhibitionism), nocturnal enuresis, and learning problems in children including those found in mental subnormality (Marks, 1978b). For all these conditions behavioural management is probably the first line to be considered today.

In many other conditions behavioural treatment may well be useful, but more controlled work is needed before we can say that it is definitely the approach of choice. Examples are in social skills problems where social skills training has made tangible advances. Obsessive thoughts sometimes respond, and impulse and habit disorders like stammering, hair pulling, tics, and problems of anger control. In appetitive disorders like obesity and anorexia there is a place for behavioural treatment and recent work suggests that behavioural approaches can help morbid grief, nightmares, marital dysfunction of certain kinds, and child abuse (baby battering) (Reavley and Gilbert, 1978). Behavioural management can also be helpful for conduct disorders in children (Yule, 1978).

It is important to note that behavioural treatment has little to offer acute schizophrenia, severe depression or hypomania, or patients who have no clear goals about what they want to get out of treatment.

In selecting patients for treatment by behavioural means it is essential to arrive at clear goals of treatment by consensual discussion, in adults at any rate, and it is very helpful to have measures of outcome based on these. Next, the patient's cooperation in treatment is essential. A lot of management is teaching the patient to help himself, and what he does between sessions as homework can be critical for success. It can be important to involve significantly others in the patient's treatment where they are involved in the pathology in some way, for example in sexual dysfunction or in many obsessive-compulsive ritualisers. The site of treatment also depends on the problem, and in compulsive ritualisers treatment may need to take place in the home at some stage.

Results of Phobic Disorders and Compulsive Rituals

Most behavioural approaches to the treatment of these conditions employ a common principle called exposure. Relief comes from the individual's continued contact with those situations which evoke his discomfort (the evoking stimuli – ES). Clinicians need to search for those cues which trigger phobias and rituals and to confront the patient, given his agreement, with these cues.

The exposure can be carried out in many ways. In desensitisation in fantasy the patient is asked to close his eyes, relax, and imagine himself slowly entering the situation in his mind's eye for a few seconds, then to relax again, then to imagine himself a bit more into the situation, and so on. Desensitisation in vivo involves asking the patient to carry out the same manoeuvres in real life rather than in fantasy.

An alternative strategy would be to ask the patient to close his eyes and imagine himself in the worst possible phobia or ritual evoking situation and to stay there in his mind's eye for up to an hour until he feels better. This is implosion or flooding in fantasy. Neither desensitisation nor flooding in fantasy are used much any longer as in vivo methods are better. In vivo methods consist of asking the patient to enter the real situations that provoke phobias and compulsions and to remain there until they get used to those situations. The more slowly this is done the more it is called desensitisation and the more rapid the approach the more it is called flooding. The usual method now is to expose the patient to the ES as rapidly as he can tolerate and to use longer rather than shorter sessions, 1½ hours being the average session duration of exposure in my unit. With this form of rapid prolonged exposure the average number of sessions required to treat phobics is about 8, obsessive-compulsives about 11.

The current trend is to concentrate on real life exposure without trying to relax the patient and without trying to deliberately increase anxiety. The important point is to maintain contact with the ES without escape. There is no need to engage in any relaxation exercises – these have been shown to be redundant for outcome. There is also no need to try any implosion. Prolonged in vivo exposure is the main modality of treatment employed. Fantasy exposure is only used when there is no easy access to the real life phobic stimuli e.g. with thunderstorm phobics and in some flying phobics.

There is now good evidence that treatment after various exposure methods yields improvement in phobics lasting up to at least 4 years and in obsessive-compulsives up to 3 years (Marks, 1978c). Improvement in phobias and rituals tend to generalise to other aspects of work and social adjustment so that patients increase the range of their leisure activities. What is not changed is the pre-

3

existing tendency of many of these patients to continue to have depressive episodes, but these seem responsive to tricyclic drugs (Marks et al, 1979).

Although we seem to help most phobics and compulsive ritualisers who are co-operative in treatment — and they are the majority — there are occasional failures, as with any treatment. The commonest reason for failure is noncompliance with exposure instructions and if the patient is not willing to carry out exposure treatment then he cannot be expected to change. The second reason for failure can be the presence of severe depression which is responsive to tricyclic drugs after which exposure treatment can be used. However, there is a strong tendency to relapse when the drugs are discontinued, and sometimes the drugs need to be taken for years. The third reason for failure, which is fortunately rare, is when patients who are compliant and not depressed nevertheless fail to habituate despite carrying out all exposure instructions. Why this is so is not clear. Recently it has become apparent that an important aspect of patients' treatment is what might be called self-exposure-homework between sessions. Therapist-assisted exposure during the treatment session is merely the start of the process which the patient has to continue himself. At the end of each session the patient and the therapist together work out goals the patient needs to achieve before the start of the next treatment session. To monitor progress towards these goals the patient keeps a special exposure diary of homework which has been carried out. A detailed description of this and the general way in which exposure is applied appears in my book 'Living with Fear' (Marks, 1978c).

Over the last few years it has also become evident that treatment often has to take place in settings outside the clinic. In many compulsive ritualisers it is necessary to treat the patients in their homes to be sure that improvement generalises from the hospital to the home. Relatives may need to be taught to withhold reassurance from patients who ritualistically request reassurance. Relatives can be excellent co-therapists in helping carry out exposure, providing the patient has agreed beforehand and the therapist has shown the relative what to do. We tell our patients that we are not curing them. Rather, we are giving them a series of coping strategies to deal with their problems, which will have a tendency to return from time to time; the important thing is for patients to nip these tendencies in the bud using the exposure principle.

Some patients manage to carry out their treatment almost entirely on their own once they are shown what to do. Others find it hard to generate therapeutic strategies until they have first carried these out with a therapist. Although they might be shown time and again how to overcome their discomfort they seem unable to apply exposure principles in the absence of the therapist. When we consider that most people have had trivial fears or rituals at some time or another and have managed to nip these in the bud before the problem grows to invade their life space, the question inevitably comes to mind whether the patients we see are those who failed to inhibit the growth of such minor phobias

4

and rituals. Maybe we should think not in terms of why phobias and rituals are acquired but rather why once these are acquired patients have failed to extinguish them. This notion resembles that about the spread of cancer. Cancer cells are regularly produced in the average organism but only spread when immunological and other defence systems fail.

The exposure principle is also applicable to problems which are not classically phobic or obsessive-compulsive. Nightmares are one sample. There are now reports of their being successfully treated by patients being persuaded to tell their story out loud and to write down the bad dream at length, preferably with triumphant endings (Marks, 1978b). Another condition which has been treated in a similar fashion is morbid grief using the method that can be called forced mourning (Ramsay, 1976). This consists of persuading the patient to come into contact with cues which remind him of the deceased, to talk about the deceased, and to carry mementoes of the deceased around with him until the pain finally goes. This can be regarded as a special form of working through grief. There is now controlled evidence that for widows at risk of developing morbid grief bereavement counselling which includes discussion of the deceased is followed by less morbidity than controlled procedures (Raphael, 1977).

Unlike compulsive rituals, obsessive thoughts are much less reliably treatable by behavioural means (Stern, 1978). There are two main approaches to this problem — exposure variants, including satiation and the opposite modality of thought-stopping. The exposure variant consisted of asking the patient to recite his thoughts at length or to write them down ad nauseam. The opposite method of thought-stopping teaches the patient to interrupt his ruminations repeatedly either by shouting 'stop', snapping an elastic band on his wrist, or by shocking himself on the wrist with a portable shock-box. Both these approaches have occasional successes but also many failures.

Social Skills Problems

Social skills (assertive or personal effectiveness) training can help socially anxious subjects by a variety of techniques that expose them to social situations. Subjects are helped to decrease their social fears and, where necessary, develop new interpersonal skills in being pleasant, assertive, or otherwise as the occasion demands. Wide exploration in this field proceeds under labels like behaviour- or role-rehearsal, encounter groups in their manifold forms, and psychodrama. The technology of changing interpersonal behaviour seems to involve a dimension additional to that required in non-personal fears.

Patient populations used in treatment studies of interpersonal problems are not usually well defined, which may account for some discrepancies in findings from various workers. Perhaps advance in this area might be more rapid if patient as well as treatment characteristics were specified in more detail. Unfortunately the phenomenology of these problems has not yet been well

5

worked out. One distinction may be between social anxiety and social skills deficits, with the former requiring treatment emphasis on exposure and habituation to those social situations that cue anxiety, and the latter needing more active social skills training. This distinction makes sense but needs to be tested.

There have been many studies of social skills training in volunteers, usually students (Hersen and Bellack, 1975), but less controlled evidence is available from studies of patients. Before reviewing the latter several volunteer studies are relevant at this stage.

Analogue Studies

Most workers with volunteers report little or no follow-up, though this is crucial for evaluation. One exception is Curran and Gilbert (1975), who treated 35 'date-anxious' students with i) systematic desensitization or ii) social skills training or iii) a minimal contact control procedure. At 6 months follow-up the social skills trained group had superior interpersonal skills to the other two groups in a role-play test of dating, though desensitized subjects had comparable anxiety-reduction.

Practice-dating. This is a promising time-saving procedure for date-anxious students described by Arkowitz and his colleagues (Arkowitz et al, 1975). Only clerical skills were necessary to arrange a program of weekly practice-dates between matched date-anxious men and women. Six dates were arranged over 6 weeks, each time with a different matched partner of the opposite sex, selected at random. Subjects were student volunteers who knew their partners were also volunteers with similar aims. They were told the aim was not to get an ideal partner but to increase dating comfort and frequency. Every week each partner was sent the name and telephone number of the dating partner for that week. The only instruction was that the meeting with the designated partner should occur before the end of the week, and in some studies written reports needed to be returned to the experimenter afterwards.

Results showed that this procedure, which requires no time from a therapist, effectively increases dating frequency of partners *outside* the experiment until 3 months follow-up (Arkowitz et al, 1975). Even at 15 months follow-up, the 60% of the sample who returned a questionnaire continued to report diminution of social avoidance and distress, and improvement of social skill and dating frequency. What was impressive was that most of the post-treatment dates and casual interactions were with fresh partners. Improvement was significantly greater than after a wait list control (Christensen et al, 1975; Kramer, 1975) or than after reading a manual with discussion for enhancing social interaction (Royce, 1975). In women improvement was related to the number of practice dates engaged on in a program which included group meetings, discussion, and behaviour rehearsal (Thomander, 1975). In this population the practice dating

6

effect was not enhanced by procedures such as i) feedback from partners after the date about what they liked and disliked about the subject, or ii) social skills training in weekly group meetings which included modelling behaviour rehearsal and homework assignments, or iii) cognitive restructuring (Royce, 1975; Kramer, 1975).

Caution is needed before extrapolating from these results to psychiatric patients with social skills deficits of a severe kind. The subjects used in these experiments engaged in at least one date a month *before* treatment (Arkowitz et al, 1975). Students who seldom dated were less attractive than those who dated often, women being less socially skilled, and men initiating fewer heterosexual interactions than their high-dating counterparts. However, low-dating men, once they were actually engaged in heterosexual interaction, had a reasonable repertoire of social skills.

Though the result of practice-dating in volunteers who already have a reasonable heterosexual repertoire does not necessarily apply to psychiatric patients with high social anxiety and minimal interpersonal skills, research with practice-dating in patients is worth undertaking.

Controlled studies in patients Argyle et al (1974) taught social skills individually to outpatients who had personality and neurotic problems. Though a combination of modelling, role-rehearsal, and videotaped feedback was not better at the end of treatment than was insight-oriented individual psychotherapy of 3 times longer duration, improvement was more stable in the social skills condition at 6 months follow-up.

In neurotic inpatients Ullrich de Muynck and Ullrich (1972) reported that 30 hours of group training in assertive skills significantly reduced self-rated insecurity at the end of treatment and 6 month follow-up. Comparable patients who were treated for 30 hours with varied methods of individual treatment not directed at social skills showed no significant changes.

Within a sample of patients comprised equally of personality disorders and schizophrenia, Goldsmith and McFall (1975) found 3 hours of individual interpersonal skills training (modelling, rehearsal, coaching, and audiofeedback) to be superior to an assessment-only control group, and to insight-oriented individual treatment. Skills training led to greater change in specific training measures, with evidence of generalisation of improvement outside treatment. However, there was no detailed follow-up.

Percell et al (1974) noted that the addition of role-rehearsal to goal-directed group discussion enhanced improvement in the assertive skills of outpatients. Role-rehearsal produced significantly greater change on self-reported assertiveness, anxiety, and self-acceptance. No follow-up was reported.

In socially inadequate outpatients, Marzillier et al (1976) compared i) 11 hours of systematic desensitisation individually, and ii) the same duration of individual social skills training consisting of role-rehearsal with therapist modelling, and audiotaped feedback, and iii) a 15-week wait-list control. Both social skills training and desensitisation patients improved significantly more than did untreated controls on the range of social contact, while social skills patients also improved more than controls on social activities. Other measures did not change differentially across conditions after treatment. At the 6 month follow-up of half the social skills patients, the increased social activity was maintained.

Another controlled study is by Shaw (1976). She treated 30 chronic social phobics (19 of them men) with 10 sessions of i) social skills training individually, including role-play, or ii) desensitisation in fantasy, or iii) flooding in fantasy. Up to 6 months follow-up patients from all three conditions improved significantly and similarly in their social anxiety, enjoyment of social situations, work, depression, tension, and fatigue.

More superiority for social skills training was reported in a rather different group of 20 patients who were socially inadequate as well as socially phobic (Trower, 1976). These patients were assigned at random to either i) desensitisation in fantasy with a social homework program, or ii) social skills training with the same homework program. Specific deficits improved with both treatments but significantly more with social skills training, which also produced more improvement of reported social difficulties and frequency of social activities up to 6 months follow-up.

Lasting generalisation of improvement outside the treatment setting is an essential criterion for evaluating a new therapeutic method. None of these studies in patients showed a clear and lasting advantage for social skills training over traditional coaching, advising, and setting of homework tasks. A controlled study by Falloon et al (1977) aimed to explore this issue.

In the work of Falloon et al (1977) 51 patients with social skills deficits completed 10 weekly sessions of 75-minute group treatment; 44 patients were followed up for a mean of 16 months. Random assignment was to one of three conditions i) cohesive group discussion during which subjects described their social behaviour, were given advice on anxiety management, and were asked to complete homework tasks between sessions. ii) A role rehearsal condition including all the foregoing plus therapist's modelling of social interactions concerning target situations. iii) A role rehearsal plus daily social homework condition had all the foregoing plus a more structured social homework programme recorded daily in a social diary. In the first 2 conditions patients kept a non-specific diary as a control.

All three conditons produced significant but incomplete improvement at the end of treatment and 16 month follow-up. The two role rehearsal conditions were significantly superior to group discussion on several measures. Patients who completed daily social homework assignments did significantly better than patients who completed control homework, suggesting that the added improvement was due to the homework rather than to compliance. Alcohol and drug abuse patients usually dropped out. The 4 schizophrenics in remission all

8

lost their improvement at follow-up, while patients with other diagnoses retained their gains to 16 month follow-up.

Falloon et al (1977) concluded that though cohesive goal directed group discussion was associated with lasting improvement in social function this effect was enhanced by modelling and role rehearsal of social interactions, and was further increased by graded social homework that involved close contact in the home environment. Though social skills training is a useful therapeutic advance, more work is needed to facilitate transfer of gains from treatment to real life situations.

With a multiple baseline design further useful results in 4 neurotic patients with social skills deficits were reported by Stravynski et al (1979). Social targets improved as skills training was introduced significantly more than did problems which were left untreated, though these too improved later presumably through generalisation, and improvement was maintained over 6 months follow-up.

One type of patient does badly with social skills training — chronic schizophrenics. All 4 in the series of Falloon et al (1977) did badly at follow-up, as did 3 treated by Liverman (1971, personal communication) in the author's ward. Until research produces better lasting results, social skills training is wasted on schizophrenics.

Mixed Neurosis

Controlled-studies of mixed neurotic patients are rare. A large controlled comparison of behavioural and psychodynamic psychotherapy was published by Sloane, Staples, Cristol, Yorkston, and Whipple (1975). They treated 94 mixed neurotic outpatients. These comprised 57 with anxiety states, 26 with personality disorders, and the remainder with a mixture of neurotic problems. Patients were assigned at random to treatment by experienced behavioural or psychoanalytic therapists, or they were placed on a four month waiting list while remaining able to telephone a psychiatrist for help if need be, and being called at intervals by an assistant to assure them they were not forgotten. Each kind of treatment condition was given by one of three therapists for a mean of 14 sessions. Ratings were mainly blind, and in two thirds of cases came from informants as well.

At 4 month follow-up patients from all three conditions improved significantly on target problems; both treatment groups improved significantly more than the waiting list control group. Only behavioural patients improved significantly on work adjustment. By 1 year follow-up most waiting list patients had also received treatment. There were now no significant differences between the 3 groups, though behavioural patients showed a trend toward more improvement on target problems than did waiting list patients. Improvement was maintained to 2 years follow-up. Those patients whose target problems improved also showed improvement in other measures of adjustment. Sympton substitution was not found.

9

Though there were few significant differences between the groups on measures of *outcome,* there were interesting differences in *process* variables in a direction opposite to what might have been anticipated. Behaviour therapists were significantly more empathic and selfcongruent and made more interpersonal contact with their patients than did psychoanalytic therapists — (these variables did not correlate with outcome). Not surprisingly, more talking was done by patients during psychoanalytic sessions and by therapists during behavioural sessions. In both treatment conditions patients who spoke longer improved more. Behavioural therapists were more directive and informative. It is thought-provoking that psychoanalytic treated patients did better where they had received fewer 'clarifications and interpretations' or were more liked by their therapists. The latter finding has often been reported elsewhere as well.

The interest of this careful study lies mainly in its process variables. Few measures of outcome showed significant differences between the 3 treatment conditions, though the trend was for treated patients to do better than waiting list patients and for patients who had 'acting out' disorders on the MMPI to do better with a behavioural approach. As most behavioural treatments have been shown to exert their effect by specific procedures for particular forms of behavioural disorder, a broad approach for a mixed bag of difficulties loaded the dice against finding significant differences, which in fact occurred. Furthermore the waiting list patients had far less therapist contact, and little expectation of improvement, merely marking time until they could receive treatment; thus even the limited superiority of the treated groups could be due to simple therapist contact, rather than to the behavioural or psychoanalytic content of the sessions. The indifferent (though statistically significant) results emphasize the importance of selecting suitable patients for behavioural psychotherapy. Most of the patients in the study of Sloane et al had anxiety states and personality disorders. As yet these have not been shown to respond especially well to behavioural rather than other treatment, despite extensive claims for anxiety-management-training in volunteers (reviewed by Marks, 1977).

Neurotic depression Much is written about the behavioural theory and treatment of depression. Depression is so common and serious as to constitute a major public health problem and several antidepressant drugs have a well established place in their treatment. Drugs have three disadvantages: 1. Improvement from them often takes several weeks to start; 2. drugs have side effects, though most patients tolerate these well; 3. some patients are not helped by drugs. When helpful, antidepressant drugs commonly need to be continued for many months or even for years, suggesting they are damping down the depressive process until it remits naturally, rather than curing the problem. On the other hand, several effective antidepressants are cheap, and little time is needed to prescribe and supervise them.

To be more useful than drugs, behavioural approaches have either 1) to be cheaper than drugs for the same amount of improvement, or 2) to produce

10

greater improvement alone or in combination with drugs, or 3) to help sufferers who do not respond to drugs or do not take them because of side effects. As yet, present behavioural approaches are not specially promising for the management of severe depression.

One idea that has been mooted is that the state known as 'learned helplessness' in animals and in man constitutes a paradigm for clinical depression (Seligman, 1977). However, it has not so far been shown that learned helplessness is associated with the concomitants of serious clinical depression such as guilt, nihilism, suicidal ideas, anorexia, and insomnia lasting at least several weeks. At the moment the common features which have been demonstrated are *brief* blue mood, decreased reaction time and problem-solving ability, and distortion of skill expectancy. Furthermore, these deficits might well be present in many psychiatric states other than depression and this remains to be tested. Because A and B share certain features C does not prove their commonality. C might also be present in D through Z. Seligman has commented (personal communication) that 'model airplanes do not need to make transatlantic flights, they only need to embody the essence of flying in an airplane'. Clinicians might reply that model airplanes cannot fly the Atlantic, and until they do they have little practical significance, as with so many other models.

Because learned helplessness diminishes after experience of mastery or success, these have been suggested as a treatment for clinical depression. However, success or mastery experiences have so far only been shown to be associated with transient improvement in mood and have not been demonstrated to be useful for severe and lasting clinical depression. Furthermore, in phobics and obsessives who improve with exposure treatments which provide many mastery experiences, the tendency to depressive spells remains unchanged (Marks, 1971; Marks et al, 1975). While it is possible that to reduce depression the mastery experiences need to be in specific areas linked to that depression, this remains to be demonstrated. Until the learned helplessness model can be shown either to produce or to alleviate clinical depression its relevance remains dubious. It may be more relevant perhaps to states of chronic apathy such as those found in certain deprived children.

There are occasional case reports of behavioural approaches producing worthwhile results in isolated cases, e.g. by contingency management (Liberman and Ruskin, 1971; Lewinsohn, 1975). A rash of controlled studies has appeared of cognitive, behavioural, and combined approaches in neurotic depression. The results are sobering.

Five studies were on patients (Harpin, 1978; Morris, 1975; Rush et al, 1977; Schmickley, 1977; Shaw, 1977). In only one was an uncontaminated comparison with controls possible at follow-up (Rush et al, 1977), and here there were no significant differences from drugs, even though drugs were given for a shorter time (3 months) than is customary with many clinicians, and the drug group had far more therapist contact. Harpin (1978) found no difference in depression

11

between a cognitive-behavioural and a waiting list condition even at the end of treatment. The other two studies had no follow-up.

Two studies were on volunteers (Gioe, 1975; Taylor and Marshall, 1977). These compared the controls with treated groups only at the end of treatment, never at follow-up. The cognitive group of Taylor and Marshall showed some relapse of depression on the Hamilton Scale at one month follow-up (their Fig. 2).

The largest clinical study to date is that of Rush et al and this deserves more detailed consideration. Forty-one unipolar severely depressed outpatients were assigned randomly to individual treatment with either cognitive behaviour therapy or imipramine 250 mg daily. Treatment sessions were given weekly to a total of 12 for the drug group and a mean of 15 for cognitive behavioural treatment. Cognitive sessions lasted 50 minutes and drug sessions only 20 minutes, so that the cognitive group had a total of 750 minutes therapist time compared with only 210 minutes time for the drug-treated group.

By the end of treatment both groups improved significantly in depression, but cognitive behaviour therapy produced significantly superior results on self-report and *non*-blind therapist and assessor ratings, and had fewer dropouts. At follow-up both groups maintained most of their improvement on self-ratings on the Beck Depression Inventory, though the cognitive group had lost some of their gains. However, differences were no longer significant between patients who completed cognitive or imipramine therapy ($p < .06$ at 3 months and $< .23$ at 6 months), though significantly more drug patients had asked for re-treatment. This is of little consequence as imipramine is cheap and requires negligible therapist time for maintenance. A weakness in the design was that imipramine was terminated after 11 weeks and not continued during follow-up, whereas many clinicians see the need to continue such medication for a longer period, though with minimal therapist contact. The point is emphasised by Beck's comment (personal communication) that patients improved again on re-treatment.

If all patients *including dropouts* are included, the cognitive therapy group had significantly lower scores at three month follow-up than the drug group ($p < .01$). Including dropouts before drugs could act is not a fair trial of drugs, though it does raise the issue of treatment acceptability. In general tricyclic drugs have high acceptability. Where they do not, psychological treatments are worth considering. However, it should be remembered that treatment adherence can be increased by simple measures like involving relatives as co-therapists to give the drug (Blackwell, 1976), and keeping a diary of tablets taken. This is worth a try before giving up drugs, unless the side effects are serious.

Another flaw in the design of Rush et al (1977) is that duration of therapist contact was far longer in the cognitive than in the imipramine patients. It is thus not clear whether the temporarily superior results of cognitive therapy were due to the specifically 'cognitive' component of the treatment, or to the substantial

12

directive therapist contact given to 'cognitive' patients. Spending 350% more therapists' time can only be justified if the results are outstandingly and lastingly better than conventional treatment with tricyclics. This was hardly the case here. Patients were taken into this trial where they surpassed a score of 20 on the Beck Depression Inventory, whose maximum is given as 40 in figure 2 of Rush et al. At 6 months follow up the mean score had decreased from 31 pretreatment to 8 for cognitive, and 12 for imipramine patients, a difference that was well within chance limits ($p < .23$) and it does not seem clinically worthwhile considering the much greater investment of time in cognitive patients. Rush et al mention several further but unpublished studies concerning the value of cognitive therapy for depression. It remains to be seen whether their designs allow more optimistic conclusions.

At the moment behavioural or cognitive methods can hardly be recommended as a routine for neurotic depression. However, there is a case for helping patients with their social problems where such are present in addition to giving them antidepressant medication. Klerman et al (1974) found that depressed women who had already improved on amitriptyline maintained this improvement more in the next year of follow-up if they continued their medication and improved in their social adjustment where they had casework. Outcome was best where they had both.

Also relevant is the finding that three potentially remedial features are associated with vulnerability of working class women to depression: lack of an intimate confidant, rearing of three or more small children unaided, and lack of employment (Harris, 1976). Help with such issues might be therapeutic.

Behavioural methods may have a contribution to make in helping patients solve life's difficulties, but it would be a pity if premature enthusiasm for 'cognitive behaviour therapy' raised unjustified hopes. More realistic would be careful exploration of the respective roles of antidepressant medication and various problem-solving approaches, separately and combined.

Sexual Dysfunction

Sexual dysfunction describes, in the male, failure of erection, premature ejaculation, and failure of ejaculation. In the female sexual dysfunction describes vaginismus and anorgasmia. The approach used by Masters and Johnson incorporates many behavioural components of what we call the sexual skills programme. Emphasis is usually on treating the couple, i.e. the patient and stable partner but there are reports of useful treatments of single partners as well. There is no need to have the elaborate strategy of a dual sex therapist team treating a couple, as one therapist is usually quite sufficient and produces comparable results.

During sex therapy it is important to analyse the problem carefully in some detail with the couple. They need to be able to communicate well with one another, and to have a vocabulary of sexual terms for this purpose. It can be helpful for them to write down their erotic fantasies to improve communications. As with any treatment, details are individually tailored for the patient's particular needs, but they do need to set aside uninterrupted time and privacy for their sexual homework exercises (LoPiccolo, 1975).

At least two principles can be seen at work in sexual skills training programmes. First performance anxiety is decreased by exposure through regular graded practice and by decreasing demand e.g. by having a ban on coitus during particular phases. Secondly, skills are trained by providing information and films and literature. Graded steps are prescribed for specific items of sexual behaviour which have to be carried out as homework. The couple gradually progress from this to more difficult tasks which might include 1) pleasuring exercises e.g. sensate focus in which the sexual partners learn to caress one another in the nude and 2) a written homework diary recording each step of sexual behaviour performed.

For many couples who are uncomfortable with one another's bodies training in the mutual caressing exercises that constitute sensate focus is essential. With these couples are first asked to avoid touching one another's genitals and subsequently engage in gentle caressing. For some couples however, sensate focus is unnecessary when they are already completely comfortable handling one another's bodies.

Particular problems require specific techniques of management. In men, for premature ejaculation the squeeze or pause method is recommended to be carried out by the wife or by the husband. There may be no advantage of the squeeze over the pause technique. Once the pause method has been satisfactorily applied during masturbation it is continued during coitus. For failure of erection, stimulation from the wife is recommended, including teasing while the penis is flaccid. For failure of ejaculation super stimulation is suggested, sometimes with a vibrator.

For primary anorgasmia in women there is now controlled evidence that directed self-masturbation techniques are useful. These are used together with a vibrator, involvement of the husband, and in more general aspects of a sexual skills training programme. For secondary anorgasmia these manoeuvres may also be useful. For vaginismus the emphasis is on gradual dilation of the vagina by using dilators or fingers. Dilation exercises are carried out first by the wife and then by the husband as well. As the dilators and fingers are inserted into the vagina the woman is also asked to contract the vaginal muscles to achieve voluntary control.

Evidence for the efficacy of sexual skills training programmes is now mounting. In general premature ejaculation and vaginismus are fairly easy to treat and anorgasmia is being treated with increasing success (Marks, 1978a). today are exhibitionists and paedophiliacs. In the treatment of these and other deviants there are two main principles. When a fear of heterosexuality is present

14

this needs to be treated as with any other sexual dysfunction. However, if no heterophobia is present — and this is true of many sexual deviants — this aspect does not need special attention.

In contrast, nearly all deviants need special measures to decrease the sexually deviant urge. One useful way is by using various forms of aversion. Though the evidence for the usefulness of electric aversion is reasonable, in recent years this form of aversion has largely been abandoned in favour of using the patient's own self-induced unpleasant fantasy as the aversive cue. This is given the rather pompous term of covert sensitisation. As an example, the patient who is tempted to expose himself is taught to think of himself being arrested in the act and this then reduces the urge. An equally good way of stopping the urge is by stinging himself by snapping an elastic band on his wrist at the same time. He could also use a portable shock box instead. The important point is for the patient to practise repeatedly first with the therapist and then by himself outside the treatment sessions in situations of gradually increasing strength of temptation. This is called cue exposure. Fairly good results can be obtained by using these methods (Marks, 1978a).

Stammering Stammering has been treated successfully in the short term by many diverse methods. Evidence is accumulating however that this improvement can be lasting with behavioural techniques and Howie and Tanner (1978) have shown that significant gains have continued to 18 months follow-up. Patients are taught special forms of breath control so that they can learn to speak only while exhaling using the diaphragm, gradually rehearsing more and more difficult phrases in increasingly anxiety-provoking situations. It can be useful to treat groups of stutterers together allowing them to gain confidence first in group conversations and then to complete speech assignments of their own between sessions paying special attention to those situations that cause them particular difficulty e.g. telephone calls, situations with large audiences etc. At follow-up stutterers have been found to be much more fluent faster and more confident than pretreatment, although their speech is not usually perfect. Even at follow-up fluency is still not automatic and stutterers have to attend to their speech fluency. The results, however, are very worthwhile.

Writers cramp and ticks have been treated successfully by various workers. Treatment involves a form of habit reversal in which as soon as the cramp or tic begins the opposite muscular movements are brought into action to inhibit the pathological movements. Although controlled data on the treatment of this condition is not available, the uncontrolled work is promising.

Problems in children Although the work discussed so far has all been done in adults many of the principles are equally applicable to children. The treatment of phobias, rituals, lack of social skills, and stammering seems to be similar for children as it is in adults. In children there is wide scope for behavioural management not only of these but also of other disorders. Enuresis has been treated very successfully by the bell and pad apparatus, though it is not yet clear

15

that this is superior to simpler rewards for dry nights. Encopresis too has been treated successfully by similar operant methods. In the management of learning problems of childhood, including those in the subnormal, contingency reward methods seem to be definitely indicated, together with modelling of the appropriate responses to be learned. Structuring of the environmental system surrounding the child can be crucial for success (Risley, 1977). Increasing attention is being paid to teaching parents and teachers how to modify their behaviour towards children for the reduction of conduct disorders and the improvement of their learning abilities (Yule, 1978). Mothers who batter their babies can also be taught how to relate more positively to their children by the modelling of maternal behaviour in a wide variety of difficult interactions with the child. Rehearsal is an integral part of this treatment (Reavley and Gilbert, 1978).

Biofeedback Although this area was introduced with great acclaim in the late 1960's, controlled studies were slow to get off the ground. The few now available have produced sobering clinical results that suggest that on the whole the 'magic box' is not especially helpful compared to simpler methods needing no equipment. The infatuation with the field may have more to do with the love of equipment and the paraphernalia of pseudoscience than with demonstrable benefits for patients. This is not to deny the scientific advances which may eventually come out of this field, but at the moment practising clinicians can largely ignore it.

In the treatment of phobic patients true biofeedback of autonomic symptoms such as heart rate has not been found to be clinically useful. In each of 2 carefully controlled studies, although biofeedback significantly decreased heart rate during exposure in vivo, this effect did not generalise to enhancing the rate of decrement of subjective anxiety, skin conductance, or respiratory rate, at least in the short term (Nunes and Marks, 1975; 1976). Intensive training did not improve results. As Lang (1975, p. 20—21) commented 'while biofeedback may achieve anxiety reduction as a placebo, its ability to inhibit anxiety directly has not yet been shown'.

The addition of EMG feedback adds little to relaxation training for the relief of generalised anxiety (Harvey et al, 1977; Lavallee et al, 1977) or of tension headaches (Haynes et al, 1975). While Philips (1977) found that tension headaches were more relieved by EMG biofeedback than by pseudobiofeedback, no comparison was made with straightforward relaxation, which is the crucial comparison for clinical practice.

In migraine headaches relaxation training had comparable effects to those of biofeedback of fingertip temperature (Blanchard et al, 1978). This type of biofeedback was slightly less good than that of vasoconstriction of extracranial arteries (Friar and Beatty, 1976) in reducing the number of major migrainous attacks, but in this study no comparison was made with non-biofeedback controls.

For drug abuse in students 2 controlled studies have examined the value of biofeedback training of alpha EEG and of EMG (Lamontagne, 1975 and 1977), but the overall results in terms of reduced drug use compared to that in controls were unimpressive, except among medium drug users in the second study.

Overall, the promise of biofeedback for behaviour therapy remains in the future if at all. It is still not generally a useful tool for today's clinician.

Ward-based Behaviour Modification Procedures

These have largely been used for the rehabilitation of chronic schizophrenics. Most of the work has consisted of contingency management, largely in the form of token economies, and a huge literature exists on the subject, with but few carefully controlled trials with follow-up. In one such trial Baker et al (1977) compared contingent with noncontingent tokens, and found that both groups of schizophrenics improved in social withdrawal, but with few symptomatic changes. The authors concluded that contingent tokens were not responsible for changes. A problem in the design was that both groups had contingent *social* reward, and this may have led to their limited gains. Paul and Lentz (1977) in a large controlled study compared traditional treatment with milieu treatment and also with social learning combined with a token economy. The behavioural method achieved marginally more gains for a slightly lower overall cost. We can conclude that so far the large research effort has not found behavioural methods to be a great advance in the management of chronic schizophrenia.

Occasional benefits have been reported for the use of token economies in individual case studies, e.g. in a phobic with chronic personality disorder (Marks, Cameron, and Silberfeld, 1970) and in an autistic compulsive ritualiser (Lindley et al, 1978). However, these programmes are expensive to mount in terms of time and energy and it is by no means clear which types of problems in adults are especially responsive to such an approach. In children, on the other hand, the approach may have much more to offer, e.g. for the management of conduct disorders, educational problems, and mental handicap.

In summary, when applied to appropriate cases, behavioural management has a great deal to offer in certain types of problems. It can be regarded as one aspect of psychiatric management which can be given successfully by a wide range of caring professionals from different backgrounds, provided that they are sensitive clinicians and familiar with the principles of practical management, which is more important than an erudite knowledge of esoteric phenomenological theory.

COMMENTARY TO CURRENT TRENDS IN BEHAVIOUR THERAPY

Andrew Mathews

Professor Marks' erudite and wide ranging review has left few areas of behavioural therapy undiscussed. In commenting on such a comprehensive survey it seems appropriate to focus on only some of the topics raised, chosen for their special theoretical and clinical importance or potential for future development. I will therefore limit myself to specific areas — all of which have been touched on already, but all of which I believe could be usefully developed further. These include the role of exposure in the treatment of phobic patients, the results of marital/sexual therapy, the status of cognitive treatment for depression, and some recent extensions of behavioural treatment into general medicine. Before dealing with these specific areas however, I would like to outline some comments on the nature of behaviour therapy and the skills required to practise it.

The Nature of Behavioural Psychotherapy

Einstein has been quoted to the effect that 'common-sense is that collection of prejudices which is acquired by the age of eighteen'. Creative scientific advances, in other words, often require the rejection of earlier 'common-sense' ideas. Rather than relying on common-sense, behavioural techniques are largely guided by objective evidence of results. It is therefore in the use of objective measurement and empirical experiment that behavioural therapy is distinguished from alternative schools of psychological treatment. Results of this methodology have often confirmed common-sense principles but not by any means invariably so. Common-sense would not obviously lead to obsessional patients being systematically contaminated with the very thing they avoid or phobic patients being flooded with fantasies of the things they most fear. Empirical study shows that contrary to early fears both procedures are usually more helpful than harmful.

If behavioural psychotherapy relies heavily on empirical findings, is there any need for theory? In the past, psychological theories (and not just theories of learning) have made vital contributions to developing new behavioural techniques and there seems no reason to suppose that this process will not continue (examples include desensitisation, modelling, operant learning, social skills training, etc.). For the clinician to remain ignorant of psychological research and theory would thus needlessly restrict the inflow of ideas and theoretical concepts necessary for treatment innovation, although such ideas must also be empirically tested in the clinic. It may not be necessary to have extensive training in psychological theory to be an effective practitioner as nurse-therapists have shown. It remains to be seen however, whether such therapists can develop new methods and adapt to new ideas in the future. As with physical medicine, new treatments sometimes evolve empirically, and before their mechanism is understood, but the doctor would hardly be justified in ignoring new concepts arising from research, whether physiological, biochemical, or psychological.

Behavioural psychotherapy may thus be defined as those treatments that are related to experimental psychological research (as opposed to psychodynamic theory) whether this is in the laboratory or the clinic, and are guided in application by the objective assessment of results.

The Role of Exposure in the Treatment of Phobias

There can be no doubt that systematic exposure to phobic situations is usually beneficial and that most successful treatments for phobias or obsessions utilise this principle. I do not think however, that the evidence yet justifies the belief that exposure alone is both necessary and sufficient for improvement to occur.

Most phobic patients have experienced exposure — often repeated exposure — to phobic situations at a time when their symptoms were developing and worsening. It would therefore be more useful to describe the *type* or *conditions* of exposure that produce improvement rather than deterioration. For example, long continuous exposure is generally better than short discrete periods of exposure, especially in the case of highly feared situations (Mathews, 1978). Even after prolonged exposure, anxiety does not diminish in some patients. In one case of my own, intense fear in a moth phobic continued for many hours during continuous exposure apparently maintained by the unpredictable fluttering of the moth used in treatment. Laboratory research suggests that anxiety levels are partly a function of the perceived controllability or predictability of aversive events so that perhaps it is important that patients themselves control the rate of exposure. Alternatively, phobic situations may need to be held constant for a time if fear is to diminish and before more intense stimuli can be tolerated. In any event, treatment of this patient was facilitated by changing to a larger but less mobile species.

19

Given a constant stimulus situation, it is true that fear nearly always declines although the rate of decline may be slower for very fearful situations. If so, then the more frightening the stimulus the longer the period of exposure required for benefit. In one study of dental phobics however, we found that long periods of imaginal flooding were beneficial only if combined with the imaginal rehearsal of coping behaviour (Mathews and Rezin, 1977). It can be seen therefore, that we need to understand much more about the mechanism of exposure before we can make the generalisation that relief always comes from continued contact with the situations that evoke fear.

Can phobic patients improve *without* exposure to the feared stimuli? This seems unlikely, and in any event it is difficult to show that improvement has occurred until patients stop avoiding phobic situations. However, there may be many different ways in which phobic avoidance can be overcome, not all of which employ exposure during actual treatment-sessions. We have recently developed an effective and highly economic treatment for agoraphobia which does not involve the therapist in exposure sessions, but provides the right conditions for patients to practise by themselves (Mathews et al, 1977). Patients are seen for discussion at home with their spouse and given detailed but simple written instructions on the method of graded practice in going out from home. We also found it useful to incorporate a brief explanation of agoraphobia together with suggestions on the limited use of tranquillisers during practice, and psychological methods of coping with panic feelings. The patients spouse is given guidance as to methods of encouraging, charting, and praising each step in graded practice. Despite the lack of direct therapist involvement with actual practice sessions patients made as much or more progress with this approach than we had previously achieved when therapists carried out flooding or graded exposure themselves. In a further controlled replication of this method, the therapist's time involvement has been cut to about 4 hours, with no loss of effectiveness (Jannoun et al, in press). In this latter study the comparison treatment used as a control procedure did not involve graded practice instructions. Although on average this alternative was significantly less effective it produced some interesting successes which may throw new light on the role of exposure.

The comparison treatment was based on the premise that avoidance could be maintained by high levels of general anxiety. If this general anxiety could be reduced by (for example) solving stressful life problems then phobic avoidance might decrease without special instructions to practice. Despite initial scepticism, in the hands of one therapist this approach proved as effective as graded practice, although in the hands of a second it was distinctly less effective. The pattern of change with the more successful therapist was interesting: at the end of treatment (4 weeks) general anxiety was reduced but avoidance behaviour was not. After 6 months follow-up however, avoidance behaviour had also reduced and had even caught up with graded practice treatment. How can

20

this unexpected result be explained? We might guess that a reduction in anxiety shifts the balance in favour of going out more and that, given time, this shows up as reduced avoidance behaviour. An updated model of agoraphobic behaviour might thus describe avoidance as the outcome of a behavioural decision process in which there are incentive factors (e.g. ability to shop, see friends, etc.) and cost factors (e.g. fear of precipitating a panic attack, social embarrassment, etc.). The probability of going out can be shifted by introducing a new incentive (e.g. pleasing the therapist or spouse) or a reduced cost (e.g. reduced expectation of panic). Of course, there is no reason not to combine both influences within one treatment. So far the evidence suggests that it is usually easier and more effective to concentrate on positive instructions and incentives for real-life exposure, as in our home practice technique. However, the finding of limited success with alternative anxiety-reduction techniques has important theoretical implications for the question of whether an exclusive emphasis on exposure is justified. Further research might therefore be profitably directed towards combinations of anxiety — management and exposure techniques.

Sexual and Marital Therapy

This has been one of the areas in which a major expansion of behavioural techniques has occurred in the last decade. The apparently successful programme described by Masters and Johnson proved difficult to use in British clinics and a less intensive and less costly procedure had to be developed. We have found that once-weekly or even less frequent attendance with couples carrying out graded exercises at home is both practical and effective.

In our own work (Mathews et al, 1976) both instructions for graded practice and discussion of the problems arising from this practice seemed to be necessary for maximum benefit. A further marginal advantage was found for a dual-sex therapy team over a single therapist. One further advantage of the team however, is that therapists feel more at ease and comfortable when working as a pair. Possibly as a result of this they produce a lower patient dropout rate under these conditions.

While some problems, such as premature ejaculation in men can be treated quite successfully with the appropriate behavioural techniques (in this case, the 'squeeze' or 'start—stop' technique of stimulation), other problems have proved more difficult. One such difficult problem is that of loss of sexual interest and enjoyment in women. Examination of the type of patient seen in our series suggests that the emphasis by Masters and Johnson on achievement of orgasm as the main criterion of success may be misleading. In the vast majority of female referrals to an NHS clinic the main complaint was of a complete loss of sexual interest and/or enjoyment with lack of orgasm as only a part of the problem. Indeed, in some patients, sexual contact may be avoided despite the occurrence of orgasm when intercourse does take place. The main components common to the treatments used with this problem include the following:

(a) A complete prohibition on intercourse and other anxiety-arousing aspects of love-making in the early stages of therapy.
(b) Instructions for practice in mutual caressing with effective communication of likes and dislikes in a relaxing atmosphere.
(c) Gradual approach to genital stimulation and intercourse at a rate controlled by the female partner.

Although self-stimulation (masturbatory training) is a useful technique with some women, for many others this remains quite unacceptable and in our experience it is counter-productive to persist with this approach if it is rejected after a reasonable period of discussion. Some preliminary evidence suggests that low doses of androgens may add to the effects of behavioural treatment alone in these problems, although this finding requires replication (Carney et al, 1978).

The precise mechanisms operating in this relatively complex treatment remain unclear. Although anxiety reduction via education, reassurance, and exposure may be seen as one component, there are several reasons for believing it is not sufficient. In many female patients anxiety is not apparent while interest and enjoyment are completely lacking. It is difficult to disentangle the effects of other aspects of the marital relationship from sexual problems, and a greater general understanding between partners may facilitate sexual response. Hence we have consistently found that very poor marital relationship ratings (i.e. independent of sexual aspects) predicted poor response to treatment. So too did a pre-treatment rating of patient's partner as 'unattractive'.

Despite the complexities involved in understanding the mechanisms of treatment within a relationship, there are now a number of controlled outcome studies which establish that behavioural methods of treating sexual dysfunction are effective. Significant superiority on at least some outcome measures have been shown over a wait list control group (Munjack et al, 1976) and over imaginal desensitisation (Carney et al, 1978). In combination with negotiated contracts specifying mutually agreed changes in behaviour going beyond sexual difficulties, these techniques have also proved successful with more general marital/sexual problems, and are as or more effective than interpretative conjoint therapy (Crowe, 1978).

When marital problems or conflict are the main target a number of studies have now substantiated early claims that behavioural treatment is effective. The main components of these methods are:

(a) Specification of marital conflict in terms of specific behaviours (general complaints such as 'he does not love me' being translated into the behavioural cues for this feeling, e.g. 'he never says I look nice' etc.).
(b) Training couples to be more specific and honest in communicating their likes and dislikes to each other.
(c) Practice in problem-solving exercises in which the couple are guided towards compromise solutions; each partner accepting changes in their own behaviour that are the subject of a written contract.

(d) Partners then keep records of success in meeting the contract terms so that this can be discussed in subsequent sessions.

Although based on a simplistic model of the marital relationship as a behavioural bargain, results of such treatment are encouraging. Probably the most convincing data so far is from Jacobson (1978) who contrasted a behavioural contracting procedure with a similarly structured non-directive treatment, and a wait-list control. Behavioural contracting proved superior both in terms of the observed positive behaviour changes and a questionnaire report of satisfaction. Comparisons with interpretive psychotherapy have not as yet produced very convincing differences, although the trend is in favour of the behavioural approach.

In view of the relationship between poor marital relationship and the outcome of treatment for sexual dysfunction, further developments may involve combining marital counselling with other treatments. Although marital improvement does not in itself change phobic or obsessional symptoms (Cobb et al, in press), such improvement is likely to make the spouse's involvement in other treatments both easier and more effective.

Cognitive Treatment of Depression

In commenting on this developing area, Professor Marks describes results so far as 'sobering' and suggests that enthusiasm for cognitive methods may raise unjustified hopes. Clearly there is as yet no unequivocal evidence that cognitive therapy is more effective than alternative methods but my own reaction is that results so far are more encouraging than sobering. The comparison with drug therapy by Rush et al (1977) is the key study since all other controlled studies are with mildly depressed volunteers. Rush et al treated severely depressed out-patients using methods developed by Beck that combine both cognitive and behavioural components. Patients are given homework tasks aimed at increasing satisfying activities, but are also taught to identify and monitor specific thoughts that appear to make their mood worse. These thoughts (typically negative self-judgements) are then tested by the patient and therapist in collaboration using such methods as systematic observation and experiment in an attempt to gather evidence to the contrary. The method can be clearly distinguished from more direct thought-manipulation techniques, such as thought-stopping, which do not attack the cognitive *content*. Cognitive therapy as described by Beck involves an interactive exchange between therapist and patient and would seem to require more specialised training and clinical skill.

The criticisms that have been advanced against the results of Rush et al include the following points:

(a) Cognitive therapy patients had more therapist time (12½ hours) than drug patients (3½ hours).

(b) At six months follow-up the superiority for cognitive therapy was no longer significant.

(c) Assessors were not blind to treatment group.

(d) Drug treatment is cheap, and more expensive alternatives must be shown to be better rather than just equivalent.

(e) Drug dosage used may not have been optimal for all patients or continued long enough.

In considering the first criticism, it may be worth bearing in mind that in earlier comparisons of imipramine and psychotherapy, using similar dosage levels, *no* significant effect of psychotherapy on measures of depression but a highly significant benefit from the drug have been found. Such studies suggest that the amount of the therapist's time in contact with the patient does not in itself have any significant influence on severe depression. With respect to the lack of significant differences at six-month follow-up, bearing in mind that 68% of drug-treated patients received further treatment in the follow-up period compared with 16% of cognitive therapy subjects, it would seem that no firm conclusions can be drawn. The lack of blind assessment is certainly regrettable, although standardised self-report measures have typically been found to correlate quite closely with independent psychiatric assessment.

Finally, even if it were true that the alternative drug treatment used was cheaper and might be further improved, this does not seem relevant to the question of whether cognitive therapy is effective or not. Cognitive therapy is moderately difficult and expensive to deliver, but it appears to do something. Drug treatments have their own disadvantages in terms of acceptability, compliance, and need for chronic administration so that a psychological alternative that is more expensive in the short term may not turn out to be so in the end. Further evaluation is clearly necessary if only because treatments found effective in the hands of enthusiastic innovators often fail to replicate, but it might reasonably be claimed that cognitive therapy today is in a similar stage of development as was exposure treatment a decade ago. The major controlled study at that time was that of Gelder, Marks and Wolff contrasting desensitisation with dynamic psychotherapy. In this comparison it was psychotherapy that took longer to complete and differences between treatments were also significant only at the end of treatment and not on follow-up. Assessors were intended to be blind but the authors stated that 'it was impossible to prevent them learning the nature of the treatment'. Self-ratings by the patient, therapist, and assessor all agreed closely however, so that this did not seem a major problem, as noted earlier. There is no intention to equate two very different studies but rather to suggest that in ten years' time the techniques of cognitive therapy may well be as established and refined as exposure treatments have now become.

Behavioural Medicine

One of the objections to the cognitive-behavioural methods discussed in the previous section is that the alternative drug treatments are more economic. It was argued that even if true, it did not imply that cognitive behavioural treatment was ineffective; but would none the less be an important consideration in favour of drugs for the busy clinician. A telling disadvantage of drug treatment however, is the problem of low compliance rates, averaging about 50% for out-patients. It is only recently that the importance of the patient's own behaviour for the success of pharmacological or other treatments has been fully appreciated, but this belated realisation has resulted in a new growing point, sometimes termed 'behavioural medicine'. This term refers to the application of behavioural methods to the problems of physical medicine; such as low compliance with medical advice, the treatment of psychosomatic disorders, and of chronic illness behaviour.

It has often been assumed that high rates of treatment adherence can easily be obtained by educating patients about the advantages of compliance and the dangers of non-compliance. However, a number of research studies have cast doubt on this assumption. In fact, raising anxiety to a high level without at the same time providing precise behavioural instructions about how risks may be reduced can sometimes be counter-productive. Haynes et al (1976) provide evidence of the relative ineffectiveness of education alone in a study of hypertensive men. Individual interviews designed to increase their knowledge of medical risks and explain the need to take medication failed to significantly increase adherence to treatment on follow-up. In a subsequent study, those men found to be non-compliant were again randomly allocated to experimental or control groups. Experimental patients were offered a brief behavioural programme involving the following components:

(1) Patients were encouraged to monitor their own BP and were asked to chart this together with a record of medication taken.
(2) Interviews were used to establish daily habits that could cue pill-taking and the medication regime was tailored so as to cause minimal disturbance in the patient's life.
(3) Self-charted records were reviewed briefly at fortnightly intervals when high compliance was praised, or the regime re-tailored if necessary.

After six months 70% of the experimental patients showed both increased compliance and decreased BP while only 11% of the controls showed similar changes. Comparable results have been reported with other patients being advised to keep to special diets or following rehabilitation programmes after myocardial infarction. It seems probable therefore, that relatively simple behavioural methods can lead to a significant increase in compliance rates, although the increased cost of these methods in professional time requirements must also be borne in mind.

On the other hand, there are some patients in whom excessive compliance with medical treatment and advice may be more harmful than beneficial. In such patients the reaction to a chronic physical complaint or handicap is that of excessive dependence on medical care; and the physician's response to such dependence may serve to reinforce illness behaviour (e.g. persistent complaints, medication demands, and helplessness). Early reports described this syndrome in a proportion of chronic pain patients, but the concept has been subsequently broadened to include a proportion of all patients with physical handicaps and psychosomatic disorders. The general programme developed by Wooley et al (1978) for a psychosomatic ward includes a number of common components:

(a) Illness behaviour is no longer reinforced by displays of excessive concern by relatives, or medication on demand from clinicians.

(b) A rehabilitation plan is negotiated with the patient who takes an active role in specifying behavioural goals which then become the main treatment target (e.g. increased activity, return to work, etc.).

(c) Steps taken towards these goals are monitored and encouraged by staff, family, and fellow patients.

Although no fully controlled trial has yet been reported, a systematic study of chronic psychosomatic patients before and after the introduction of such a behavioural programme in a ward setting provides strong grounds for optimism (Wooley et al, 1978). Following the programme, patients showed significant reductions in physical complaints and increases in reported achievements, which were partially maintained at one year follow-up. Surprisingly, the presenting diagnosis was not obviously related to outcome but patients without intact families were significantly more likely to relapse while those returning to families either maintained or improved their functioning during follow-up.

In a final example of behavioural medicine there are some instances when medical care may itself constitute a stressful life-event as is the case with major surgery. It has long been established that recovery from surgery tends to be more rapid if patients are adequately prepared psychologically for the after-effects of surgery. Recent research provides additional evidence that training in cognitive-coping methods may be as, or more effective in reducing the adverse consequences of medical stress. These methods involve an initial discussion to establish which aspects of the forthcoming event are stressful for the patient and then to encourage the rehearsal of alternative anxiety-relieving thoughts about the same events. For example, depending on individual preferences patients could learn to relax and focus on the beneficial aspects of a stay in hospital or on positive thoughts about the skill of the hospital staff to counteract fearful thoughts. Although similar cognitive techniques (termed anxiety management training) have been advocated with anxious psychiatric patients, there have been no controlled clinical studies in this population. The best evidence that anxiety management training helps to reduce stress thus comes from studies of surgery or similar medical procedures (Langer et al, 1975; Kendall et al, 1979), where it has been shown to reduce both subjective anxiety and pain as well as decreasing the hospital stay and analgesics required.

As indicated in the introduction this commentary has been deliberately selective and has ignored large areas in which behavioural treatments have much to offer. I hope however, to have shown that the behavioural approach is far from being narrowly confined by its origins in conditioning theory; but is in the process of healthy expansion guided on the one hand by psychological research and on the other by controlled clinical enquiry. As to future prospects, I anticipate that the coming decade will see an accelerating rate of application to interpersonal problems, disorders of mood, and the many psychological aspects of general medicine.

COMMENTARY ON CURRENT TRENDS IN BEHAVIOUR THERAPY

Anthony Bedford

In addition to Professor Marks' thorough and comprehensive summary about which Professor Mathews rightly comments that few areas of Behavioural Therapy were left undiscussed, we have now heard Professor Mathews' own detailed and topical analysis of a number of important and controversial areas of the review article. In the face of this, it would seem to be superfluous, and indeed rather difficult, to add a great deal of any merit to the points already covered. Furthermore, in common I suspect with a number of my colleagues involved in commenting on later review papers, I find it impossible to suggest that specifically clinical applications have been less than adequately covered.

It would, however, perhaps be helpful to expand on other areas covered by the review, some of which have a somewhat parochial aspect from our viewpoint and in particular, behaviour modification procedures based in institutional settings. I should like to extend this to a discussion of design in clinical research into behaviour modification and some more general issues in this field. Some brief specific points about biofeedback and its excursions into medical psychology may also usefully be made.

Behaviour Modification

In view of the very wide application and enormous (and expanding) literature in the area of ward based behaviour modification procedures as well as (not least) this hospital's particular involvement with these methods, it would be worth expanding on Professor Marks' review comments in this area. Recent submissions to the DHSS for the formulation of ethical guidelines for behaviour modification suggest that 40% of hospitals use these methods, the majority being for chronic psychiatric patients.

Token economy programmes specifically seem to have occupied a fairly steady 8% of behaviour therapy literature (Ciminero et al, 1978) in the period

28

1970–1976, the highest figure for a specific approach behind desensitisation, modelling/behaviour rehearsal, and positive reinforcement. In spite of this, and in spite of the implications involved in such a large therapeutic effort, it is the case that very few good controlled evaluations of token economy procedures in particular, or behaviour modification programmes in general, have been carried out.

One example of such an evaluation which has given rise to a number of articles by Hall, Baker and others, and which was discussed by Professor Marks, has been carried out in a traditional setting with chronic schizophrenic patients. The essential novelty of this approach is that it has tried to use a standard experimental group vs. control design (and done so), rather than intra subject comparisons, or experimental within-group designs as in Ayllon and Azrins' (1968) original work.

Hall et al (1977) have summarised, with reference to a large number of sources, the various methodological issues that need to be satisfied for token economy research, and have proceeded to carry out an experiment on a 12-month treatment phase with long term follow-up, which contains adequate measures or controls for all these factors. The result has been to isolate the actual procedure of contingent token payment for analysis and it has been found wanting. It is the case that contingent social reinforcement was used in both control and experimental groups, but the study would have lost any scientific credibility without this. Unfortunately, what is relevant scientifically is not always so from a clinical point of view and there are numerous features of interest in this study unrelated to the main finding of no significant difference overall between token and control groups. For example, the most useful measures in two relevant therapeutic areas show continuing improvement after treatment. These were the social embarrassment and social withdrawal factors of the Wing Ward Behaviour scale and two psychiatric scales. Three of these showed no improvement during the main study. An explanation for this is not immediately forthcoming, but the authors produce the quite modest assertion that 'the research programme did not maximise therapeutic effectiveness as far as symptomatic change is concerned'. Speculation as to the cause of the finding is somewhat unproductive, but the relevance is undeniable: most of the early evidence on chronic schizophrenics indicated failure of behaviour after removal of behavioural pressures (e.g. Ayllon and Azrin, 1968) and although many studies claim response maintenance (e.g. Heap et al, 1970) the precise role of the reinforcement contingencies in these measures is not clear (Kazdin and Bootzin, 1972). One tends to be forced to the conclusion in this case that maintenance of therapeutic change was achieved by continuity of social and ward pressures (Paul, 1969a). Marks et al (1968) indicate, in examining controlled studies, that the more active the control treatment the less marked is the superiority of the token approach: in this case, the apportioned effect of tokens appears to have been non-significant as regards behavioural level overall though they affected the

29

rate of acquisition of behaviour. Hall et al (1977) themselves specified the factors they felt to be responsible for therapeutic changes, which included social reinforcement, nurse-patient relationship, informational feedback on performance, nursing attitudes and expectations, and levels of social stimulation. None of this, however, is an explanation for the subsequent *improvement* in scales which showed no change during the treatment period.

The experiment does cast some doubt on what exactly is going on in ordinary uncontrolled token economy programmes. On the one hand no one is surprised that contingent social reinforcement is effective in producing therapeutic change but on the other, no one is surprised that non-contingent social stimulation produces change (Wing and Brown, 1970). A considerable amount of evidence has accumulated that non-target behaviours, which have no contingent relationship to tokens, change under the influence of a token programme, frequently in areas that have apparently little direct relationship to the targeted behaviour (e.g. Maley et al, 1973; Gripp and Magaro, 1974): conversely, behaviours which are apparently related show no change (e.g. Ferritor et al, 1972).

These findings again are not unduly remarkable when viewed from a non-operant point of view, but only when tokens are considered as specific secondary reinforcers in an operant system.

If it is accepted that token economy programmes do have some positive effect frequently over and above milieu and traditional treatments (e.g. Olson and Greenberg, 1972; Paul and Lenz, 1977) it is by no means clear on what theoretical foundation this is based. Hall et al (1977) provide a comprehensive list of what every token economy programme should have (except tokens) and these amount in sum to environmental stimulation, both physical and social, some form of structured prompted goal orientated and rewarded purposive framework, and optimism (from Staff). Kazdin (1975) points out that until relatively recently token economies were explained by operant principles: failures were failures in implementation. He goes on to suggest that work by Winkler and others (e.g. Winkler, 1971) shows that patient performance in a token economy depends at least in part upon notions from economic theory. He cites firstly the 'consumption schedule' describing the relationship between income and expenditure — individuals who have low income spend a greater proportion of that income than individuals with high income; secondly, 'Engels Law' that as income increases the proportion of total expenditure spent on urgent needs decreases, whereas expenditure on luxuries increases; thirdly, the responsiveness of consumer demand to price changes ('the elasticity of a demand curve').

This economic model appears to provide the sort of specific testable hypotheses that are required for analysis of token systems. Consumption schedules imply that at least three methods of increasing token earning behaviours and token income are available: prices of back-up reinforcers can be increased, value of tokens can be decreased, and the range of back-up reinforcers can be increased. Turning to demand characteristics in response to price change, the generally inelastic nature of necessities — that is, that a price increase tends to reduce demand relatively little for these items — would suggest that the price of necessities relative to luxuries should be high to stimulate spending. This type of prediction can be usefully made and tested, whereas operant principles, although making useful predictions about contingencies and rate and style of reinforcement, fail in this as regards expenditure, earnings, and performance. It is clear, however, that the economic model is only a model and that the underlying principles are still not clearly elucidated from an operant point of view.

A number of questions emerge from this, some of which I hope to consider separately. The first, and clinically most important, relates to aim: to what extent can what we know now about behaviour modification of this type be applied in different areas in an efficacious manner? The second, and generally more important, has to do with the foundation of behaviour modification overall, and methodology: in what way is this type of programme to be investigated usefully in the future, and to what extent can specific factors be isolated using traditional experimental design? Furthermore, how far can behavioural treatment now be considered from the viewpoint of operant approaches alone?

The situation is illustrated by a recent uncontrolled study by Elliott et al (1979) that looked at the relative importance of social reinforcement and other token related variables in maintaining improvements brought about by the token system. This concluded in a paragraph that is worth quoting in full: 'Perhaps the greatest importance of the complete token system is that it is this total regime and this alone that provides a clear structure within which nurses can function to bring about continued improvement. Although social reinforcement may theoretically be all that is required for behaviour change, this study suggests that without a more rigid structured system like the full token economy 'package' such behaviour change is not in evidence.'

It seems clear that clinical applications and research into token economies part company at this point. The same thing was also suggested ten years ago (Paul, 1969b). Unfortunately, Yates (1970) concluded in a major review that 'behaviour therapy is fundamentally distinguishable from other therapeutic efforts by one mark only: the application of the experimental method to the understanding and modification of abnormalities of behaviour'. These problems relate to a longstanding debate on the subject of design in clinical research which has general applications to behaviour therapy, and which I should like to consider somewhat later in this discussion.

Some issues relating to procedural aspects of token economies such as generalisation and maintenance might be usefully looked at in relation to developments of these methods in groups other than chronic psychiatric patients.

31

Token Economy Programmes with Other Groups

After the initial development of token economy programmes for use with chronic psychiatric in-patients, there has been a rapid proliferation of such programmes in institutions and in the community, many applied to non-psychiatric patients and indeed many to normal individuals. The particular population that I should like to discuss is adolescent delinquents, a group in whose treatment token economies have played a particularly large part. The trend appears to have started in the late 1960's, especially in the USA and in Canada and the first major programme was the Case Project (Cohen, Filipczak and Bis, 1968). This utilised a token economy in an institutional setting for young offenders aged 13—19. The main emphasis was on academic, social, and self-help skills; effectiveness in these areas earned tokens to be exchanged for what were essentially luxuries and privileges. Of 41 boys spending an average of eight months in the programme, 56% had committed further offences at three-year follow-up as opposed to 76% of a control group, while standardised achievement test improvements had been maintained.

The Kansas Achievement Place programme (Phillips et al, 1971) aimed to modify and develop the social abilities of young delinquents and attempted to achieve generalisation of this to their natural environment. This has been the model for a large number of other token economy programmes, including ones in this country (e.g. Brown, 1977). The mainstay of the system are the 'teaching parents' who are responsible for the development and maintenance of a behavioural treatment programme in a family setting.

Most of the North American programmes provide a fairly extensive range of basic amenities rather than allow these to be earned: this may well be the result of the Wyatt vs. Stickney case in 1972 which laid down that American law would not tolerate forced patient labour devoid of demonstrable therapeutic purpose. Without going into the details of the extensions of this precedent, the result is the barring of privileges being made conditional on the performance of work within a hospital and, to quote the legal analysis, 'that the items and activities that are emerging as absolute rights are the very same items and activities that behavioural psychologists would employ as reinforcers — that is "contingent rights"'' (Wexler, 1973). Presumably, the delinquent programmes carry over from the in-patient psychiatric systems since most delinquents would not be categorised as 'patients' and would therefore presumably not be subject to the Wyatt ruling.

The programmes used in this Hospital employ a three-pronged system: a basic token economy with tokens delivered non-contingently on a regular time schedule, individual contingent behaviour modification programmes, and a comprehensive social skills training system. This fits with Bandura's (1969) suggestion that the three components necessary for the application of reinforcement principles in a treatment setting were an incentive system, contingent consequences, and a means of establishing appropriate behaviour. The incentive system in this case is set at a level at which earnings buy everything from meals to leave away from the Hospital.

One of the most useful newer developments in token economy programmes is the application of peer group pressures; this has been used in a number of different environments (particularly schools) and has proved to be effective in the control of behaviour. This brings us to the most vexed question of all throughout all behaviour modification programmes, that of response maintenance and transfer. There is no doubt that some results in this area have been alarming. Our own findings with young schizophrenics suggest that, although behaviour is acquired rapidly it is also lost rapidly (cf. Hall et al, 1977) but preliminary findings on behaviour disordered young people look somewhat different. To generalise this to a delinquent group in particular would be inappropriate as the evidence for slow but more maintained learning under a token system is best shown in a group of behaviour disordered individuals whose disturbance is in the context of either organic or developmental impairment. Kazdin (1975) stresses nine factors some of which have been shown to aid response generalisation. These include intermittency and fading of tokens and replacement by social reinforcement, manipulation of reinforcement delay and, interestingly, the use of self (or covert) reinforcement with self-instruction moving towards self-control and cognitive approaches to behaviour control.

In purely practical terms it again appears that token economies provide a useful structure in which to carry a particular approach: in this case, the replacement of maladaptive behaviour based on the acquisition of self-care and social skills. This compared exactly with the conclusion mentioned earlier in Elliott et al's (1979) study on chronic schizophrenics: neither would deny the utility of the package but it is doubtful whether any unitary operant model can explain what is going on within it.

Since the same methodological problems arise across the whole range of institutional behaviour modification systems, it might now be appropriate to turn to a problem affecting all aspects of behavioural treatments.

Methodology and Design in Clinical Research

The key to the experimental issues that I would like to raise can be summarised in two points: firstly, the one mentioned earlier (Yates, 1970) and echoed by many others that the distinguishing characteristic of behaviour therapy is the experimental scientific approach in both analogue and clinical studies and secondly, that a necessity exists for finding a theoretical basis that is capable of generating testable hypotheses. As has been discussed earlier, operant theory has been unfruitful in a number of aspects of token economy research and, whilst it may be profitable at this stage to view token programmes in terms of other models (such as the economic one), this is not going to be helpful in the long run from a theoretical point of view.

Good behaviour therapy practice, therefore, is not intended to be merely a case of providing a control group for every eventuality but of trying to weld a clinical treatment procedure into a theoretical background and to test hypotheses relating to the background.

The fundamental theoretical basis of behaviour therapy in general has been and in the main still is learning theory but the elaborations of this have not remained at a wholly operational level. Insofar as Eysenck's (1967) theory makes multi-level predictions from socio-psychiatric through conditioning to physiological bases it has had enormous heuristic value in the analysis and treatment of behaviour disorders. In the area of the psychophysiological bases of neurotic behaviour disorder this theory has been the only serious contender for many years until Grays' (1975) contribution that has tied in and together a number of loose ends and has extended the range of the theory further into neurophysiology. There is little doubt, in my view, that the future of behaviour therapy is intimately connected with the development of such unifying theories and the evidence to support them. This particular theory has an enormous and central quality covering, as it does, the mechanisms of the learning process, and the laws of learning elaborated as early as Hull and Spence (e.g. Spence, 1956), and carrying on through to the Russian work (e.g. Zhorov and Yermolayeva-Tomina, 1972). In spite of this, however, it is not in itself sufficiently elaborated to cover the entire range of behavioural applications and so leaves gaps at both the sociopsychiatric end (thus applications) and at the neurophysiological end. Supposing that this particular Unifying Theory is temporarily espoused, to what extent can clinical methodology be tailored to have at least some connection with a central basis? Eysenck (1971) has stated that the apparent oversimplification and partial nature of the theory of behaviour therapy 'is an inevitable price to be paid for attempting to approach this field scientifically' and indeed the argument of scientific vs unscientific is beginning to rank with nature vs nurture as a sterile controversy. What is required, in extension of a point made previously, is a clinical research methodology that allows reliable and relevant data gathering (thus not just relating X and Y because it provides an aura of scientific credibility) and allows such data to be utilised in a theoretical model.

Yates (1976) compares three research strategies in some detail: these include factorial group design, operant therapy techniques, and the experimental study of the single case. On balance, he concludes that the last of these is most useful for practising behaviour therapists in that it supplies a general methodology applicable to all presenting problems but that all the methods have merits and disadvantages. Cochrane and Sobol (1976) in a thoughtful analysis of behaviour therapy research provide a breakdown of 118 studies by therapeutic technique and problem area taken from four behaviour therapy Journals for 1973. The major division is into operant methodology and another, but traditional design. Unfortunately, a heavy reliance is placed on analogue studies and studies of social-interactive behaviours. The former may well not adequately reflect a clinical entity (Bernstein and Paul, 1971) and seems to place 'hard' behavioural techniques at a disadvantage to 'soft' techniques, whereas clinical studies appear to generate the opposite impression. Borkovec and Rachman (1979) justify analogue studies at least partly on the grounds of the utility of these studies in their own right but acknowledge generality of results as a relevant issue on clinical grounds.

Cochrane and Sobol's (1976) article ends with a lengthy summary of recommendation for design and reporting of behaviour therapy experiments most of which almost every clinician would find acceptable and equally most of which ignored in the reporting of studies: the recommendations relate, in the main, to the traditional or operant designs used in the majority of studies examined.

In summary, the conclusions to be drawn seem to be that a number of methods are rigorous and acceptable for within-study design. Of these, the single case methodology as originally developed by M B Shapiro (e.g. Shapiro, 1961) is the most effective way available to a clinician to be able to make a research contribution to the elucidation of a specific clinical issue; it differs from operant design in that control is not merely being demonstrated over a piece of behaviour but more importantly that the *way* in which control is achieved conforms to an initially generated hypothesis.

Until such time as the Unifying Theory and the developments of neuropsychology mesh to put behaviour research entirely out of business clinicians will need a personal methodology as well as the more traditional factorial group design, and it would therefore appear not to be possible satisfactorily to spread one methodology across the behaviour therapy board. For the continuity of this form of treatment as a specific entity, the single case method may eventually prove to be the differentiating factor; furthermore, a point well made by Yule and Hemsley (1977) in a review of single case technique in medical psychology it is necessary, in moving behaviour therapy into new areas such as this, to provide a tight individual framework within which to develop without losing sight of the original objectives.

Biofeedback, Relaxation and Medical Psychology

I should like to conclude with some short and selective remarks directed towards biofeedback (to which the final sentences of the previous section have particular relevance) and towards the use of relaxation techniques.

Professor Marks' comments on biofeedback are largely well made as there is no doubt that this area has been disappointing. Nevertheless, in spite of the vast number of poorly controlled and inadequate studies some evidence is beginning to accumulate that at least the principle of feeding back biological information to an individual can be of assistance. Almost all the useful applications are highly specific — the opposite end of the spectrum from, for example EEG biofeedback. An example of this is the neuromuscular retraining of foot drop in stroke patients. Burnside (1979), in re-assessing and replicating adequately Basmajian et al's (1975) methodologically unsound study, appears to have concluded that the procedure genuinely does work, and encopresis has been treated by improvement of sphincter control using biofeedback (Engel et al, 1974). A similar result was obtained by Kohlenberg (1973) who used biofeedback with reinforcement of successful responses. A further excursion into medical psychology, again related to biofeedback, is a summary of a series of studies by Engel and others (Engel, 1977) in which he argues cogently for the application of operant conditioning techniques to the control and analysis of cardiovascular function in non-psychiatric patients. This is in direct distinction to the very unsatisfactory results obtained in anxious patients and perhaps stresses the relevance of fine focus in the biofeedback procedure.

Relaxation (progressive or otherwise) is enjoying a new lease of life after having been shown to be non-essential in desensitisation. Applications include cue-controlled relaxation in the control of psychomotor seizures (Wells et al, 1978), the development of a 'relaxation response' for use in anxiety management, and the possibility that prolonged relaxation training may have very different effects from the brief process normally used. As yet, only case studies seem to be available (e.g. Boudreau, 1972) but no doubt a controlled study will soon be forthcoming.

All these areas are on the developing fringe of behaviour therapy and offer new and challenging applications. It is to be hoped that sobriety will prevail in the methodology with which such new applications are researched.

RESPONSE TO COMMENTARIES BY PROFESSOR MATTHEWS AND MR. BEDFORD

Isaac Marks

I would like to say how much I enjoyed the discussion papers of Professor Matthews and Mr. Bedford, I found them enormously interesting and am only sorry there is not much to disagree with. I agree with most of the points made though sometimes with a slight difference in emphasis. I agree fully with the need for objective measurements not only in behavioural treatment, but in health care in general and medicine in particular. Certainly, this is one of the hallmarks of behavioural treatment as it is of a lot of other forms of therapy. We certainly need to have theories for innovation but we need constructive, useful theories and bad theory can be a great impediment to progress. I would like to submit that we have had a lot of awful theory in this field for quite a long time. It is now time to discard these in favour of something more realistic. Many of these theories are, in fact, quite irrelevant to the clinicians daily practise with patients and a lot of them perhaps merely give us the feeling that we know what we are doing. Many are mythologies, religions at whose altars we are worshipping without much relevance to clinical practice.

Certainly in behavioural treatment, the clinician does not need to have a high level of knowledge of the so-called theoretical basis in order to be an effective therapist. The question is whether less theoretically trained therapists can get results. Professor Matthews is absolutely correct in saying that we need theory for innovation; we cannot innovate and really develop the subject on a scientific basis without having reasonable theories. My answer to the question 'Can a clinician without extensive theoretical training get good results?' is yes, yes and yes again, but to the question 'Will people accept this evidence that para-professionals and others get good results?' — my answer is no, no and no again! There is a great deal of evidence over the whole world now, not only in psychiatry of behaviour therapy in particular, that para-professionals can get results as easily as those obtained by people with MD's and PhD's. A recent survey of the reading habits of 257 behaviour therapists showed that 79% of them read the journal 'Behaviour Therapy'. In fact, experimental journals are rarely read by practising clinicians so that the actual behaviour of behaviour therapists does not suggest that they use much theoretical knowledge.

On the subject of lay therapists who do a lot of excellent work without much theoretical training – a group in Philadelphia looked at the treatment of obesity. The subjects were very obese people treated in groups by behavioural programmes. Groups treated by lay therapists who had only a few weeks instruction were compared with groups treated by fully trained psychologists. The drop out rate for the lay therapists was significantly lower than in the groups treated by the PhD trained psychologists; you can draw your own conclusions from that. Generally we do not get *better* results from lay therapists, but we do find they tend to get as good results as the professional therapists.

We now have powerful evidence that phobic and obsessive compulsives, those with sexual dysfunction, sexual deviants and acute hospital psychiatric patients respond as well to treatment by lay therapists and medical auxiliaries as to treatment by professionals. If use is to be made of lay therapists in this kind of way there are all sorts of implications for the structure of the Health Service.

I would like to give you an illustration of a case treated innovatively in the wards at the moment by a nurse. By the time I came to the ward round the nurse had already worked out a programme, without previous instruction. This was a case unique in my experience, and perhaps in any of your experiences. This was a lady of 24 years who was sent to me as never having had a normal bowel action in her life. She had had manual evacuation of faeces performed under anaesthetic on numerous occasions. She had been investigated for Hirschsprung's disease and had had so many contacts with doctors of various kinds, that she had an enormously thick wad of notes. This lady came into the ward and she was admitted with the idea that maybe a behaviour programme might help. She had been in hospital for a few days by the time I saw her for the first time on a ward round, and by then the nurse on the ward had already, on her own initiative, worked out a programme of treatment which was very innovative because this was a totally new case. Now, three months later, the patient consistently maintained normal bowel actions for the first time in her life.

We have found repeatedly that therapists trained without a highfalutin' theoretical base can be very good innovative clinicians. Of course, this varies, as it does for all clinicians and some of our nurse-therapists are more innovative than others.

As regards the bases for behaviour modification, Kozdin emphasised the current determinants of behaviour rather than the ancient history of what happened with Mum, Dad and Siblings. Emphasis is on overt behaviour change. Specific target problems are defined and treatment is measured by what's happening with the patient. First let us take the point that Professor Matthews made, that exposure may not always be necessary for successful treatment of phobias and compulsions. There are quite a number of exceptions to this rule, exceptions where a non-exposure condition results in phobia – or ritual-reduction. Most of us are aware of cases where sudden wild abreaction of all emotions, not just fear, results in the patient losing his phobias and rituals. Such events cannot be construed as a straight exposure treatment and the explanation as to why such patients improve is not known. We can speculate, but then, regularly, antidepressants with depressed phobics and ritualisers can reduce their phobias and rituals without any exposure at all.

In a study shortly to appear in the British Journal of Psychiatry we looked at compulsive ritualisers who had behavioural treatment, and in addition had Chlomipramine or placebo. We dichotomised them according to their pre-treatment on the Wakefield and Hamilton rating scales for depression. These patients were not primary depressives, but a group of ritualisers with a scatter of depression scores at the start of treatment. The group that had some depression at the start did significantly better on Chlomipramine than did the placebo group, both before behavioural treatments were brought in and especially afterwards. Chlomipramine thus conferred an advantage before exposure was introduced – it conferred even more advantage afterwards. The non-depressive sub-group did not derive any advantage from taking Chlomipramine, so here's a demonstration of a non-exposure treatment helping to make a significant reduction in phobias and rituals. Why should this be so – who knows?

Clearly the exposure hypothesis is not the start and end of all phobic- and ritual-reduction. We need to modify the exposure therapy. What we need to do is set up a table concerning the two kinds of exposure which occur. On the one hand there is sensitising exposure which is what most patients describe when they come to us giving a history of contact with a phobic situation from which they escape and then get worse. Secondly, there is the habituating exposure which usually occurs in treatment in which patients are exposed to phobic or ritual evoking stimuli in a way which is habituating, and with this most patients tend to get better. So what are the differences between sensitising and habituating exposure? One possible difference is that in sensitising exposure contact is more brief and in habituating exposure contact is more prolonged. Gradually we should be able to work out an equation that predicts whether exposure will desensitise or habituate and that is one of the big theoretical tasks that lies ahead.

Professor Matthews is to be congratulated on his emphasis on home treatment. Certainly this is a direction in which we need to go, not only for phobics and ritualisers but for all kinds of therapy including sex therapy. I liked very much that phrase about 'we can regard the process as a behavioural decision that the patient has to make between the incentives to go out and meet the fears and the costs of so doing'. I think that that encompasses a whole lot of what we know about the situation.

Let us now switch to some of the comments on the sexual disorders. There was that important comment he made namely 'the absence of pleasure in patients with sexual dysfunction is not necessarily due just to anxiety, but has other causes as well'. A question which arises is why poor marital relationship leads to poor outcome with sex therapy. Is this solely because non-compliance is far more likely, or do other factors operate as well?

With respect to the cognitive therapy of depression, I am more sobered than intoxicated by the results and would be delighted to see some controlled results with follow-up that would make me change my mind. It might be that in ten or twenty years' time cognitive therapies of various kinds may have a lot to offer for depression, but as a practising clinician I would certainly not teach it to the average therapist of any professional background at the moment, I would prefer to wait and see how worthwhile the model turns out to be. Model aeroplanes are intriguing but generally don't fly the Atlantic and I would not recommend people to fly in model aeroplanes but rather to wait until a Boeing 747 was available. We are no way in sight of 747's yet. If I were asked to crystal gaze, it seems to me that the term cognitive therapy is a slight misnomer for where we should be going. Perhaps we should be going for a more general problem-solving approach. I am thinking now of the kinds of results that Weissman et al got with depressives. They found that this approach helped patients to reduce the social difficulties in their lives and seemed to have the consequence of reducing relapse in depression. If we think of George Brown's work with working-class Mums who get depressed when life events are confined with specific vulnerability factors. It would seem to be a logical approach to help such people solve their daily problems by developing their problem-solving skills and I would prefer to go down that road rather than the one that cognitive therapists have taken.

There is a study done by Harpin in my unit, which is not yet published, with depressed patients in whom drugs had failed. He found no significant improvement in mood from a cognitive behavioural approach in seriously depressed chronic patients. It might be argued that cognitive therapy at present is like desensitisation in fantasy, behavioural psychotherapy would be far less interesting than it is now. It was the development of exposure in vivo that led to the real pay-off with phobias and rituals. It may be that cognitive methods will have changed into something radically different before we see real clinical results. With respect to developments in behavioural medicine these are important, I fully agree, and hope that there will be far more in this line. There are now studies reported by Stunkard et al, concerning three towns in California with populations of some 10,000 to 20,000 people. One town constituted a control group. The study involved subjects at risk for hypertension and coronary artery disease. In the control town the incidence of coronaries from the pre-treatment to the post-treatment phase of the follow-up, actually went up slightly over two years. A second town had what one might call a behavioural medicine approach. On the radio, TV and newspaper an educational programme was launched into reducing risk factors, in addition high risk subjects were identified who smoked, had a high-fat diet or were hypertensive. These subjects had individual interviews having behavioural programmes to reduce their smoking, take their anti-hypertensive medication, reduce the fat and salt intake in their diet. After the programme there was a significant drop in the amount of coronary heart disease and hypertension which tended to flatten out in year two. In the third town there was also education by mass media (radio, TV and newspapers) about how to regulate smoking and diet which could affect heart disease, but this third group had no individual interviews of high risk individuals. By the end of the follow-up period of one year, the town mass media instructions alone also had had significant effect but less than in the second town. At year three the second and third towns were comparable. For the whole cohort, the average increase in life expectancy was about five years and in reviewing this work Stunkard comments that all improvements in medicine and health since the beginning of this century in this age group has had four years increase in life expectancy. This little programme of mass media instruction produced a five year increase. There is a whole lot of scope for behavioural medicine in many better ways.

Lastly, we come to the comments about behaviour therapy in institutional settings. So far it does appear to me that maximum therapeutic input of token economies has produced only marginal gains. In future, it might be more profitable to take the direction indicated in the study by Liberman in California where an attempt was made to reduce family emotionality. In view of the ideas that high emotionality produces high relapse rates in schizophrenics, one might consider training families to reduce their level of emotional stress. A promising approach that has already been proved was used by Fairweather et al where they ran an operant conditioning programme in mental hospitals. They found the initial results were very disappointing once the patients were discharged, but when the approach was changed to try to prepare patients for group living before discharge by training them as a group who knew they were going to be discharged, however, into a group home that they could run themselves, the rate of relapse or readmission was far lower and the patients became much more self-sustaining, and took their own medication. These results are more impressive than those of any from token economies. It might well be that token economies have more to offer, as Mr. Bedford was saying, with behaviourally disordered young people rather than with schizophrenics. There may be a large field for exploration here.

References

Argyle, M, Bryant, B and Trower, P (1974) Social Skills Training and Psychotherapy: A comparative study. *Psychol. Med., 4*, 435
Arkowitz, H, Christensen, A and Royce, S (1975) Practice Dating as Treatment of College Dating Inhibitions. *Behav. Res. and Ther., 13*, 321
Ayllon, T and Azrin, HN (1968) *The Token Economy: A Motivational System for Therapy.* New York: Appleton

Baker, R, Hall, JN, Hutchinson, K and Bridge, G (1977) Symptom Changes in Chronic Schizophrenic Patients on a Token Economy: A controlled experiment. *Brit. J. Psychiat., 131,* 381–393

Bandura, A (1969) *Principles of Behaviour Modification.* New York: Holt

Basmajian, JV, Kukulka, CG, Narayan, MG and Takebe, K (1975) Biofeedback Treatment of Foot-drop compared with Standard Rehabilitation Technique. *Archives of Physical Medicine and Rehabilitation, 56,* 231–236

Bernstein, DA and Paul, GL (1971) Some Comments on Therapy Analogue Research with Small Animal 'Phobias'. *Journal of Behaviour Therapy and Experimental Psychiatry, 2,* 225–237

Blackwell, B (1976) Treatment Adherence. *Brit. J. Psychiat., 129,* 513–531

Blanchard, EB, Theobald, DE et al (1978) Temperature Biofeedback in the Treatment of Migraine Headaches. *Arch. Gen. Psychiat., 35,* 581–8

Borkovec, T and Rachman, S (1979) The Utility of Analogue Research. *Behaviour Research and Therapy,* Vol. 17, No. 3, 253–263

Boudreau, L (1972) Transcendental Meditation nd Yoga as Reciprocal Inhibitors. *Behaviour Therapy and Experimental Psychiatry, 3,* 97–98

Brown, B (1977) Gilbey House: A token economy management scheme in a residential school for adolescent boys in trouble. *B.A.B.P. Bulletin,* Vol. 5, No. 3, 79–89

Burnside, IG (1979) Electromyograph Feedback in the Remobilisation of Stroke Patients. Conference Proceedings of International Conference on Psychology and Medicine, Swansea

Carney, A, Bancroft, J and Mathews, A (1978) Combination of hormonal and psychological treatment for female sexual unresponsiveness: A comparative study. *British Journal of Psychiatry, 133,* 339–46

Christensen, A, Arkowitz, H and Anderson, J (1975) Practice Dating as Treatment of College Dating Inhibitions. *Behav. Res. and Ther., 13,* 321

Ciminero, AR, Doleys, DM, Williams, CL (1978) Journal Literature on Behaviour Therapy 1970–1976: Analysis of the subject characteristics, target behaviours and treatment techniques. *Journal of Behaviour Therapy and Experimental Psychiatry,* Vol. 9, No. 4, 301–309

Cobb, J, McDonald, R, Marks, I and Stern, R Which behavioural approach? Marital or exposure treatment for combined marital and phobic-obsessive problems. (In Press)

Cochrane, R and Sobol, MP (1976) Myth and Methodology in Behaviour Therapy Research. In: *Theoretical and Experimental Bases of the Behaviour Therapies.* (Eds MP Feldman and A Broadhurst). London: Wiley

Cohen, HC, Filipczak, JA and Bis, JS (1968) Case Project: In: *Research in Psychiatry,* Vol. 3. (Ed J Schlien). Washington: A.P.A.

Crowe, M (1978) Conjoint Marital Therapy: A controlled outcome study. *Psychological Medicine, 8,* 623–636

Curran, JP and Gilbert, FS (1975) A Test of the Relative Effectiveness of a Systematic Desensitization Program and an Interpersonal Skills Training Program with Date Anxious Subjects. *Behaviour Therapy, 6,* 510

Elliott, PA, Barlow, F, Hooper, A and Kingerlee, PE (1979) Maintaining Patients' Improvements in a Token Economy. *Behaviour Research and Therapy,* Vol. 17, No. 4, 355–369

Engel, BT (1977) Operant Conditioning of Cardiovascular Function: A behavioural analysis. In: *Contributions to Medical Psychology,* Vol. 1. (Ed S Rachman). Oxford: Pergamon

Engel, BT, Nikoomanesh, P and Schuster, MM (1974) Operant Conditioning of REctosphincteric Responses in the Treatment of Faecal Incontinence. *New England Journal of Medicine 290,* 646–649

Eysenck, HJ (1967) *The Biological Basis of Personality.* CC Thomas, Springfield, Illinois

Eysenck, HJ (1971) Behaviour Therapy as a Scientific Discipline. *Journal of Consulting and Clinical Psychology 36,* 314–319

Falloon, IRH, Lindley, R, McDonald, R and Marks IM (1977) Social Skills Training of Outpatient Groups: A controlled study of rehearsal and homework. *Brit. J. Psychiat., 131,* 599–609

Ferritor, DE, Buckholdt, D, Hamblin, RL and Smith, L (1972) The Non-effects of Contingent Reinforcement for Attending Behaviour on Work Accomplished. *Journal of Applied Behaviour Analysis, 5,* 7–17

Friar, LR and Beatty, J (1976) Migraine: Management of trained control of basoconstriction. *J. Consult. Clin. Psychol., 44,* 46–53

Gioe, VJ (1975) Cognitive Modification and Positive Group Experience as a Treatment for Depression. PhD Dissertation, Temple University

Goldsmith, JB and McFall, RM (1975) Development and Evaluation of an Interpersonal Skill Training Program for Psychiatric Inpatients. *J. Abn. Psychol., 84,* 5

Gray, JA (1975) *Elements of a Two Process Theory of Learning.* London: A.P.

Gripp, RF and Magaro, PA (1974) The Token Economy Programme in the Psychiatric Hospital: A review and analysis. *Behaviour Research and Therapy,* Vol. 12, 205–228

Hall, JN, Baker, RD and Hutchinson, K (1977) A Controlled Evaluation of Token Economy Procedures with Chronic Schizophrenic Patents. *Behaviour Research and Therapy,* Vol. 15, No. 3, 261–285

Harpin, E (1978) A Psychosocial Treatment of Depression. PhD Dissertation, Department of Psychology, State University of New York

Harris, T (1976) Social Factors in Neurosis, with Special Reference to Depression. Chapter in Van Praag, HM (Ed). *Research in Neurosis.* Bohn, Schellema and Holkenna, Utrecht

Harvey, DC, Rowan, D and Ross, D (1977) Relaxation Training: 'Is your magic box really necessary?' Paper to BABP, Keele, July

Haynes, R, Sackett, D, Gibson, E, Taylor, D, Hackett, B, Roberts, R and Johnson, A (1976) Improvement of Medication Compliance in Uncontrolled Hypertension. *The Lancet.* June 12th, 1265–1268

Haynes, SN, Griffin, P, Mooney, D and Parise, M (1975) EMG Biofeedback and Relaxation Instructions in the Treatment of *Behaviour Therapy, 6,* 672–678

Heap, RF, Boblitt, WE, Moore, CH and Hord, JE (1970) Behaviour – Milieu Therapy with Chronic Neuropsychiatric Patients. *Journal of Abnormal Psychology, 76,* 349–354

Hersen, M and Bellack, AS (1975) Social Skills Training for Chronic Psychiatric Patients. Rationale, research findings and future directions. *Comp. Psychiat., 17,* 559

Jacobson, NS (1978) Specific and Nonspecific Factors in a Behavioural Approach to Marital Discord. *Journal of Consulting and Clinical Psychology, 46,* 442–452

Jannoun, L, Mumby, M, Catalan, J and Gelder, M A Home-Based Treatment Programme for Agoraphobia: Replication and controlled evaluation. (In Press)

Kazdin, AE (1975) Recent Advances in Token Economy Research. In: *Progress in Behaviour Modification,* Vol. 1. (Eds M Hersen, RM Eisler and PM Miller). New York: A.P.

Kazdin, E and Bootzin, RR (1972) The Token Economy: An evaluative review. *Journal of Applied Behavioural Analysis, 5,* 343–372

Kendall, P, Williams, L, Pechacek, T, Graham, L, Shisslak, C, Herzoff, N (1979) Cognitive Behavioural and Patient Education Interventions in Cardiac Catheterization Procedures: the Pado Alto medical psychology project. *Journal of Consulting and Clinical Psychology, 47,* 49–58

Klerman, GL, Dimascio, A, Weissman, M, Prusoff, B and Paykel, ES (1974) Treatment of Depression by Drugs and Psychotherapy. *American Journal of Psychiatry, 131,* 2

Kohlenberg, RJ (1973) Operant Conditioning of Human and Sphincter Pressure. *JOurnal of Applied Behavioural Analysis, 6,* 201–208

Kramer, SR (1975) Effectiveness of Behaviour Rehearsal and Practice Dating to Heterosexual Social Interaction. PhD Dissertation, University of Texas at Austin

Lamontagne, Y, Hand, I, Annable, L and Gagnon, MA (1975) Physiological and Psychological Effects of Alpha and EMG Feedback Training with College Drug Users. *Canad. Psychiat. Assoc. J., 20,* 337–349

Lamontagne, Y, Beausejour, R, Annable, L and Tetreault, L (1977) Alpha and EMG Feedback Training in the Prevention of Drug Abuse. *Canad. Psychiat. Assoc. J., 22,* 301–310

Lang, PJ (1975) Acquisition of Heart Rate Control. Chapter in Fowles, DC (Ed). Columbia University Press, 20–21

Langer, E, Janis, I and Wolfer, J (1975) Reduction of Psychological Stress in Surgical Patients. *Journal of Experimental Social Psychology, 11,* 155–165

Lavallee, Y, Lamontagne, Y, Pinard, G, Annable, L and Tetreault, L (1977) Effects of EMG Feedback, Diagepam and their Combination on Chronic Anxiety. *J. Psychosom. Res., 21,* 65–71

Lewinsohn, PM (1975) The Behavioural Study of Treatment of Depression. Chapter in Hersen, R et al (Eds). *Progress in Behaviour Modification,* Vol. 1, 19164. New York: Academic

Liberman, R and Ruskin, DE (1971) Depression: A behavioural formulation. *Archives of Gen. Psychiatry, 24,* 515–523

Lindley, P, Marks, I, Philpott, R and Snowden, J (1978) Treatment of Obsessive-Compulsive Neurosis with History of Childhood Autism. *Brit. J. Psychiat., 130,* 592–7

LoPiccolo, J (1975) Direct Treatment of Sexual Dysfunction. Chapter in Money, J and Musaph, J (Eds). *Handbook of Exology,* Amsterdam: APS Biological and Medical Press

Maley, RF, Feldman, GL and Ruskin, RS (1973) Evaluation of Patient Improvement in a Token Economy Treatment Programme. *Journal of Abnormal Psychology, 82,* pp. 141–144

Marks, IM, Cameron, PM and Silberfeld, M (1970) Operant Therapy for an Abnormal Personality. *Brit. Med. J., 1,* 647–648

Marks, IM (1971) Phobic Disorders 4 years after Treatment. *Brit. J. Psychiat., 118,* 683–8

Marks, IM (1977) Exposure Treatments. In: *Behaviour Modification,* 2nd Edition. (Ed S Agras). Little, Brown and Co

Marks, IM (1978a) Behavioural Psychotherapy of Adult Neurosis. In: *Handbook of Psychotherapy and Behaviour Change,* 2nd Edition. (Eds SL Garfield and AE Bergin). John Wiley and Sons

Marks, IM (1978b) Rehearsal Relief of Nightmares, and their Relationship to Rituals, Depression and Temporal Lobe Pathology. *Brit. J. Psychiat., 133,* 461–465

Marks, IM (1978c) *Living with Fear.* McGraw-Hill

Marks, IM, Hodgson, R and Rachman, S (1975) Treatment of Chronic Obsessive-Compulsive Neurosis by in vovo Exposure: A two-year follow-up and issues in treatment. *Brit. J. Psychiat., 127,* 349

Marks, IM, Hallam, RS, Connolly, J and Philpott, R (1977) *Nursing in Behavioural Psychotherapy: An advanced clinical role for nurses.* Royal College of Nursing, Henrietta Place, London

Marks, IM, Bird, J and Lindley, P (1978) Behavioural Nurse Therapists. *Behavioural Psychotherapy, 6,* 25–36

Marks, IM et al (1979) Clomipramine and Exposure for Compulsive Rituals. Submitted for Publication

Marks, J, Sonoda, B and Schalock, R (1968) Reinforcement vs Relationship: Relationship Therapy for Schizophrenics. *Journal of Abnormal Psychology, 73,* 379–402

Marzillier, JS, Lambert, C and Kellett, J (1976) A Controlled Evaluation of Systematic Desensitization and Social Skills Training for Socially Inadequate Psychiatric Patients. *Behav. Res. and Ther., 14,* 225

Mathews, A (1978) Fear REduction Research and Clinical Phobias. *Psychological Bulletin, 85,* 390–404

Mathews, A and Rezin, V (1977) Treatment of Dental Fears by Imaginal Flooding and Rehearsal of Coping Behaviour. *Behaviour Research and Therapy, 15,* 321–328

Mathews, A, Teasdale, J, Mumby, M, Johnston, D and Shaw, P (1977) A Home-Based Treatment Program for Agoraphobia. *Behaviour Therapy, 8,* 915–924

Mathews, A, Bancroft, J, Whitehead, A, Hackman, A, Julien, D, Bancroft, J, Gath, D and Shaw, P (1976) The Behavioural Treatment of Sexual Inadequacy: A comparative study. *Behaviour Research and Therapy, 14,* 427–436

Morris, NE (1975) A Group Self-Instruction Method for the Treatment of Depressed Outpatients. PhD Dissertation, University of Toronto

Munjack, D, Cristol, A, Goldstein, A, Phillips, D, Goldberg, Whipple, K, Staples, F and Kanno, P (1976) Behavioural Treatment of Orgasmic Dysfunction: A controlled study. *British Journal of Psychiatry, 129,* 349–353

Nunes, J and Marks, IM (1975) Feedback of True Heart Rate during Exposure in vivo. *Arch. Gen. Psychiat., 32,* 933

Nunes, J and Marks, IM (1976) Feedback of True Heart Rate during Exposure in vivo. Partial replication with methodological improvement. *Arch. Gen. Psychiat., 33,* 1346—1350

Olson, RP and Greenberg, DF (1972) Effects of Contingency Contracting and Decision Making Groups with Chronic Mental Patients. *Journal of Consulting and Clinical Psychology, 38,* 376—383

Paul, GL (1969a) Chronic Mental Patient: Current Status — Future Directions. *Psychological Bulletin, 71,* 81—94

Paul, GL (1969b) Behaviour Modification Research: Design and Tactics. In: *Behaviour Therapy: Appraisal and Status.* (Ed CM Franks). New York: McGraw-Hill

Paul, GL and Lentz, RJ (1977) *Psychosocial Treatment of Chronic Mental Patients: Milieu vs Social Learning Programs.* Harvard Univ. Press

Percell, LP, Berwick, PT and Beigel, A (1974) The Effects of Assertive Training on Self-Concept and Anxiety. *Arch. Gen. Psychiat., 31,* 502

Philips, C (1977) The Modification of Tension Headache using EMG Biofeedback. *Behav. Res. and Ther., 15,* 119—129

Phillips, EL, Phillips, EA, Fixsen, DL and Wolf, MM (1971) Achievement Place: The Modification of the Behaviours of pre Delinquent Boys within a Token Economy. *Journal of Applied Behaviour Analysis, 4,* 45—59

Ramsay, R (1976) Treatment of Grief. Paper to meeting of EABT, Spetsae, Greece and CBS film

Raphael, B (1977) Prevention Intervention with the Recently Bereaved. *Arch. Gen. Psychiat., 34,* 1450—4

Reavley, W and Gilbert, M (1978) Child Abuse. Talk given at Institute of Psychiatry, London

Risley, TR (1977) The Social Context of Self-Control. Chapter (p. 71—81) in Stuart, RB (Ed): *Behavioural Self-Management.* Brunner/Marel, NY

Royce, WS (1975) Practice and Feedback as Treatment for Social Isolation. PhD Dissertation, University of Oregon

Rush, AJ, Beck, ST, Kovacs, M and Hollon, S (1977) Comparative Efficacy of Cognitive Theory and Pharmacotherapy in the Treatment of Depressed Outpatients. *Cognitive Therapy, 1,* I, 17—37

Schmickley, VC and Johnson, RG (1977) Cognitive Therapy and Research. I. A self-managed cognitive-behavioural treatment for depression

Seligman, M (1977) In: *Psychopathology,* (Eds J Maser and M Seligman). San Francisco: WH Freeman and Co

Shapiro, MB (1961) The Single Case in Fundamental Clinical Psychological Research. *British Journal of Medical Psychology, 34,* 255—262

Shaw, BF (1977) A Comparison of Cognitive Therapy and Behaviour Therapy in the Treatment of Depression. *J. Cons. Psychol., 45,* 543—51

Shaw, P (1976) Three Behaviour Therapies in the Treatment of Social Phobia. Paper to Annual Meeting of BABP, Exeter, July

Sloane, RB, Staples, FR, Cristol, AH, Yorkston, NJ and Whipple, K (1975) *Psychotherapy versus Behaviour Therapy.* Harvard University Press, London

Spence, KW (1956) *Behaviour Theory and Conditioning.* Yale University Press, Connecticut

Stern, RS (1978) Treatment of Obsessive Thoughts: Three Pilot Studies. Paper to European Association of Behaviour Therapy, Vienna

Taylor, FG and Marshall, WL (1977) A Cognitive Behavioural Therapy for Depression. *Cognitive Therapy and Research, 1,* March

Thomander, LD (1975) The Treatment of Dating Problems: Practice Dating Dyenbic Interaction Group Discussion. PhD Dissertation, Michigan State University

Trower, P (1976) Treatment of Social Failure: Effect of Imaginal and Practical Techniques on Two Kinds of Social Problems. Paper to BABP Annual Meeting, Exeter, July

Ullrich de Muynck, R and Ullrich, R (1972) The Effectiveness of a Standardised Assertive-Training Program. Paper presented at the 2nd Annual Conference of the European Association of Behaviour Therapy, Wexford, Eire, September

Wells, KC, Turner, SM, Bellock, AS, Hersen, M (1978) Effects of Cue-Controlled Relaxation on Psychomotor Seizures: An Experimental Analysis. *Behaviour Research and Therapy,* Vol. 16, No. 1, 51–55

Wexler, DB (1973) Token and Taboo: Behaviour Modification, Token Economies and the Law. *California Law Review, 61,* 81–109

Winkler, RC (1971) The Relevance of Economic Theory and Technology of Token Reinforcement Systems. *Behaviour Research and Therapy, 9,* 81–88

Wooley, S, Blackwell, B and Winget, C (1978) A Learning Theory Model of Chronic Illness Behaviour: Theory, treatment and research. *Psychosomatic Medicine, 40,* 379–401

Yates, AJ (1970) *Behaviour Therapy.* New York: Wiley

Yates, AJ (1976) Research Methods in Behaviour Modification. In: *Progress in Behaviour Modification,* Vol. 2. (Eds M Hersen, RM Eisler and PM Miller). New York: AP

Yule, W (1978) Teaching Parents and Teachers. Talk given at Institute of Psychiatry, London

Yule, W and Hemsley, D (1977) Single Case Methodology in Medical Psychology. In: *Contributions to Medical Psychology,* Vol. 1. (Ed S Rachman). Oxford: Pergamon

Zhorov, PA and Yermolayeva-Tomina, LB (1972) Concerning the Relation between Extraversion and Strength of the Nervous System. In: *Biological Bases of Individual Behaviour.* (Eds V Neblitsyn and JA Gray). New York: AP

CURRENT TRENDS IN NEUROPHARMACOLOGY AND PSYCHOPHARMACOLOGY

David Grahame-Smith

The intention of this paper is to pick out certain topics of interest in the clinical pharmacology of psychotropic drugs, to examine some of their basic clinical and pharmacological effects and the relevance of these to their therapeutic action and to the understanding of the abnormalities of brain function present in mental illness and its correction. Lastly this paper aims to consider the relationship between the pharmacokinetic properties, the pharmacodynamic actions, and the therapeutic effects of certain psychotropic drugs with particular reference to the individualisation of dosage schedules and the clinical monitoring of psychotropic drug therapy.

The implications of neuropharmacology in the consideration of cerebral mechanisms of mood and behaviour

It is exceedingly difficult at present to see how the intimate biochemical and pharmacological functioning of the human brain in vivo can be directly investigated. A good deal of the hypothesising that implicates one neurotransmitter or another in the abnormal functioning of the brain which underlies manic-depressive disease and schizophrenia is based on the knowledge of the pharmacological actions of drugs which, largely serendipitously, have been found to have a beneficial effect on these conditions.

Drugs are exogenous molecules that interact with endogenous molecules and set in train a sequence of events by which a biological process is manipulated. When this molecular interaction is put to therapeutic ends a disordered physiological process is either returned to normal or altered in such a way that the symptoms or manifestations of the disease are ameliorated.

Two points follow from this that are relevant to the biology of normal and abnormal mental function which, although self-evident, are nonetheless worth stating:

1. Whatever the rationale for the use of the drug in mental illness, if the drug can be shown by a clinical trial to produce a benefit, then at some level a

47

potentially definable biological process is involved. This does not help very much because it is tantamount to saying that you must have a brain to be mad.

2. It is reasonable to suppose that an understanding of the actions of the drug, whether from studies in man, animals, intact organs, cells, particles, or at the molecular level, might give some insight into the pathological processes involved in the mental illness. There are two corollaries to this which have been used by those interested in this field. *First* when drugs worsen or change the quality of mental illness the study of the actions of such drugs may give insight into the underlying processes (e.g. studies on amino-acid administration in schizophrenia; see Grahame-Smith, 1973).

It is this kind of reasoning which has caused so much attention to be focused upon the role of the brain monoamines noradrenaline, dopamine, and 5-hydroxytryptamine in the mechanisms underlying schizophrenia (Grahame-Smith, 1973; Snyder et al, 1974), manic depressive disease (Schildkraut, 1969; Shopsin et al, 1974; Van Praag, 1974), and the mental syndromes produced by reserpine and psychotomimetic drugs.

TABLE 1(a). Some current shorthand hypotheses concerning the role of monoaminergic function in the causation of mental illness based upon the mode of action of psychotropic drugs

Drugs	Illness	Possible mechanism of action	Shorthand 'aetiological' conclusions
Phenothiazines Butyrophenones Thioxanthenes	Schizophrenia Mania	Dopamine receptor blockade (see Snyder, 1974)	Overactivity of dopaminergic systems
Tricyclic anti-depressants	Depression	Inhibition of presynaptic monoamine reuptake → increased monoaminergic function (see Iversen, 1973)	Decreased monoaminergic function
Monoamine oxidase inhibitors	Depression	Decreased metabolism of monoamines → increased monoaminergic function (see Iversen, 1973)	Decreased monoaminergic function
Lithium	Prophylaxis of manic depressive disease	Increased functional activity of 5-HT (see Green & Grahame-Smith, 1975)	Disturbance in 5-HT function
ECT	Depression	Increased sensitivity to behavioural actions of 5-HT and dopamine (Green & Grahame-Smith, 1976)	Decreased 5-HT or dopamine function or 'sensitivity'

TABLE 1(b). Drugs 'mimicking' certain aspects of mental illness, their mode of action, and conclusions on aetiology

Drug	Clinical effects	Action	Conclusions
Reserpine	Depression	Depletion of brain monoamines (see Iversen, 1973)	Depression 'due to' decreased monoaminergic function
LSD	'Psychotic symptions	5-HT agonist/antagonist (see Grahame-Smith, 1973)	Aspects of schizophrenia due to 5-HT dysfunction
Amphetamine	Syndrome-like paranoid schizophrenia	Dopamine release (see Snyder et al, 1974)	Aspects of schizophrenia due to dopaminergic overactivity

Tables 1a and 1b show some general current hypotheses concerning the pharmacological actions of some of the drugs used in the treatment of mental illness or which produce mental syndromes together with the over-simplified but quite widely held beliefs linking their pharmacological actions to the aetiology of the mental illnesses. The tables do an injustice to the arguments and open-mindedness of the workers propounding the hypotheses but it is these shorthand conclusions that get taken up into the general body of knowledge and pervade our thinking and thus they need critical examination.

There is a serious flaw in this whole approach which might be explained by an artificial analogy. Suppose we knew as little about the pathophysiology of heart failure as we do of brain function in mental illness. Suppose too that by serendipity a powerful diuretic was discovered and used empirically and with benefit in this uncharted syndrome of 'heart failure'. If the mode of action of this drug was then investigated, the investigations would reveal that its action was on the kidney and the conclusion would be drawn quite wrongly that the syndrome of 'heart failure' was due to a *primary* disturbance in renal tubular sodium excretion. We know, of course, this renal tubular functional change is a 'normal' response to the altered haemodynamic state produced by the heart failure and although a renal abnormality is involved, excessive and undivided attention upon it would distract from the primary cause of heart failure.

Consider schizophrenia in this light. There is a very impressive correlation between the ability of phenothiazines and other neuroleptics to block the actions of dopamine in the brain and their antipsychotic potency. In addition the similarity between amphetamine psychosis and paranoid schizophrenia coupled with the actions of amphetamine in releasing brain dopamine also fits into this picture. This has led to the proposition of a 'dopamine hypotheses' for the causation of schizophrenia (see Snyder et al, 1974). It is difficult to be sure exactly what is meant by 'the dopamine hypotheses' of schizophrenia except that it implies that somehow or other a disturbance or 'an overactivity' of dopaminergic neuronal function is involved. This may be so but it would be naive at this stage to consider it a primary disturbance. Theoretically such a disturbance could occur by any of the mechanisms shown in Table 2.

TABLE 2. Possible mechanisms by which an 'overactivity' of dopaminergic function could occur in schizophrenia

1. By an 'overactivity' of a neuronal system relaying through a dopaminergic system, which then itself would be 'overactive' though secondarily so.
2. By decreased function of a system normally inhibiting dopamine function.
3. By an increased firing rate of dopaminergic neurones.
4. By increased synaptic function.
   (a) Increased synthesis
   (b) Increased release
   (c) Decreased metabolism
   (d) Decreased reuptake
5. By increased post-synaptic responses to dopamine
   (a) Increased dopamine receptor sensitivity
   (b) Increased neuronal responses to dopamine
      (i) Changes in biochemical amplification of dopamine's action
      (ii) Changes in neuronal circuitry relaying dopaminergic function.

The neuroleptics could equally well be acting at a secondary level (Grahame-Smith, 1973). Curare would prevent any physical violence ensuing from a schizophrenic paranoid delusion but it would be foolish therefore to invoke a 'peripheral cholinergic hypotheses' as the cause of paranoid schizophrenia. There is nothing in the indirect evidence culled from drug studies that implicates dopaminergic mechanisms in schizophrenia which convincingly shows that an abnormality in dopaminergic function is a *primary* aetiological factor. Indeed, just as the kidney during heart failure responds in a normal physiological manner to the change in the haemodynamic state produced by heart failure, it might be that the dopaminergic systems in the brain are over-functioning as a normal response to some other more fundamental disturbance. The neuroleptics would then dampen down this over-activity without affecting the primary disturbance. This is rather destructive reasoning, particularly when there are few ideas as to what the primary disturbance might be. One can speculate upon two other possibilities. First, one can imagine a disturbance of sub-cortical systems lying at an even more 'primitive' level than the monoaminergic systems but requiring monoaminergic systems for its linkage to cortical functions. Second, a subtle neurohumoral mechanism acting within the brain which alters in a diffuse way the function of monoaminergic systems or the reactivity of neuronal systems to their action.

These are not entirely idle speculations for there are now precedents upon which they may be based. In regard to the first speculation it has been shown that in rats the syndrome of a distinctive form of hyperactivity produced by

50

increasing brain 5-HT levels or by central 5-HT agonists depends for its expression upon brain dopaminergic function. If one interferes with the dopaminergic function pharmacologically either by decreasing brain dopamine levels or by pharmacologically blocking the action of brain dopamine then the pharmacological stimulation of 5-HT receptors no longer brings about the abnormal hyperactive behaviour (see Green and Grahame-Smith, 1974a; Heal et al, 1976). The precedence is therefore set for the dopaminergic function in some way to play a linking or permissive role in the expression of behavioural syndromes produced by the abnormal function of non-dopaminergic pathways.

The second speculation is more hazy but is based upon the effects which small polypeptides, such as thyrotrophin releasing hormone (TRH) (Green and Grahame-Smith, 1974b), melanocyte stimulating hormone, release inhibitory factor (MIF) (Plotnikoff et al, 1972), inhibitors of brain protein synthesis such as cycloheximide, and perhaps ECT have on the behaviour of rats and mice. These effects involve changes in the hyperactivity syndromes produced by raising brain 5-HT levels or by the administration of 5-HT agonists, the hyperactivity syndrome produced by raising brain dopamine levels with L-dopa and a monoamine oxidase inhibitor, pentylenetetrazol produced convulsions, pentobarbital induced sleeping time, and the turning behaviour produced by dopaminergic influences in rats with unilateral nigrostriatal lesions. TRH potentiates the hyperactivity syndromes without having much effect on monoamine synthesis and turnover and shortens pentobarbital induced sleeping time. Cycloheximide on the other hand does the opposite (Green et al, 1976). The actions of TRH on these behavioural syndromes are not mediated by its action on the pituitary to release TSH since its behavioural actions occur in hypophysectomised rats. These phenomena suggest that polypeptides like TRH and MIF may in some way modulate the activity of monoaminergic systems or the response of other neuronal systems to their actions. Inhibitors of protein synthesis like cycloheximide could act either by preventing the synthesis of some neuromodulating polypeptides or by preventing either the release of monoamines or by mediating their action. The changes in brain function brought about by electroconvulsive shock in animals, which is discussed a little later, is also suggestive of a rather diffuse change in the function of monoaminergic systems or in the reactivity of neuronal systems to their action. However unclear the picture may be at the moment there is sufficient evidence to consider systems internal to the brain, possibly mediated by polypeptides, which modulate neuronal activity in monoaminergic systems or systems influenced by them.* If this turns out to be the case then an abnormality in such a neurohumoral control mechanism could result in overactivity or underactivity of the neuronal systems such as those subserved by the monoamines. The cyclic nature of manic-depressive disease, the latency of action of tricyclic

* See section on neuropeptides

antidepressants, the waxing and waning of several psychiatric syndromes, the usual requirement of a course of ECT, are phenomena the time course of which might be explained by gradual biochemical and pharmacological changes requiring more primary changes in protein/polypeptide synthesis.

One can apply the same types of argument to the actions of tricyclic antidepressants, monoamine oxidase inhibitors, and the known effect of reserpine in producing monoamine depletion in the brain, and then to the 'serotonin' or 'noradrenaline' hypotheses of manic-depressive disease. Here again the primacy of the involvement of monoaminergic systems in the aetiology of such conditions is based upon rather shaky evidence. The evidence culled from the action of antidepressive drugs could be equally applied to a monoaminergic function of the secondary level mediating some other primary disturbance. Such abnormalities in CSF monoamine metabolites in depression as have been demonstrated, particularly the low levels of 5-HIAA and its decreased rise on the administration of probenecid (see Van Praag, 1974 and 1977), need not necessarily imply a primary abnormality in monoaminergic function. However, Van Praag's work (1977) showed that 5-HT can alleviate the depressive syndrome and this effect was potentiated by clomipramine (a relatively selective inhibitor of 5-HT reuptake) and that a negative correlation between 5-HT turnover in the CNS and the therapeutic effect of chlorimipramine does go some way towards implicating an abnormality in 5-HT function of a primary rather than a secondary nature. There are though, criticisms of a biochemical nature which can be levelled at the significance of monoamine metabolism (such as 5-HIAA in the CSF [Green and Grahame-Smith, 1975; Bulat, 1977]). Be that as it may, the work which Van Praag has done (Van Praag, 1977) and the work done by Asberg, Traskman and Thonen (1976) does suggest that whatever the reason, there might be alterations in CSF 5-HIAA during depression. Van Praag and his colleagues showed that within a group of patients with endogenous depression the rise in 5-HIAA in response to probenecid was decreased in about 40% of patients. Asberg and her colleagues have shown a bimodal distribution of 5-HIAA in the CSF in depressed patients, one group having very low CSF 5-HIAA levels and the other group more normal levels. In the group with low CSF 5-HIAA levels Asberg and her colleagues showed that the lower the level the worse the depression, and indeed that the incidence of suicide of a violent form was increased in those with the lowest 5-HIAA levels. These findings are extremely important since they suggest that there is a group of endogenous depressives with abnormal 5-HT function/metabolism. It remains to be seen whether this is a primary or secondary phenomenon.

Recently there have been some encouraging studies of the biochemistry of the post-mortem brain, particularly of schizophrenic brain. Monoamine neurotransmitters and their metabolites have been measured in various sites. In addition, new radio ligand binding techniques have been applied to see if there were any changes in dopamine receptors. Although the neurotransmitter and metabolite concentration changes are very much a matter of controversy there is a tantalising possibility, still not definitely proven, that there might be an increase in the number of dopamine receptors in certain brain areas. An influence of chronic neuroleptic treatment, which in animals increases the number of brain dopamine receptors, has not been excluded absolutely.

So much of current psychopharmacology research and therapeutic practice is based upon monoaminergic mechanisms that it is well to ask the question: 'What do these mechanisms do?'

Moore (1971) has summed it up succinctly in a general way: 'Highly integrated neural functions such as those involving thought processes, which are generally considered to take place in cortical structures, may be modified by primitive, chronically active sub-cortical neuronal systems (e.g. limbic and reticular activating systems). Accordingly a dysfunction of these delicately balanced primitive systems may result in derangement of mental processes and behaviour.'

Because we know so little of the functional neuro-anatomy of human thought processes, mood, and behaviour, it is necessary to play the game of association between the effects of drugs in man, the known actions of drugs, the functional neuro-anatomy of animal behaviour, and the effects of drugs with known actions on animal behaviour and to try by this game, by intuitive reasoning and with a fair share of serendipity to come out with some sensible answers. Crucial to all these considerations is the mode of action of the relevant drugs. Green and Grahame-Smith (1976a) have summarised their findings on the mode of action of drugs affecting the processes regulating the functional activity of brain 5-HT lithium, phenytoin, reserpine, phenothiazines, tricyclic antidepressants, dopamine depletors, inhibitors of brain protein synthesis, and electroconvulsive shock which can all be shown to affect the hyperactivity syndrome in rats produced by raising brain 5-HT levels through the administration of a tryptophan and a monoamine oxidase inhibitor or of 5-HT agonists. It is possible to dissect out whether the drugs effect the synthesis, compartmentation, release, reuptake, and immediate post-synaptic action, or the function of other neuronal pathways mediating or permitting the immediate postsynaptic action of 5-HT to be expressed as a behavioural response.

One of the interesting and more recent findings in neuropharmacological work is that the chronic effects of drugs appear different to and involve unsuspected pharmacological actions on monoamine metabolism and function when compared with the acute effects of those drugs. For instance acute chlorpromazine administration to animals undoubtedly blocks the action of dopamine in the brain and inhibits the hyperactivity syndromes produced by increasing the brain 5-HT or the dopamine function. Chronic chlorpromazine treatment however leads to a situation in which, when the chlorpromazine is stopped, the hyperactivity syndrome produced by increasing the brain 5-HT or the dopamine function is enhanced suggesting that 5-HT receptor or dopamine receptor supersensitivity has been induced by chronic pharmacological

53

inhibition. There is an interesting contrast between the effects of chronic chlorpromazine and chronic haloperidol administration. Chronic chlorpromazine administration enhances both 5-HT-induced and dopamine-induced behavioural responses whilst chronic haloperidol enhances only dopamine-induced behavioural responses. This suggests that given acutely chlorpromazine blocks both 5-HT and dopamine whereas haloperidol blocks only dopamine. Clinically many psychiatrists recognise the therapeutic differences between chlorpromazine and haloperidol in psychosis.

Another example of the chronic effect of treatment on the brain involves recent findings on electroconvulsive shock (ECS) in rats.

Repeated electroconvulsive shock (ECS) in rats enhances the behavioural responses to increased brain 5-hydroxytryptamine (5-HT), dopamine (DA), and probably noradrenaline (NA) agonist activity (Modigh, 1975; Evans et al, 1976). This enhancement of monoamine action has been found in several model systems: (see Grahame-Smith et al, 1978).

1. The hyperactivity syndrome in rats produced by raising brain 5-HT or by 5-HT agonists.
2. The hyperactivity syndrome in rats produced by raising brain DA or by DA agonists.
3. The rotational behaviour produced by either amphetamine (ipsilateral turning) or apomorphine (contralateral turning) in rats with unilateral nigrostriatal lesions.
4. The hyperactivity produced by apomorphine and clonidine (?noradrenaline agonist activity) in mice (Modigh, 1975).
5. The increased secretion of growth hormone produced by apomorphine (Modigh, 1977).

Note that in all of these experiments the behavioural responses were tested 24 hours after the last shock.

The time course of the effects of ECS are interesting. For the enhancement of monoamine function to occur, a shock a day for at least six days is needed (routinely we give a shock a day for 10 days). Recently though, Costain et al have found that monoamine responses are enhanced by a 'clinical' regimen of ECS (i.e. one shock daily on Monday, Wednesday and Friday for three consecutive weeks).

After a shock a day for ten days the enhanced behavioural responses to 5-HT agonist activity were still present three days after the cessation of shocks and lasted for a total of six to seven days.

Subconvulsive ECS (90 v for one sec) given in otherwise comparable manner to convulsive ECS (150 v, 50 cycles/sec, sinusoidal for one sec) does not produce enhanced responses to monoamine agonist activity.

Green (1978) has shown that flurothyl (Indoklon), a convulsive gas which has been used as an alternative to ECT in the treatment of depression, produces changes in brain monoamine mediated behavioural responses similar to those produced by ECS.

Overall there are rather minor biochemical changes in the synthesis, turnover, and reuptake of the monoamines which certainly do not explain the marked changes in monoamine induced behavioural responses. Largely by exclusion, it seems that ECS produces some change post-synaptically and the questions that arise are:

1. Does ECS produce increased post-synaptic receptor sensitivity to the brain monoamines? Preliminary evidence from our own laboratory and that of Deakin, Owen and Crow suggest that this is not the mechanism.
2. Does ECS alter the activity of the neuronal systems modulating the through-put resultant upon the stimulation of post-synaptic monoamine receptors?
3. Does ECS release neuromodulatory substances within the brain such that the reactivity of neuronal systems stimulated by primary monoamine stimuli is increased? There is at present no evidence on this.

Grahame-Smith et al (1978) have discussed the relevance of this work on ECS to the clinical effects of ECT and the neuropharmacology of depression. The action of ECS to enhance brain monoamine function fits in generally with the known pharmacological actions of tricyclic antidepressants and monoamine oxidase inhibitors and considering all the evidence so far it would be a cruel joke on nature's part if the increase in the functional activity of brain monoamines produced by repeated ECS did not have something to do with their therapeutic effect in depression. It is of some importance to find out how ECS produces these effects because it may be possible to substitute drug therapy for ECT and to produce similar biological changes with less hazard and perhaps fewer side effects.

The effects of repeated administration of neuroleptics, lithium, and now ECS force one to consider the role that 'adaptative' changes in brain function play in both the therapeutic and adverse effects of these therapies. For instance tardive dyskinesia induced by chronic neuroleptic therapy might be dependent upon the dopamine receptor sensitivity induced by chronic dopamine receptor blockade. It is difficult to know whether the latency of onset of the action of lithium in mania and of tricyclic antidepressants in depression is due to the time they take to reach a pharmacokinetic steady-state or due to delayed effects which these drugs might have.

This is particularly important in considering the links between the pharmacokinetic, pharmacodynamic, and therapeutic phases of psychotropic drug therapy. If a drug actually produces its therapeutic effect by its early acute pharmacological action (A), (i.e. A therapeutic effect) then hopefully this set of conditions is fairly easy to analyse. But if the acute pharmacological action (A) leads to chronic 'adaptive' pharmacological actions (C) which are responsible for the therapeutic effect (i.e. A + C therapeutic effect), then this situation becomes much more difficult to analyse.

55

The Individualisation of Psychotropic Drug Therapy: Monitoring Techniques

The sequence of events which occurs between the administration of a drug and its therapeutic effect is extraordinarily complex. The sequence is diagrammatically depicted in Figure 1.

FIGURE 1. Processes occurring on drug administration

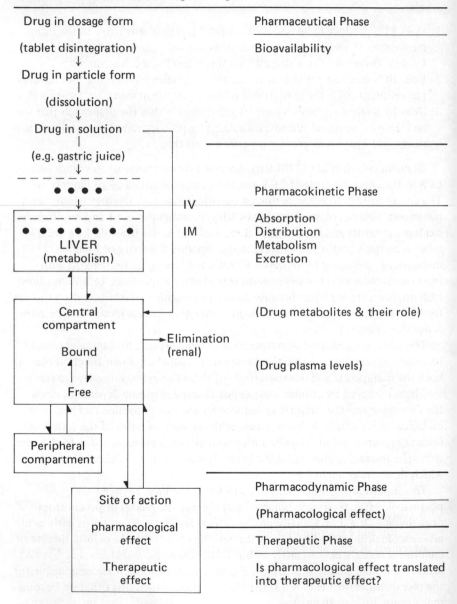

This sequence, which is at the core of the discussion that follows, ignores one extremely important factor: that of patient compliance with prescription drug therapy. Blackwell (1973) has looked at this problem and identified certain factors associated with noncompliance. He identified psychiatric disease as a particular problem because it may erode the capacity to cooperate and therapy is often prolonged.

In a study of patients with schizophrenia, Richards (1964) found that those who refused medication expressed unfavourable feelings towards authority. There is little doubt that, if the patients have hostility towards the psychiatrist and a lack of insight into their illness, compliance is likely to be disastrously poor.

Multiple medications and frequent dose regimens generally foster poor compliance. The drug treatment should be as simple as possible. The setting in which drugs are prescribed and administered influences compliance. Blackwell (1973) quotes several studies showing that amongst psychiatric patients lack of compliance is worse in out-patients than in in-patients.

What can be done about non-compliance? Firstly the treatment must be kept as simple as possible and compatible with the patient's everyday habits. The current trend of prescribing tricyclic antidepressants as one dose at night is an example of this. Undoubtedly, chronic neuroleptic therapy in schizophrenia has been aided by the introduction of depot neuroleptics which are given every 1–3 weeks by injection under supervision. The most important thing is that the physician is aware of the problem of non-compliance as a cause of failure of therapy and that he is then prepared to go into this as a possibility and to follow this up with appropriate action to overcome it. One cause of non-compliance which is not often appreciated is the adverse effects of drugs.

Many physicians and psychiatrists do not bother to explain to patients the nature of the drug they are receiving. It is no wonder that patients do not co-operate well. Several other ways of improving patient compliance have been discussed by Blackwell (1973). The point of emphasising this matter is that sophisticated consideration of the clinical pharmacology of psychotropic drugs is only relevant if the patient is taking the treatment.

Returning to Figure 1, bioavailability, though important, will not be discussed here. The rest of the sequence can be broken down into three phases (see Grahame-Smith, 1977a):

1. Pharmacokinetic Phase

This involves the study and understanding of the absorption, distribution, metabolism, and excretion of drugs. This phase is described through the measurement of drug and metabolite concentrations in blood and/or urine over periods of time after dosing. The proper mathematical description of plasma drug concentration/time curves can tell one a great deal about the disposition of the relevant drug in relation to its pharmacological effect (Greenblatt and Koch-Weser, 1975). These aspects in regard to psychotropic drugs have been dealt with in some detail by Lader (1976). The pharmacokinetic behaviour of a drug or its metabolites in blood is of major importance in determining its effect because however many structural and metabolic barriers drug molecules have to pass the concentration of a drug at its site of action must have the blood concentration as one of its major determinants. The relationship between the blood concentration with time and the pharmacological effect may be a complex one, so complex that it can be difficult to sort out, but logically a relationship must always exist if only we knew how to analyse it properly.

By study of the pharmacokinetic phase inter-individual variability in regard to absorption, distribution, metabolism, and excretion of drugs can be defined and the contributions such studies have made to our understanding of the variability of responses to drugs is very considerable.

2. Pharmacodynamic and Therapeutic Phases

The pharmacodynamic phase is concerned with understanding of the pharmacological effects of the drug and however ignorant one may be of the mode of action of psychotropic drugs their actions in relation to their therapeutic effects is still of prime importance and must be interposed between the pharmacokinetic phase and the therapeutic phase. The pharmacodynamic phase is very complex for psychotropic drugs because the parent drug and its metabolites must pass the blood-brain barrier and sometimes neuronal membranes to affect intraneuronal mechanisms. In many cases these multiple barriers through which drugs pass, by passive or active transport mechanisms, obscure the relationship between the plasma level and the therapeutic effect.

Some non-psychotropic drug actions are superficially simple, for example simple pharmacological antagonists such as β-adrenoceptor blocking agents and morphine antagonists. Other drugs have much more complex actions involving cascades of biochemical and pharmacological events and such indeed may be the case for many psychotropic agents. In terms of their effects in relation to time some drugs are 'on/off' and the degree of effect closely follows the blood level and in terms of its intoxicant effect alcohol is one of these.

Some drugs are 'hit and run'. This phenomenon can occur in two ways. First the drug may bind and continue to act (i.e. not immediately reversible) despite a falling blood level (irreversible monoamine oxidase inhibitors); the second mechanism by which this effect may be brought about is when the drug sets in train a sequence of pharmacological effects which take time to run down (one suspects that this might be the case with tricyclic antidepressants and neuroleptics though it is difficult to be sure). With such drugs the relationship between blood levels and pharmacological effects may be difficult to sort out and subject to great variation in the clinical situation. Although it is difficult to

58

be certain, one suspects that many cases of schizophrenia unresponsive to neuroleptic drug therapy are unresponsive not because the drug is not producing a pharmacological effect but because the disease process is unresponsive to the pharmacological effect of the drug. While our understanding of the neurochemical and neuropharmacological bases of mental illness and the true mode of action of psychotropic drugs is so incomplete it would be foolish to think that just because one achieves a certain pharmacological effect in the brain that the mental illness is going to recover. For instance, however much of a positive ino-tropic effect is feasible with non-toxic doses of digitalis the degree of such an effect might be insufficient to bring about an appreciable therapeutic benefit in some cases of severe cardiac failure. It is also debatable as to how much of an improvement in mortality and morbidity occurs by lowering the blood glucose with oral hypoglycaemics in mild mature-onset diabetes. I merely wish to point out that on occasions one can certainly produce a pharmacological effect without necessarily achieving therapeutic benefit. One cannot help feeling that when depression is truly unresponsive to adequate doses of tricyclic antidepressants and schizophrenia is unresponsive to neuroleptics that the therapy is probably inappropriate and reflects our lack of understanding of the aetiological process responsible for the condition and/or our ignorance of the mode of action of the drugs.

The investigation and the sorting out of the pharmacokinetic, pharmacodynamic, and therapeutic phases and their linkage in psychotropic drug therapy is of importance in two ways. First it has practical benefit in helping to individualise drug therapy for a particular patient. Secondly it leads to a greater understanding of the actions of drugs in the clinical situation and through this provides clues to the disordered brain function underlying the mental illness.

Individualisation of Tricyclic Antidepressant Drug Therapy

There is something of a controversy at present about the relationship between the plasma concentrations of tricyclic antidepressants and their therapeutic effects in depression.

Some points are worth emphasising:

1. What holds for one tricyclic antidepressant need not hold for another. There are differences in metabolic pathways, pharmacokinetic properties, and pharmacological actions between members of this class of drugs.
2. Diagnostic criteria between studies should be comparable. It is generally agreed that tricyclic antidepressant drug therapy is most effective in classic 'endogenous' depression and less so in 'reactive' depression. Since a relationship between plasma concentration of a drug and its therapeutic effect is only likely to be seen in 'responsive' patients there is little point, from the purist's angle, in studying the relationship in patients who do not respond.

3. Qualitative and quantitative precision of measurement of the drugs and their metabolites in plasma is of crucial importance.

One of the reasons for interest in this problem is the very wide difference in plasma levels of nortriptyline, amitryptyline, and imipramine found in patients receiving the same doses of these drugs in a steady state plasma level (Asberg, 1974). This is largely due to genetic differences in metabolic capacity resulting in differences in the rate of the elimination of the drugs from the body (Sjoqvist, 1975). There has been discussion of the role which plasma protein binding might have in accounting for inter-individual differences in response since only the 'free' fraction of drug in the plasma is likely to be pharmacologically active. Desmethylimipramine, for instance, is about 90% bound to plasma proteins and a 10% decrease in binding would increase the pharmacologically active fraction by 100%. Sjoqvist and his colleagues (Sjoqvist, 1975), however, looked at this aspect by comparing the total plasma concentration of desmethylimipramine with the ability of the plasma to inhibit noradrenaline uptake by rat brain slices. There was a very good correlation suggesting that, generally, differences in plasma protein binding are not an important factor.

TABLE 3. Relationship between Nortriptyline plasma concentration and therapeutic effect.

Study	Conclusion	Comment
1. Asberg 1971	Best results obtained with levels 50 – 140 ng/ml >140 ng/ml response less <50 ng/ml response less	Endogenous depression. Treatment period only two weeks. Other drugs also given.
2. Kragh-Sorensen, Asberg and Eggert-Hansen, 1973.	>170 ng/ml response poor.	Endogenous depressions (fairly severe). 4 weeks
3. Kragh-Sorensen et al 1976a	>180 ng/ml poor response Reduction of level → improvement.	Endogenous depression. 4 weeks
4. Ziegler et al 1976a	Best results 50 – 140 ng/ml >140 – 260 ng/ml results not so good, particularly at 3 – 6 weeks	'Depressed' patients. 6 weeks
5. Lyle et al 1974	No correlation or upper therapeutic level found	'Depressed'
6. Burrows, Davies and Scoggins, 1972; Burrows et al, 1974.	No correlation or upper therapeutic level found No correlation.	'Depressed' Kragh-Sorensen et al (1976b). Mixed groups of depressives. No severe depressives. Fluctuations in plasma levels considerable

Nortriptyline

Table 3 lists the investigations done with conclusions and comments. It can be seen that in four studies there is evidence that at the least there is a 'therapeutic window' for nortriptyline in which a therapeutic response is likely to occur, i.e. with a 'steady state' plasma level of about 50–140 ng/ml. Below 50 ng/ml a therapeutic response is unlikely. Patients with levels > 140 ng/ml are less likely to do so well but when the dosage is reduced and the plasma level falls to within the therapeutic window they improve again. It has been suggested that at high concentrations nortriptyline might block catecholamine receptors which could hypothetically account for the fall-off of the therapeutic effect at high plasma levels.

Three studies have not shown any correlation between plasma levels and clinical response. These have been criticised on several counts (see Kragh-Sørensen et al, 1976b). My own impression from reviewing these studies is that in those investigations in which a 'therapeutic window' effect has been found the conclusion is valid and it should be possible to replicate the results if the trial methodology and choice of patients is similar. In this field it is essential to compare like-studies.

Amitriptyline

The situation in regard to amitriptyline is no less confused. Table 4 lists two studies showing some correlation of plasma levels with therapeutic response, in one with both amitriptyline and nortriptyline (its metabolite) and in the other amitriptyline alone. In a more recent study Coppen (1978) has been unable to confirm some previous results.

Certainly no 'therapeutic window' has been found for amitriptyline as has been for nortriptyline alone. Looking at the evidence on amitriptyline so far it is clear that further carefully designed studies are needed to clear up the matter. From what has been presented up till now it seems that the measurement of

TABLE 4. Relationship between amitriptyline plasma concentration and therapeutic effect

Study	Conclusion	Comment
Braithwaite et al (1972)	Linear positive correlation. Amitriptyline 20 – 278 ng/ml. Nortriptyline 20 – 228 ng/ml.	Measured. Amitriptyline & Nortriptyline 'Depressive' illness undefined.
Ziegler et al	Response positively correlated with amitriptyline level, not with nortriptyline.	Outpatient depressives.
Coppen (1977)	No correlations found of plasma levels with therapeutic effect. Good correlation of nortriptyline level with decreased tyramine effect.	Multicentre WHO study. Primary depressive illness. Six weeks administration.

61

plasma amitriptyline (and nortriptyline) levels as a fine guide to amitriptyline therapy is not going to add a great deal.

Imipramine (see Table 5)

The early study by Walter (1971) measuring only imipramine fluorometrically suggested a narrow range of levels with a correlation between plasma level and clinical response. Gram et al (1976) and Glassman et al (1977) have gone into the matter in much greater detail. These studies show that on a fixed dose of imipramine the plasma levels of imipramine and desipramine vary considerably. However, although a precise correlation between the plasma level of imipramine and/or desipramine and the response may not be possible, there is a good indication that there is a therapeutic range at levels below which a response is unlikely and that 33% of patients may not get into that therapeutic range associated with the highest response rate on a fixed dosage schedule of 3.5 mg/kg/day (Glassman et al, 1977). Gram et al (1976) make the points that the imipramine/desipramine ratio may be important, that the compounds may have separate effects, and that their ratio is variable from patient to patient and that this is also a source of potential variability in influencing the outcome.

What is to be made of all this?

1. The studies on nortriptyline showing a therapeutic window (or curvilinear relationship between plasma level and therapeutic response) look reliable. Without access to plasma level determinations the advice given by Asberg (1976) is useful. A standard dose of nortriptyline of 50 mg t.d.s. produces therapeutic plasma levels in about 65% of patients. If in three weeks there is no response,

TABLE 5. Relationship between imipramine plasma levels and therapeutic response

Study	Conclusion	Comments
Walter (1971)	Imipramine (only). Range 2.5 − 7.1 ng/ml. Positive correlation.	Endogenous depression. Fluometric assay.
Gram et al (1976)	Responders plasma levels imipramine ⩾45 ng/ml and desipramine >75 ng/ml. No fall off at high levels.	Endogenous depression. Placebo period followed by clinical evaluation on treatment at 5 − 6 weeks.
Glassman et al (1977)	Positive correlation (r = 0.48). Pooled imipramine and desipramine plasma levels. Response rate poor with plasma level 150 ng/ml. Response rate improved in range 150 − 200 ng/ml. Plateaux about 250 ng/ml. No fall off in effect with high plasma levels.	Depressed. Unipolar delusional patients − no correlation between plasma level and clinical response. In males with high plasma levels, good response.

lower the dose to 25 mg t.d.s. (since it is most probable that the level is too high). Wait one week and if no effect, raise the dose to 75 mg t.d.s. If still no response change to another antidepressant agent; she suggests chlorimipramine.

2. A case can be made for measuring plasma imipramine and desipramine levels in patients treated with imipramine to ensure that they are in the therapeutic range (i.e. combined levels between 150–250 ng/ml)

3. The situation with regard to amitriptyline is difficult and more work is needed to clarify the matter.

4. There are now several studies showing excellent correlations between the inhibition of the tyramine pressor response and the plasma level from anitriptyline measured as (nortriptyline) and nortriptyline, yet the actual correlations with the therapeutic response in depression are usually rather weak. A similar lack of correlations has been recorded with inhibition of 5-HT platelet uptake by tricyclic antidepressants. This means that the peripheral pharmacodynamic effect does not mirror the central effect through which the therapeutic response is mediated. This points to either pharmacokinetic differences existing between the compartment housing the peripheral sympathetic nervous system and the brain compartment *or* to pharmacodynamic differences, i.e. is the mechanism by which tricyclic antidepressants effectively produce their antidepressant effects really inhibition of monoamine re-uptake? If inhibition of monoamine re-uptake is not the mechanism by which the tricyclic antidepressant drugs effectively produce their therapeutic action and if this depends upon longer term complex changes in monoamine turnover, metabolism, or changes in receptor sensitivity, and so on, then simple relationships between plasma levels and therapeutic response are unlikely to be found. I believe that the work that has been done in this field suggests that such a complexity does exist and that much more work is needed to verify or refute the hypotheses that inhibition of monoamine re-uptake is the mechanism by which these drugs act to relieve depression. If another mechanism is discovered it would change our thinking about the likely relationships between the pharmacokinetic properties of the drugs and what at present are believed to be their important pharmacodynamic effects.

Individualisation of Neuroleptic Drug Therapy in Schizophrenia

The variability in response to neuroleptic drug therapy in schizophrenia is well known. Is this variability due to the differences in the pharmacokinetic handling of the drug, in its pharmacodynamic effects, or in the link between its pharmacodynamic effects and the therapeutic action?

A major difficulty in the identification of pharmacological factors that might account for some of the observed variability in drug response in schizophrenia (as in depression) is that patients do not form uniform groups. It may be thought that in some patients clinical improvement does bear a good relationship to adequate plasma levels and central pharmacodynamic effects. Other patients may remit or remain well without medication, the natural course of the illness being the main determinant. Others may prove resistant to therapy however adequate the plasma levels and the pharmacodynamic effects of the drugs at present being used. Again, as with antidepressants this heterogenicity may obscure the factors relating drug prescription to therapeutic response.

Another important complicating factor is that, in general, factors which are of prognostic value for the natural course of schizophrenia bear a similar relationship to the outcome of drug treatment, but neither prognostic factors nor environmental factors such as social stresses or family influences explain in a satisfactory way the wide variation in the clinical course of treated patients. In schizophrenia certain clinical factors have been shown to be associated with a good response to treatment (Leff and Wing, 1971) and certain psychosocial factors are associated with an increased risk of relapse (Vaughn and Leff, 1976). The point here is that the disturbance in brain function (whatever that may be!) in schizophrenia, the drug used to treat it, and the influence of environmental factors on that disturbed brain function all interact, certainly in the context of long term out-patient therapy. We have hardly begun to sort these interactions out.

Most of the work on plasma levels in neuroleptic drugs has been carried out with chlorpromazine. In a series of early studies Curry, Davis and Janowsky (1970) showed that there were wide variations in the plasma levels of chlorpromazine in patients receiving the same dose, though within patients, dosage and plasma levels varied in a consistent way. In a later study Sakalis et al (1972) showed, however, that intra-individual consistency was poor in a group of acutely ill psychotic patients who were monitored during the early phases of treatment. The low correlation between dosage and plasma levels has been widely confirmed (Rivera-Calimlim et al, 1976; Wiles et al, 1976); the overall relationship between dosage and plasma levels is, however, not simple and Wiles et al (1976) have suggested that though plasma chlorpromazine levels increase with dosage up to a daily dose of 400 mg, patients receiving larger doses had a lower mean plasma level of chlorpromazine – this confirmed similar findings reported by MacKay, Healey and Baker (1974) with chlorpromazine and Martensson and Roos (1974) with thioridazine.

The variability in the relationship between plasma levels and dosage is also accompanied by a variability in the relationship between plasma levels of chlorpromazine and its clinical effects. Most workers report a plasma level range of 0 to 110 mg/ml in patients receiving conventional doses of chlorpromazine by mouth; there does not appear to be a 'therapeutic range' of levels for patients receiving chlorpromazine. A number of studies (Curry et al, 1970; Rivera-Calimlim, Castanida and Lasagna, 1973; MacKay et al, 1974; Kolakowska et al, 1976; Rivera-Calimlim et al, 1976; Wiles et al, 1976) have shown that clinical improvement in both acute and chronic schizophrenic patients treated with chlorpromazine was associated with a wide range of plasma levels; furthermore there were no significant differences between the plasma levels of patients who responded and patients who did not.

However, results have not been uniformly negative. Sakalis et al (1972) showed that the clinical changes in the first fortnight of treatment in acute patients were related to plasma chlorpromazine levels although this correlation was not maintained throughout treatment. Rivera-Calimlim et al (1976) showed a relationship between plasma chlorpromazine levels and clinical improvement for certain symptoms of schizophrenia and suggested that a plasma level range of 50—300 ng/ml was associated with improvement in thought disorder and paranoid ideation but not with some negative symptoms of schizophrenia such as withdrawal, retardation, blunting of affect, and somatic concern. This suggests that it might be possible to show a relationship between plasma levels of a neuroleptic drug and certain aspects of a patient's symptomatology which would have been masked by a lack of correlation between the plasma levels and a global clinical response.

Plasma levels of chlorpromazine have also been shown to correlate positively with plasma levels of prolactin which may be an indication of the dopamine blocking action of chlorpromazine in the hypothalamus (Kolakowska et al, 1975; Wiles et al, 1976). In addition, extrapyramidal side effects have been shown to be associated with higher levels of plasma chlorpromazine and prolactin in acutely ill schizophrenic patients (Wiles et al, 1976) though this relationship did not hold in chronic patients (Kolakowska et al, 1976).

The search for active metabolites has suggested that metabolic pathways might be important in determining the outcome of treatment with neuroleptic drugs. Sakalis et al (1974) and MacKay et al (1974) have reported higher levels of a pharmacologically active metabolite of chlorpromazine, 7-hydroxychlorpromazine, in patients who had improved clinically. Wiles et al (1976) found that acutely ill patients who failed to respond to treatment had a greater proportion of chlorpromazine sulphoxide, a pharmacologically inactive metabolite, in plasma samples taken just before a dose. Chlorpromazine has a multiplicity of metabolites and these studies have been concerned with only a few; it is therefore difficult to show a positive relationship between only a fraction of what could be the total amount of pharmacologically active drugs and metabolites and any clinical changes.

Relationships between plasma levels and clinical changes after a single dose of the drug may not necessarily be observed after multiple doses or during long term treatment, either as a result of the persistance and accumulation of the drug in the body, the development of tolerance, or changes in other factors influencing the disease process. Tolerance is a particularly interesting phenomenon and clinical observation has suggested that long term administration of neuroleptic drugs leads to the development of tolerance to some of the side effects. Tolerance could be due to pharmacokinetic factors or to changes in the sensitivity of those areas of the brain affected by the drug. The relationship observed between plasma chlorpromazine levels, extrapyramidal side effects, and prolactin levels in acute patients does not hold for chronic patients and no relationship could be shown between plasma levels of chlorpromazine, plasma levels of prolactin, or extrapyramidal side effects in chronic patients who had been receiving chlorpromazine for a prolonged period (Kolakowska et al, 1976). Both prolactin levels and extrapyramidal side effects are related to the dopamine blocking effects of neuroleptics in the brain and the finding that these indices of dopamine blockade in chronic patients were lower than in acute patients in spite of similar plasma levels would suggest that there could be an acquired tolerance to some of the dopamine blocking effects of neuroleptic drugs without any apparent interference in their capacity to maintain their therapeutic activity. One wonders whether these aspects of tolerance might be related to the *increased* sensitivity of animals to the behavioural effects of central 5-HT and dopamine action after long term neuroleptic drug administration (Heal et al, 1976), perhaps indicating receptor supersensitivity subsequent to receptor block.

In animals the effects of neuroleptic drugs on dopamine turnover in the brain are also different during acute and chronic treatment; Wiesel et al (1975) showed that, while a single dose of chlorpromazine led to increases in levels of homovanillic acid (HVA) in the rat striatum which correlated with plasma and brain levels of the drug, HVA levels after repeated dosage correlated only with brain levels and not with plasma levels. There is evidence that the effects of repeated administration of neuroleptics vary between one area of the brain and another and this could explain why tolerance to extrapyramidal side effects can occur without any lessening in therapeutic effects. Sayers et al (1975) have shown that repeated administration of chlorpromazine produces smaller rises in HVA in the caudate nucleus than a single dose given acutely, while others (Bowers and Rozitis, 1974) have shown no difference between the effects of acute and chronic chlorpromazine treatment on HVA levels in the limbic system and in the hypothalamus.

In man, Goodwin, Post and Sack (1975) showed an increase in HVA in cerebrospinal fluid in patients shortly after the start of phenothiazine treatment but not in patients who had been on phenothiazines for more than five weeks.

These studies confirm the clinical impression that there is a dissociation between the therapeutic effects of neuroleptic drugs and their capacity to produce extrapyramidal side effects; they also suggest important implications for the prescription of anti-cholinergic drugs in the management of drug-induced extrapyramidal side effects in patients on chronic treatment. There is some evidence that some anti-cholinergic drugs lead to a reduction in plasma levels of chlorpromazine (Rivera-Calimlim et al, 1976), perhaps by interfering with absorptive mechanisms but this finding has not been confirmed by others (Wiles et al, 1976); it has also been shown (Singh and Smith, 1973) that anticholinergic drugs prescribed during acute treatment occasionally leads to a therapeutic reversal with an exacerbation of symptoms. It is also well known that withdrawal of anti-parkinsonian drugs carries very little risk of a recurrence of parkinsonian symptoms (Orlov et al, 1971) and that the routine long term prescription of these drugs can increase the intensity and duration of dyskinetic symptoms in tardive dyskinesia and sometimes lower the threshold for the manifestation of tardive dyskinesia (Klawans and Rubovits, 1974).

A large number of factors are known to affect the relationship between plasma levels of a drug and clinical changes and these have been reviewed elsewhere (Curry, 1974). With chlorpromazine, such factors as the presence of the drug were shown to affect the concentration of chlorpromazine in plasma (Curry et al, 1970). As chlorpromazine is 95–98% bound to plasma proteins and as this binding is reversible and has been shown to vary in the interval between doses, variations in binding could theoretically also lead to fluctuations in plasma level concentrations and non-linear relationships between levels and clinical effects.

Similar non-linear relationships between plasma levels and therapeutic effects have been shown with thioridazine (Martensson and Roos, 1974). Forsman et al (1974) have recently developed a gas-chromatographic method for determining plasma levels of haloperidol and have shown a 1–10 fold variation in serum levels in patients on the same dose and, as with other neuroleptics, it has been difficult to identify a therapeutic range which might serve as a guide to treatment.

There have been no reports so far relating plasma levels of the long acting depot neuroleptic preparations to therapeutic effects. This is because it has proved difficult to develop an assay sensitive enough to measure the very low plasma levels obtained with these drugs. It is possible that inter-individual variability in plasma levels may be less of a problem with these drugs than with other neuroleptics as they are administered parenterally. A sensitive radio immunoassay for fluphenazine is now available (Wiles and Franklin, 1977) and preliminary results on a small group of patients receiving usual maintenance doses of fluphenazine decanoate (Modecate) suggests that patients on different dose regimens show a narrow range of plasma levels (1–3 ng/ml) with very little change within patients between one injection cycle and the next (Wiles et al, in preparation).

The absence of a linear relationship between plasma levels of chlorpromazine and other neuroleptic drugs and therapeutic responses has led to a series of studies relating the concentration of phenothiazines in red blood cells to therapeutic responses. Garver et al (1976) showed that acute extrapyramidal side effects of butaperazine, a piperazine phenothiazine, were more clearly related to the quantities of the drug bound to red cells than to plasma levels. In a more recent study (Garver et al, 1977) butaperazine bound to red cells was also found to correlate more closely with the therapeutic effects of the drug

67

than the plasma levels. The rationale for measuring red-cell-bound drug was based upon the possibility that the factors which affected the accumulation of a drug in a red blood cell might be similar to those affecting the passage of a drug into the brain and its localisation at relevant receptor sites in the central nervous system.

Pharmacodynamic Approaches

The problem of measuring some 'physical' effect of a psychotropic drug on the human brain is difficult.

Advances in the understanding of hypothalamic-pituitary control mechanisms have made possible the investigation of neuroendocrine function in psychiatric illness and in its treatment by psychotropic drugs. Although the involvement of monoamines in the circuitry controlling hypothalamic-pituitary function is not precisely understood, several investigations are nevertheless proceeding along certain empirical lines, making certain reasonable assumptions, and with appropriate neuroendocrine challenge tests they are attempting to define certain characteristic neuroendocrine abnormalities in spontaneous mental illness and to detect neuroendocrine changes brought about by drugs.

One brief aside might be of interest. For years it has been thought that the 'stress' of psychiatric illness might be responsible for the endocrine abnormalities seen *or* that endocrine disease was the primary cause of certain mental syndromes.

> i.e.:

Mental illness ⟶ 'stress' ⟶ endocrine disorder

> or

Endocrine disorder ⟶ mental illness

Now it seems that thinking is moving towards considering a 'brain disease' that on the one hand might result in mental abnormalities and on the other in endocrine abnormalities,

> i.e.

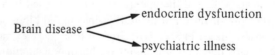

Brain disease ⟨ endocrine dysfunction / psychiatric illness

This can be tied into putative disorders of monoamine function in the following way:

68

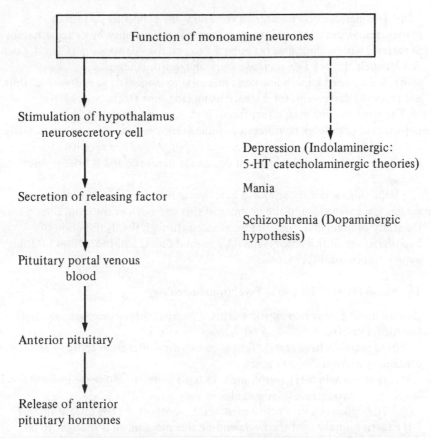

Function of monoamine neurones

Stimulation of hypothalamus
neurosecretory cell

Depression (Indolaminergic:
5-HT catecholaminergic theories)

Secretion of releasing factor

Mania

Schizophrenia (Dopaminergic
hypothesis)

Pituitary portal venous
blood

Anterior pituitary

Release of anterior
pituitary hormones

Some shorthand statements about monoaminergic regulation of pituitary hormone secretion can be made:
1. Dopamine and its agonists stimulate growth hormone release.
2. Dopamine and its agonists inhibit prolactin secretion.
3. α-adrenoceptor agonists stimulate growth hormone release.
4. α-adrenoceptor agonists stimulate ACTH release.

Quite safe neuroendocrine challenge tests are now available for experimental use, e.g.:
1. Apomorphine ⟶ Growth hormone release   (Dopamine agonist)
2. Amphetamine ⟶ Growth hormone release   (Dopamine + α agonist)
3. Clonidine ⟶ Growth hormone release   (α*-agonist)
4. Methylamphetamine → ACTH → corticosteroid   (?α receptor)
5. Hypoglycaemia   GH and ACTH   (?α ?5-HT ?ACh)

The two most striking abnormalities, in my view, yet found in psychiatric illness are:

*α-adrenoceptor

a) The increased corticosteroid secretion, the abnormal pattern of corticosteroid secretion, and its relative non-suppressibility by dexamethasone in patients with endogenous (as opposed to reactive) depression. (Carroll, Curtis and Mendels, 1976.) This is classic work and worth reading.

b) A decreased growth hormone response to α-agonists in endogenous (but not reactive) depression, for instance using clonidine (Matussek, 1978).

The most striking drug effect found is the rise in prolactin accompanying dopamine blockade by neuroleptics. Some work has been done to try to relate the rise in prolactin levels to therapeutic responses and the severity of extrapyramidal signs as an index of dopamine blockade and is briefly described on page 25.

I hope this extremely brief and inadequate mention of neuroendocrine studies gives some idea of the promise of this approach at the clinical level for the study of brain abnormalities manifested through the dysfunction of hypothalamic control accompanied by mental illness and the actions of drugs upon neurotransmitter systems.

The Blood Platelet: Its Use in Psychopharmacology

(For an up-to-date review of some aspects of what follows see Gaetano and Garattini (1978)).

Blood platelets have certain functions not dissimilar from those of serotonin-containing nerve ending/synapses.

1. They contain 5-HT (serotonin). In both platelets and nerve endings this is largely bound to intracellular granules or vesicles.

2. They possess a very active membrane transport for the inward flux of 5-HT (active uptake). At the nerve ending this mechanism is thought to be partly responsible for the termination of the pharmacological effect of 5-HT.

3. They possess on their membranes receptors for 5-HT, noradrenaline (α), isoprenaline (β). 5-HT and noradrenaline both provoke platelet aggregation and β-adrenoceptor agonists − like isoprenaline − inhibit platelet aggregation by stimulating the membrane adenylate cyclase with increases in intraplatelet cyclic AMP levels. Whether these receptors are like so-called presynaptic or post-synaptic receptors is not yet clear.

The platelet monoamine receptors can be demonstrated not only by the aggregation responses they mediate but also by radio ligand binding techniques.

4. They contain monoamine oxidase, an enzyme which metabolises monoamines.

The following are examples of how these properties of the platelet have been used to probe the 'biological concomitants' of psychiatric disorders and their treatment with psychotic drugs.

1. *Platelet monoamine oxidase activity has been used to:*
a) Monitor the effect of monoamine oxidase inhibitors in patients.

b) As a possible genetic marker for schizophrenia (the results are very unclear).

2. *Platelet 5-HT uptake has been studied in:*
a) Patients with endogenous depression in whom decreased uptake has been demonstrated by two groups (Tuomisto in Finland and Coppen in Britain).

b) Patients taking tricyclic antidepressants which, with various potencies, block the uptake of 5-HT. Relationships have been found between the plasma level of tricyclic antidepressant and the blockade of uptake but these are not mirrored by clinical improvement.

3. Platelet aggregation responses to monoamines have not been studied much in the psychopharmacological field.

An initial study in Oxford did originally seem to suggest that enhanced 5-HT platelet aggregation responses occurred in patients on chlorpromazine, thioridazine, and fluphenazine therapy and that these responses might possibly be used to monitor certain aspects of drug therapy. An attempt to replicate these findings recently has failed and the matter will have to be re-examined. (See Boullin et al, 1978 and Boullin et al, 1975.)

Some Recent Developments of Interest Depot Neuroleptics

The long-acting depot neuroleptic drugs are now firmly established as the maintenance treatment of choice in schizophrenia (Hirsch et al, 1973). Intramuscular administration ensures that patients receive the drugs and thus bypasses problems of absorption from the gut and first-pass metabolism in the liver (Adamson, et al, 1973). Of the two preparations in common use, fluphenazine decanoate (Modecate) and flupenthixol decanoate (Depixol), the latter is reputed to carry a lesser risk of causing the depression which was reported in some patients receiving fluphenazine (de Alarcon and Carney, 1969). Penfluridol, a diphenylbutypiperidine derivative related to pimzide (Orap) and fluspirilene (Redeptin), differs from other long-acting neuroleptics in that it is administered by mouth and clinical studies (Gallant et al, 1974) indicate that it provides safe and adequate control of symptoms in schizophrenic patients. Until recently it has not been possible to examine the pharmacokinetics of these compounds as 'therapeutic' plasma levels are very low and proved difficult to measure; a radioimmunoassay has now been developed that allows the detection of very low levels of fluphenazine in plasma (Wiles and Franklin, 1977) and preliminary results indicate that the range of 'therapeutic' levels is a relatively narrow one and the patients on different but effective dose regimens shared the same range of levels suggesting that clinicians were prescribing the drug in a way that produced steady plasma levels within a narrow range (Wiles et al – in preparation). The precise relationship between dosage, plasma levels, therapeutic, and unwanted effects has still to be explored. On clinical grounds anti-psychotoxic effects and extrapyramidal side-effects appear to be dose dependent,

71

but effective dose regimes show a wide scatter (Johnson, 1975). A comprehensive review of the practical matters involved in the use of depot neuroleptics in schizophrenia has been provided by Johnson (1977).

Propranolol in Schizophrenia

Atsmon, Blum and Fischl (1972) noted that when large doses of propranolol were given to reduce tachycardia and the blood pressure in a patient with acute porphyria, the psychotic features associated with the syndrome disappeared. Steiner et al (1972) went on to show that symptoms in schizophrenic patients remitted when propranolol was given in increasing dosage every two to three hours. In a pilot study Yorkston et al (1974) reported marked improvement in an impressive proportion of schizophrenic patients treated with propranolol. The same group (Yorkston et al, 1976) have confirmed and extended their findings in a larger group of schizophrenic patients. They found that while the drug was effective in controlling schizophrenic symptoms it was less effective in treating relapses. The dose of propranolol used ranged from 160 mg daily to 3000 mg daily and the average maintenance dose was 500 mg/daily. Acute toxic effects were a problem early on in these studies but improved monitoring of patients decreased the incidence of acute toxic effects and so far no chronic toxic effects have been observed. Apart from potentially improving the therapy of schizophrenia these trials also raise questions about the mode of action of propranolol and secondary implications concerning the abnormalities in the brain that underlie schizophrenic illness.

Green and Grahame-Smith (1976b) found that in rats (±)-propranolol (40 mg/kg i.p.) inhibited the hyperactivity syndrome resultant upon increasing the functional activity of brain 5-HT but did not inhibit the hyperactivity produced by increasing the functional activity of dopamine. This action of (±)-propranolol racemate was found to be due to (−)-propranolol (i.e. the β-blocking isomer). (Weinstock and Schechter, 1975.)

Green and Grahame-Smith (in preparation) have now studied a series of β-adrenergic blocking agents for their activity in blocking 5-HT induced hyperactivity syndromes in the rat. Several β-adrenergic blocking agents block 5-HT induced hyperactivity and in more recent experiments it has been shown that β-adrenergic blocking agents have no effect on another model for the functional activity of dopamine in brain, i.e. the rat with a unilateral nigrostriatal lesion in which rotational behaviour occurs with dopamine agonist treatment. It is uncertain yet as to whether the features that distinguish those β-blocking agents which do inhibit 5-HT induced hyperactivity from those which do not is due to the ease with which the former enter the brain or whether there is some intrinsic specificity of action in regard to this effect.

Middlemiss, Blakebrough and Leather (1977) have recently shown that (−)-propranolol inhibits the specific binding of 5-HT to brain membranes, perhaps indicating that propranolol can block the binding of 5-HT to brain receptor sites.

72

If the conclusions are correct that propranolol inhibits central 5-HT neurotransmission or its behavioural effects in some way and if future studies confirm its efficacy in the treatment of schizophrenia there are several implications. The dopamine receptor blocking action of neuroleptics, as their mechanism of action qua antipsychotic drugs, is one of the corner stones of the so-called 'dopamine hypotheses' of the causation of schizophrenia. If propranolol inhibits the central effects of 5-HT but not dopamine and if it is effective through this mechanism in schizophrenia then this points indirectly to an involvement of 5-HT as well as dopamine in this condition. If indeed 5-HT mechanisms are involved at a higher organisational level than dopaminergic mechanisms then the action of current neuroleptics could still be explained by their action on dopaminergic mechanisms since the central functional activity of 5-HT, at least as far as the hyperactivity syndrome is concerned, is crucially dependent upon intact dopaminergic mechanisms for its behavioural expression (Green and Grahame-Smith, 1976a).

Neuropeptides

An increasing number of peptides are being discovered in the brain and spinal cord. Several peptides thought to be sited in the gastrointestinal tract have been found in the brain. Other peptides thought to be hypothalamic and in one way or another to influence pituitary function are found in other anatomical sites within the CNS. Then, of course, we have the recent discovery of the endorphins and encephalins to consider.

This is far too big a subject to be dealt with in any detail in this paper and the reader is referred to the book edited by Hughes (1978).

However, some general information is of relevance to the immediate future of the development of psychopharmacology since several neuropeptides or their analogues are already in clinical trials for the treatment of memory loss, pain, and depression.

Thyrotropin releasing hormone (TRH), which is found in sites other than the hypothalamus, causes behavioural changes in animals, and probably functions as a neurotransmitter or neuromodulator influencing dopamine release in certain sites has already had trials, largely unsuccessful in the treatment of depression.

Other orthodox 'neuroendocrine' polypeptides now thought to have roles outside the endocrine system are luteinising hormone-releasing hormone (LHRH) and growth hormone-release-inhibiting hormone (somatostatin).

More surprisingly gastrin, cholecystokinin, and vasoactive intestinal peptide have also been found in the brain.

Substance P is now thought to function as an excitatory central neurotransmitter.

Neurotensin is a peptide found in nerve endings in various regional sites in the brain, the highest concentrations being in the hypothalamus. Receptors for it exist in the brain as judged by the binding of I^{125}-neurotensin. Its function is as yet unknown.

Vasopressin is behaviourally a fascinating peptide which has dramatic effects on conditioned avoidance behaviour in rats quite separate from its action on renal water clearance. There are several anecdotal reports purporting to show its efficacy in amnesia syndromes; I am doubtful of this, but time will tell.

Of the other peptides mentioned TRH, melanocyte stimulating hormone release-inhibiting factor (MSH-IF) somatostatin, LHRH, substance P, and neurotensin can all be demonstrated to have behavioural effects or effects upon behavioural changes produced by other drugs in animals although the dose, time of administration, and route of administration are important.

Endorphins and Encephalins (see Hughes, 1978)

The discoveries of the encephalins and then the endorphins have been the most exciting events in neuropharmacology recently.

Structurally there are four related classes of compounds:

1. β-lipotropin with a sequence of $1-91$ aminoacids.
2. Endorphins composed of $61-76$, $61-77$, or $61-91$ sequences of β-lipotropin.
3. Met-encephalin $61-65$ sequence of β-lipotropin.
4. Leu-encephalin which is Leu^{65}-β-lipotropin $_{61-65}$.

The two encephalins are present in many areas of the CNS. The endorphins are found mainly in the pituitary. β-lipotropin is located in the pituitary. The amino acid sequences in β-lipotropin are able to give rise to ACTH peptides, MSH peptides, the endorphins, and met-encephalin though not (directly) leu-encephalin although it is suggested that some related lipotropin may be found which may do so.

Most is known about the smaller peptides, the encephalins. It is now known that opiate receptors exist in the brain in synaptic membranes. A high density of these receptors occurs in the anterior amygdala and the periaqueductal grey matter, this latter is probably important in the analgesic effect of morphine. It is thought that opiates bind to these receptors and thereby produce their effects. Naloxone, a specific opiate antagonist, also binds to these receptors. The encephalins also bind to these receptors and compete with morphine and naloxone in this respect. The encephalins also have actions like morphine on classic pharmacological tests such as the inhibition of the electrically worked contractions of guinea pig ilea and the reduction of the release of acetyl choline.

The distribution of encephalins at the macro and microsequal level and studies of their neuropharmacological actions suggests that they probably act as neurotransmitters and that they modulate the release of acetyl choline and other neurotransmitter agents.

The precise physiological roles of the endorphins and encephalins have not yet been discovered nor, so far, has their discovery led to a convincing explanation for opiate addiction. Already though, there are reports of raised CSF levels of endorphins/encephalins in schizophrenia and depression. There are also anecdotal reports of the abolition of schizophrenic hallucinations by naloxone.

There is a great deal of research going on in this subject at all levels, from molecules to the disease and pieces of information are coming in every week. The next few years will clarify the situation.

Conclusion

In this paper I have tried to mix molecular neuropharmacology, experimental animal behavioural neuropharmacology, applied neurochemistry, the clinical pharmacology of psychotropic drugs, and the practicalities of psychotropic drug therapy. If it has resulted in a pot-pourri then so be it, but because the human brain is so difficult to reach we must be prepared to go from the test tube and experimental animal to man and back again to the laboratory and gradually build up comparative data. I think this approach is working quite well. It is important for practising psychiatrists to understand this line of research so that they can contribute not only to the practical therapy but, through their clinical observation of the effects of drugs, to the understanding of the neuropharmacology itself.

COMMENTARY ON CURRENT TRENDS IN NEUROPHARMACOLOGY AND PSYCHOPHARMACOLOGY

Paul Bridges

With contributions to increase the understanding of the psychoses in particular, psychiatrists are being overtaken by colleagues in various branches of neurochemistry. Tremendous advances in treatment have been primarily contributed to by psychopharmacology. We probably now tend to underestimate the fundamental discoveries that occurred in the 1950s when the foundations of modern psychopharmacology were laid in a very decisive way. Not only were effective drugs discovered but totally new drug actions were revealed. For example, the benzodiazepines have proved effective in states of anxiety, and their anxiolytic action occurs with very little sedation at the usual doses, quite unlike the barbiturates with which anti-anxiety activity is associated with considerable sedation. Then again, the neuroleptics were found to have quite specific antipsychotic activity and chlorpromazine was the first drug discovered with this action, which was previously unknown and presumably not even guessed at. Then two types of antidepressants were discovered each with very different chemical formulae but sharing a common and, at that time, entirely novel activity. They were not stimulants as the currently available amphetamines were and for the first time a specific antidepressive activity was apparent.

From the discovery of these drugs and from the subsequent increasingly successful neurochemical investigations has come the very considerable amount of information that we now have about the actions of the drugs and we are, by inference, able to consider hypotheses about the causes of mania, endogenous depression, and schizophrenia. Professor Grahame-Smith rightly points out that our current hypotheses probably do not explain the fundamental biochemical characteristics of the illnesses, but they give us a good beginning to improve knowledge. It is probably because the preparations act at different biochemical levels, as it were, that they appear to vary in their specificity. The anti-psychotic group tend to be generally similarly effective for both mania and schizophrenia,

76

while the quite wide range of antidepressant drugs that we now have (falling into a number of groups each with quite different chemical structures and seeming to have different modes of action) all appear valuable quite specifically for what is presumably a related group of illnesses that we loosely describe as endogenous depression.

Indeed, looked at rather fancifully it could be claimed that an atypical depressive illness can be diagnosed more reliably from its response to antidepressant medication than from a careful psychiatric examination. Of course, this is an over-simplification but there is some truth in the point. If an illness is found to respond decisively to an antidepressant, even although the presentation is one of obsessional neurosis then there are good grounds for saying that that particular case of obsessional illness is likely to have much in common biochemically with a typical case of endogenous depression.

So the present need is for more sophisticated theories about the clinical characteristics and presentations of psychiatric disorders so that we may, among other things, come to be able to relate diagnostic sub-groups to responses to particular drugs. For example, it is known that secondary amine tricyclic antidepressants tend preferentially to affect the uptake of noradrenaline while tertiary amine preparations tend more to affect serotonin. It could therefore be that some forms of depressive illness respond better to one type of antidepressant than another. It must be admitted that there is so far little clinical evidence that different members of the tricyclic group relate therapeutically to specific clinical presentations except that typical cases of depression in general are more likely to respond to these drugs, and it has been suggested that illnesses responding to monoamine oxidase inhibitors have other clinical characteristics than those likely to be helped by the tricyclics, the presentations will be more atypical and with prominent anxiety.

So the present situation appears to be that there is a large body of purely clinical knowledge built up from observation of psychiatric patients over the years, with information about associated (and hitherto relatively ineffective) attempts at treatment. Then on the other hand there has comparatively recently been a rapid accumulation of scientific knowledge largely derived from animal work and developed from the basic observations that particular groups of drugs appear to be effective in particular types of illness. Unfortunately, there is almost no direct relationship so far between the available clinical experience and the scientific findings. A potential link may occur in relation to plasma levels of antidepressants. For example, the so-called 'therapeutic window' could be of considerable clinical importance but many clinicians find the concept difficult to accept because common experience is that resistant illnesses tend to respond to higher doses, sometimes very considerably higher. Indeed, such a potential relationship could be counter-productive clinically. As we know so little about the relevance of blood levels of medication to the illnesses that are being treated, the physician may be inhibited from raising doses to possible effective levels because an empirical rule concerning therapeutic levels is being broken. Indeed, it could be that this is a case where scientific knowledge should remain separated from clinical decisions until we are much surer of the relationships between the two.

However, there does seem one very convincing area where objective scientific information has strongly confirmed clinical practice and that is work on electroconvulsive shock (ECS) given to rats (Grahame-Smith, Green and Costain, 1978). It is postulated that the treatment of human affective disorder requires enhanced activity of brain monoamines and it has been shown that ECS given to rats does not enhance behavioural responses to increased brain serotonin unless a convulsion is produced (sub-convulsive shocks being ineffective) and when several shocks are given confined to one day only. The clinical practice of requiring more than one treatment, that treatment should continue to be given a few days apart, and that a convulsion is necessary are all confirmed, surely not merely by chance. Furthermore, this same experimental model has shown that an effect is not produced by a period of anoxia, nor by the muscle relaxant alone, nor when the shock is given to the feet and there is no central effect. Thus, a purely scientific study, without immediate clinical associations has confirmed and established empirically the therapeutic need that a convulsion must occur. It has also justified the exact form that clinical practice has, over the years, come to take simply as a result of experience.

From the clinical side, the major problem is that we have so far no reliable and objective manifestation of any psychiatric illness and further effort is very much required in this direction. An essential link with scientific work must be the detection of some aspect of the presumed metabolic abnormality in patients with functional psychoses.

Nosology is an important starting point and the problem of the classification of depression constitutes a very good example of the special difficulties that relate to diagnosis in psychiatry.

Kendell (1968 and 1976) has produced distinguished research reports and commentaries on the problems of classifying depressive illnesses. Lewis (1971) managed, as was so often the case, to find all the hypothetical proposals unacceptable in logic. The whole point is that psychiatry is an unnervingly imprecise subject but clinical psychiatrists must, nonetheless, continue to live with this and do their best to continue to evolve hypotheses in the hope that evidence supporting one or other will appear.

The essence of the problem concerns the controversy as to whether depression is either a single experience or involves two or more conditions. This has very important research implications because should there in fact be two forms of depression, perhaps one with a biochemical abnormality (?endogenous) and perhaps one without (?neurotic), it could be difficult to locate the presenting abnormality if the sample contained relatively large numbers of patients whose metabolism was normal but where this possibility was not anticipated. The relationship between what may be called 'endogenous' and 'neurotic' depression has also been reviewed by Kilch et al (1972).

Another associated controversy concerns the relationship between anxiety and depression. Some states of anxiety respond very effectively to antidepressant medication and from points made above the pharmacological implication is that some anxiety states strongly resemble depressive illnesses in the characteristic of having a relatively specific response to a drug that we call an antidepressant. It should be noted that the best definition of an antidepressant is not a drug used for the treatment of depression, it is more accurately considered as a drug that increases the activity of one or more central neurotransmitter monoamines. The relationship between anxiety states and depressive illnesses has been considered by Roth et al (1972) and by Pollitt and Young (1971).

There has been much speculation but what is now wanted is an attempt to try to isolate sub-types of illness not so much on clinical grounds but by metabolic means and in this process the response to treatment may be of decisive importance. As Bridges (1976) has pointed out there was once a symptom-disease of 'dropsy' and this was broken down by the discovery of the therapeutic value in this condition of the foxglove with its digitalis content, although the significance was not at the time realised. Cases came to be divided into those where digitalis was effective which we now know to be of cardiac origin and cases where it was ineffective which were of renal or other causes. Subsequently a true physiological classification of oedema was developed.

Evidence from the past like this tends to refute the possibility that depression can be regarded as a continuum because groups of depressed people show so many different characteristics connected with reactivity, symptomatology, genetic relations, pattern of recurrence and response to treatment. Bridges (1976) also pointed out the analogy with 'breathlessness' as a continuum: 'Breathlessness might be considered either as a continuum or consisting of several separate experiences of respiratory difficulty, but there are nonetheless all kinds of different implications in the breathlessness of a fit person after strenuous exercise, of someone with cardiac insufficiency after mild exertion, and of a patient with pneumothorax at rest. In none of these circumstances would a disease-concept called 'dyspnoea' be of any clinical value, although it could be postulated that the first was obviously 'reactive', the second due to an inability to cope with a specific stress, and the third "endogenous"!'

If we call a condition depression then we expect depressed mood to be the predominant presentation. The illness of 'endogenous depression' may well be essentially a hypothalamic disturbance as suggested by Pollitt (1965) and with this concept in mind depressed mood, although a common manifestation, need not be the essential characteristic of the illness. The implications are important because if there is a fundamental hypothalamic disturbance present then we are dealing with an illness perhaps with more in common with endocrinology than

79

with psychiatry, as it tends to be regarded at present. The evidence of such an abnormality comes from metabolic studies mentioned below and, to some extent, from the considerable effectiveness of physical treatments of many kinds – medication, ECT, and psychosurgery (Bridges and Bartlett, 1977). After all, anxiety is also a prominent presentation of thyrotoxicosis but in this illness relatively little attention needs to be given to the psychological implications of the anxiety and nearly all the clinical involvement concerns correction of the abnormal thyroid function. Dependence on traditional diagnostic schemes is considerably reduced by means of the present state examination (Wing, Cooper and Sartourius, 1974) which could be particularly useful in attempts to relate physical findings to clinical observations.

Some progress on the lines suggested has been taking place and many of the studies have been mentioned by Professor Grahame-Smith. Perhaps of special importance, in relation to the identification of a particular form of depressive illness, is what comes from the work of Carroll and Curtis (1976) describing a simple endocrinological test that differentiates depressed patients from those who are not depressed, namely, a failure of cortisol suppression by dexamethasone. The theoretical aspects of this, implicating an abnormality of the hypothalamic-pituitary-adrenocortical system, have been discussed by Carroll, Curtis and Mendals (1976).

The possibility that the level of the excretory product of serotonin, 5-hydroxyindolacetic acid in lumbar cerebrospinal fluid, could indicate the presence of depression with sufficient clinical relevance for the value to act as a suicidal predictor when particularly low, has been suggested by Asberg, Traskman and Thoren (1976). Quite recently a clear distinction has been shown by Gold, Pottash, Davies et al (1979) between patients with bipolar depression and those with unipolar illnesses by observing the response of thyrotropin-stimulating hormones to thyrotropin-releasing hormone. Schildkraut, Orsulak, Schatzberg et al (1978) have comprehensively studied catecholamine metabolism in an attempt to provide a biochemical classification of depressive disorders.

Many of these studies have inevitably shown a number of anomalies which are difficult to explain. However, there are two basic lines of thought that can be pursued. In a paper by Bonham-Carter, Sandler, Goodwin et al (1978) a single dose of tryamine was given to a group of severely depressed patients and free and total tyramine output values were measured in two successive three-hour collections following ingestion. The depressed patients showed significantly decreased excretion of conjugated tyramine in the first three hours compared with control subjects. The severely depressed group had modified psychosurgery a week after the test and the test was repeated one year post-operatively when, despite the fact that half the patients had made an excellent recovery, the same proportion with the metabolic abnormality was found. Thus, there is support for the view that the treatments we have available for depression do not necessarily correct the basic pathology but in some way modify the manifestation of the illness. So we have to be aware of the possible occurrence of, firstly, metabolic phenomena that are secondary and that may have an association with clinical presentation such as depression, or anxiety, or obsessional symptoms. Then perhaps we should also seek a more basic pathology that may be less necessarily related to clinical aspects, so far as we are aware of the significance of them at the moment.

The genetics of the functional psychoses are complex and this is another aspect to be taken into account as shown by Schlesser and Winokur (1979) in which the association of failure of cortisol suppression following dexamethasone occurred more often in patients with a family history of depressive illness. Andreasen and Winokur (1979) have further studied classification on the basis of family history and also on the course of the illness.

The so-called and much maligned 'medical model' undoubtedly does not have universal relevance in psychiatry but there are areas where clinical and scientific problems cannot be effectively elucidated without drawing on traditional scientific and medical experiences and methods.

COMMENTARY ON CURRENT TRENDS IN
NEUROPHARMACOLOGY AND PSYCHOPHARMACOLOGY

Peter Eames

I Introduction

It is no enviable task to try to bring out for discussion points from Professor
Grahame-Smith's paper: it is both comprehensive and clinically relevant. I am
forced to a good deal of repetition, therefore, but I shall attempt at least to pick
up some of what are to me the meatier crumbs and look at them from a slightly
different viewpoint and with an inevitably different (if only because more
naive) perspective. Uppermost in my mind, of course, will be a wish to relate
pharmacological information to clinical experiences and needs and perhaps even
to try to formulate some practical strategies and tactics.

However, if Professor Grahame-Smith can be happy enough for his paper to
'come out as a pot-pourri' I can scarcely apologise enough for the fact that this
discussion comes out more like a mess of pottage!

II Three New Viewpoints

To begin with I want to suggest three particular ways of looking at
psychopharmacological phenomena which seem to me to have emerged only
fairly recently and yet seem to be of very considerable importance. They are:

First, that most drugs affecting the brain have chronic effects which are
different from their acute effects; second, that most drugs which affect
neurological and psychological phenomena do so *because* they are manipulating
neuro-regulators; and third, that these effects are less likely to be due directly to
the changes in a *particular* neuro-regulator activity than to the result of changes
in *balance* between converging neuro-regulatory systems.

(i) Acute and Chronic Effects

The two latter points are so interconnected as to demand joint consideration, but the question of balance also has implications about acute and chronic effects. These have been discussed a good deal by Professor Grahame-Smith. The sorts of adjustments of balance, within and between systems, that produce these changes seem very definitely to include changes in receptor sensitivity, quite probably relating to changes in the numbers of post-synaptic receptor-sites. It even appears that, at least in some brain areas, such numerical changes can occur quite quickly and it has been argued, for example that some inherent timing-circuits (or 'neurobiological clocks', if you will) may work by the see-saw waxing and waning of the number of active receptors under the impact of consequent lessening and increasing cellular response (Friedhoff and Miller, 1979). Another sort of adjustment is likely to involve protein metabolism, and a third is the re-adjustment of other interacting neuro-regulating systems in the face of an alteration in the overall balance.

The importance of the emergence of chronic effects should perhaps have been more obvious all along in the case of the anti-depressants in view of the well-recognised delay in the onset of their therapeutic action and has certainly forced itself on us in no uncertain way with the phenothiazines as a result of the problem of tardive dyskinesias. There is another apparently more subtle example in an almost universal phenomenon that has a number of important clinical implications. We all have the frequent experience of seeing that almost any drug acting on the brain induces sedation in the first few days of use. Commonplace though this is, and although manufacturers and textbook-writers generally do refer to 'sedation' as a so-called 'side-effect', the usual transience of the sedation rarely gets a mention. To my mind, the most absurd example is chlormethiazole, a drug that many of us use in quite impressively large doses during alcohol withdrawal: we regularly see patients after three or four days (and still taking as much as 3 grams a day or more) participating in an alert and lively fashion in group discussions and the like; yet chlormethiazole is described in the manufacturers' literature as 'a sedative hypnotic' and this description is dutifully reproduced in most textbooks. What can be the cause of such a paradox? It appears that the manufacturers' statements are based on the results of acute studies in animals. They rarely perform 'chronic' behavioural studies which, they say, are usually done by the universities. In fact, with many drugs, no such 'chronic' studies are done at all. This hardly seems sufficient excuse for failing to take cognisance of clear clinical evidence.

This general issue is also of importance to the problem of compliance. Professor Grahame-Smith suggests that a common cause of lack of compliance is that doctors do not explain to patients the nature of the drugs they are given. Perhaps just as important is not explaining what initial transient side-effects may occur. It is sometimes argued that this is likely to increase the incidence of the side-effects. This may, I suppose, be of some importance as a variable in a study of side-effects; but in practical therapeutics compliance is of very much greater importance and experience suggests, and theoretical considerations of the impact of unpleasant surprises would predict, that patients will put up with irritating effects which they *know* to expect and are *reassured* will be transient. My own most persuasive experience of this sort is that I have yet to have a patient refuse to persist with clomipramine in spite of very frequent, and I believe very unpleasant, unwanted effects during the first week or two of treatment.

(ii) Neuroregulators

I should now like to consider the question of neuroregulators. (It seems to be current practice to use this term to refer to both neurotransmitters – produced by neurones and released at synapses – and neuromodulators – produced in various sites and disseminated producing effects 'at a distance'.)

It was obviously an enormous blessing suddenly to be in possession of drugs like chlorpromazine and the antidepressants that for all their faults, actually made it possible to influence the course of illness. To say that their discoveries were serendipitous is perhaps only to say that they came about not through factors concerned with the drugs' pharmacokinetics or pharmacodynamics but with their empirically observable therapeutic effects. But the subsequent attempts to find out how the drugs worked were most important steps leading towards the great burgeoning of knowledge about neurochemistry and brain function that we are faced with today. What also has become apparent – again something which perhaps we should have predicted long ago in a practical way – is that our psychoactive drugs have their effects by acting upon neurotransmitter systems. In the past four years interest has been focused increasingly on a whole new level of chemical control, the neuromodulators. Although many of the peptides involved have been known for a long time (particularly the hormone-releasing hormones and some of the pituitary hormones like vasopressin and ACTH), the discovery of the encephalins and endorphins opened up the whole field, and knowledge and ideas about the functional structure, so to speak, of the brain have gained enormously from the development of a conceptual framework within which, for example new perspectives have arisen on the longer-known peptides. There is thus an emerging picture of multiple systems in brain function, systems which interact, and the resultants of whose interacting activities determine mental and behavioural outcomes. There is interaction – final common 'pathing' so to speak; there is feedback regulation; and there is intrinsic regulation, for example, of the types involved in the chronic effects which we have discussed. It seems inevitable, therefore, that it must take more than a simple quantitative change in a single neurotransmitter's formation, release, destruction, or re-uptake to bring about a sustained change in the outcome (namely behaviour) since the whole system is so circumscribed with re-adjustment mechanisms. At the same time, since the systems interact (among other ways) through chains and even cascades of neurones producing different neurotransmitters and are modulated, presumably, by the resultants of the differing actions of a number of neuromodulators it must be possible for the same behavioural changes to result from several entirely different single chemical changes. (It may be helpful to liken this situation to the case of genetically determined hypothyroidism: whichever of the enzymes of the chain of synthesis is affected the same clinical hypothyroid state results.)

All this great but ordered complexity has a number of implications for research into the nature of the changes in mental illnesses and, indeed, for their treatment.

In the first place, if say, schizophrenia is really 'the schizophrenias' — not in Bleuler's sense of similar but different syndromes but in the sense of different chemical lesions leading to the same (or very similar) behavioural effects — then the evaluation of the efficacy of various drug treatments must take account of that possibility. In recent years, there have been both positive and negative reports of treatment of schizophrenia with propranolol, baclofen, vasopressin, and even beta-endorphin. If it were true that these various substances were very effective but only in certain chemical (but not necessarily clinical) subgroups of patients then the usual sorts of statistical analyses employed to examine the effects could well lead to overall 'negative' results. If, instead, analysis focused on those individuals who did appear to respond, there might be two possible advances. First, there might develop a treatment approach involving successive trials of treatment starting perhaps with the drug must frequently producing improvement or perhaps with the one which produced a 'yes/no' answer most quickly. Second, from the research point of view, this could amount to using drugs as scalpels with which to dissect out the different sub-groups that could then be looked at more closely for possible clinical differences using the usual tools of phenomenology, psychophysiology, and so on. In this way we might be able to learn how to predict which treatment should be the first choice for any particular patient. (This is something of a reversal of the established approach to such problems.) Such an approach would demand, of course, that the drugs used be of considerable safety. The closer the drugs used are to being natural neuroregulators or their precursors the more likely is this safety to be achieved.

My second point is connected both directly and in the sense of being at least as heretical. If we are looking for safe and effective treatments then we should consider the possibility that in evaluating new treatments we might look not for some statistically just significant effect but for an effect of sufficient magnitude that it hits us in the eye. It seems to me that there is a good argument for conducting studies of the clinical effects of really new drugs with the intention of accepting only really obvious and dramatic improvements as valid. Of course this is open to the risk of confusing the effects of natural history but if it is done against a background of the expectation of finding 'chemical sub-groups' and if the research implications of such expectation are taken seriously then there is little risk of being led seriously astray by this sort of approach.

Thirdly, in this new era of many possibilities and known dangers attached to established treatments the idea of drugs as scalpels seems capable of creating a new ethic (if that is not too pompous a word) whereby collections of careful studies of the treatment of single cases properly conducted assessing the effects of relatively safe if experimental drugs might acquire a new respectability. Again, the less 'synthetic' the drugs assessed the less multiple their effects are likely to be and thus the safer they will be to experiment with. Perhaps this 'new ethic' will also demand that we become, whilst we explore it, 'naturopaths all'.

Like all vaguely heretical approaches, however, this will certainly demand the acceptance of certain responsibilities. For example, there is the responsibility of making careful observations and keeping careful records and looking at them all again in attempts to fit the pieces together. But above all we should heed the advice of Professor Grahame-Smith when he tells us that 'It is important for practising psychiatrists to understand current lines of psychopharmacological research so that they can contribute through clinical observation to the understanding of neuropharmacology and not just to practical therapy'.

I might add, perhaps in a rather defensive manner, that the idea of taking a qualitative rather than a 'statistical' approach is one that has spread through various disciplines in recent years. My own first recollection of a public plea for such an approach is Lord Platt's Harveian Oration of 1967, 'Medical Science: Master of Servant' (Platt, 1967). Since then, the army of educational psychologists previously dedicated to opposing the concept of specific learning disabilities has taken an interest in observing how children approach test materials rather than just what results they can score. And the fairly new breakaway specialty within psychology, namely neuropsychology, makes observation of an individual's test performance the very centre of its approach to assessment (Wood, 1979). As clinical psychiatrists we could do much worse than to take pains to follow this sort of lead.

For those who have an interest in this type of experimental approach to treatment I have tried to produce, as an aid, a tabulated version of several of the currently available texts of psychopharmacology, summarising presently available drugs of relative safety and their places in what seems to be the scheme of things synaptic. Table 6 covers only drugs interacting with major known neurotransmitters — so far I have not been able to force myself to the task of extending it to neuromodulators. (There is just one general comment I would like to make about it; there seem to be very few neurotransmitters which are clearly 'excitatory' and far too many which are 'inhibitory': there is increasing evidence for a number of very simple amino-acids as neurotransmitters — glutamic acid, glycine, and so on and no doubt the vast amount of research directed towards these substances will shortly fill out the picture.)

TABLE 6. Drugs manipulating centrally acting neurotransmitters

| Neurotransmitters | Drugs affecting Synthesis and Storage | | Breakdown-blocking drugs | Drugs affecting Receptors | | Drugs enhancing effects by blocking uptake mechanisms |
	Precursors	'Reducers'		Analogues and 'Releasers'	Blockers	
Acetylcholine + (muscarinic)	lecithin choline deanol	hemicholinium*	physostigmine	oxotremorine arecoline	atropine benzhexol benztropine tricyclics (high doses)	atropine (small amounts)
Noradrenaline − (+)	phenylalanine tyrosine L-dopa	α-methyl-p-tyrosine* disulfiram reserpine tetrabenazine lithium (oxypertine)	M.A.O.I.s thujaplicin* tropolone*	Indirect Sympathomimetics: phenylethylamine amphetamine tyramine pemoline octopamine clonidine	beta-blockers propranolol (prostaglandin-E)* (dihomo-γ-linolenic acid)	amphetamine cocaine tricyclics (desip. > imip. > clomip.)
Dopamine − (+)	phenylalanine tyrosine L-dopa	α-methyl-p-tyrosine* reserpine tetrabenazine lithium-hydroxybutyrate* (oxypertine)	M.A.O.I.s thujaplicin* tropolone*	Indirect Sympathomimetics apomorphine piribedil	phenothiazines thioxanthenes butyrophenones pimozide sulpiride (P.G.E.1)* (D.H.L.A.)	amphetamine (high dose) cocaine benztropine
5-hydroxytryptamine −	L-tryptophan 5-hydroxytryptophan	valine leucine reserpine tetrabenazine lithium	M.A.O.I.s	dimethyltryptamine* bufotenine* (L.S.D.)* pimozide	cyproheptadine methysergide pizotifen (L.S.D.)* (propranolol) phenothiazines	tryptamine α-methyltryptamine* tricyclics (clomip. > imip. > desip.)
γ-amino-butyric acid −	glutamic acid (pyridoxine)	thiosemicarbazide*	sodium valproate (benzodiazepines) (D-cycloserine)	muscimol* baclofen (benzodiazepines)	picrotoxin* bicuculline*	

*Not readily available clinically.   ( ) Not certain action, or very complex actions.

87

III Some Practical Implications of Current Psychopharmacology

I should now like to change tack and go on to consider three particular areas of current interest — at least to me.

(i) Serum Levels

First I should like to consider the question of the use of serum levels in monitoring treatment. The evidence reviewed by Professor Grahame-Smith on the correlations between serum levels of antidepressants and their clinical effect seems to be far from encouraging. Even a few years ago nortriptyline must have stood fairly low in the order of antidepressant popularity, and with the flood of newer, often quite different drugs for this purpose, it has doubtless sunk much lower. Yet it seems that this is the only drug for which evidence of a predictable relationship is at all persuasive. It is only fair to point out that there is another factor, less creditable perhaps, but intensely practical: serum levels of a wide range of drugs are not readily available to the majority of clinicians and even the simple matter of taking and sending samples, especially in bulging psychiatric out-patient departments, is simple only in concept. (This is a situation bearing some similarity to that of the use of bacteriological studies before the prescribing of antibiotics — the almost universally accepted principle is very widely sacrificed to expedience and nowhere more than in the busy and difficult setting of general practice where, after all, most infections are dealt with.) With these rather large problems, both scientific and everyday, I seriously doubt that the use of serum levels in monitoring treatment will find much general acceptance. It is possible that they may come into standard use in a more restricted way, for example in attempts to elucidate drug-resistance. (The general question was recently reviewed in a Leading Article in the British Medical Journal with rather similar conclusions.)

On the other hand, the research which has been done has provoked valuable ideas about strategies for drug usage. Professor Grahame-Smith has quoted Asberg's advice on nortriptyline. As another example, not long ago, at the meeting of the British Association for Psychopharmacology Dr. William Sargent was advocating the use of lithium without serum-level control by the expedient of increasing the dose until tremor and vomiting appeared and then dropping it by one dosage step. I am not necessarily advocating such a strategy (though the game of sending simultaneous samples from the same patient to different laboratories — or even to the same laboratory, but with different labels — usually produces results sufficient to shake, or at least nudge, one's faith in the scientific practice). But I do want to make the point that strategies of this type can be proposed only because there exists the relevant knowledge about the relationships between serum levels and therapeutic effects. So I want to suggest that as clinicians we should be aware of what these sorts of sophisticated studies show and put our minds to the problem of formulating strategies for many more of the commonly used psychoactive drugs and then of testing these strategies empirically in clinical settings. There is a potential catch, of course: unless this sort of approach is used fairly widely there are likely to be difficulties in persuading reputable journals to publish such results and without wide dissemination the strategies would lose a great deal of their point.

The situation with serum levels and the phenothiazines seems even more fraught, not only with the problems of multiple and insufficiently characterised metabolites, but also with the peculiarities of distribution and fate. The very lengthy persistence in brain tissue of chlorpromazine (attested not only by animal studies but also by the clinical feature of much delayed relapse after the end of lengthy treatment) raises the possibility of rapid 'fixing' to explain the failure of large doses to produce higher serum levels. I confess I know of no clear study demonstrating a relationship between higher doses and greater clinical effect but clinical experience certainly suggests it. The nearest to a proper study I have seen with data presented informally by Wagemaker showing that the planned aggressive use of rapidly increasing doses of chlorpromazine (up to 2 grams in 24 hours) greatly decreased the time to disappearance of florid signs in acute schizophrenics compared with the use of more commonly employed dosages.

(ii) Anticholinergic Drugs

I should like next to pursue and extend some of the points made by Professor Grahame-Smith about anticholinergic drugs. It is now eight years since the first very clear demonstration that a majority of patients taking phenothiazines long-term have no more extrapyramidal symptoms and signs without anticholinergic drugs than with them (Orlov et al, 1971). For at least five years it has been known that the concurrent use of these two groups of drugs increases the probability of the development of tardive dyskinesias (Klawans and Rubovits, 1974). In spite of this, the habit of prescribing anticholinergics from the start of, and throughout, phenothiazine treatment appears to be very widespread. Obviously there is considerable need to solve, not only the problems of doctor-patient communication but also the problems of researcher-clinician communication. It is clear that the appropriate general strategy should be to reserve anticholinergics for use when extrapyramidal problems actually appear and only for brief *reviewed* use at that. Further, there should be careful exploration of the values of the various different anticholinergic drugs now in use in order to establish the most suitable — or, rather, the least unsuitable. (It seems to be relatively little known, for example, that the safest and quickest means of treating *acute* dystonic reactions is intravenous diazepam.) All anticholinergics, of course, block receptors of acetylcholine; but benztropine, the increasing use of which appears to have reached us from America (as can be seen perhaps from the fact that it costs about ten times as much as benzhexol!) also blocks dopamine re-uptake and therefore militates against the main therapeutic actions of the phenothiazines. If other 'anticholinergics' have the

89

same effect to any degree this may be at least one factor explaining some experimental findings showing that anticholinergic drugs reverse the therapeutic effects of neuroleptics on 'adaptive behaviour' and 'social participation' (Singh and Lal, 1978) and also analogous effects demonstrated in animal work. Another factor may be revealed by the suggestions that anticholinergic drugs may reduce blood levels of chlorpromazine, and may exacerbate the symptoms during acute treatment with it. (It is perhaps of particular interest here that it is only in the acute early phase of treatment that therapeutic response to chlorpromazine shows a correlation with serum levels.) However (as reviewed by Singh and Lal) it is clear that cholinergic blockade *itself* tends to increase schizophrenic symptoms particularly by interfering with habituation — this may be a good example of the perturbation of a balance by interfering with either of two contributing factors (in this case decreased cholinergic activity or increased dopaminergic activity).

Thus there are many good reasons for being very sparing in the use of anticholinergic drugs during phenothiazine treatment. How to turn this idea into truly standard practice is altogether another matter.

(iii) Schedules of Administration

Finally, I should like to look at the question of schedules of administration. The pharmacokinetic considerations discussed by Professor Grahame-Smith in relation to variability of responses in different individuals also have implications for establishing the most fruitful and appropriate ways of using our drugs. We might start from the fact that the pharmacokinetics of the drug determine how often it need be given (in a particular dose) in order to achieve a particular serum concentration — though perhaps we should subsume all the complex and largely unknown details of drug-distribution and its influence on the time/blood-concentration relationship by talking rather of 'body concentration'. Next, we need to try to relate the necessary pharmacokinetic data on any particular drug to the 'body concentration' needed for therapeutic effect.

As an example, consider amitriptyline: there appears to be little difference in the therapeutic effect, or the delay in achieving it, whether this drug is used in divided doses or in a single daily dose of the same daily amount so the distribution necessary for the same pharmacodynamic effect is presumably achieved by either schedule (and incidentally, this must be so regardless of what the *serum*-levels are doing). On the other hand, although diazepam has a very long half-life and a strong tendency therefore to accummulate, nevertheless, as far as its anxiolytic action is concerned there seems little doubt that regular divided doses are necessary if consistent sedation and even overt intoxication are to be avoided. Where there is a choice of equally effective schedules the next step is to consider how the goal of compliance can best be reached and the evidence (to no-one's surprise) shows that the simpler and less frequent the schedule the more likely is compliance. (This is very fully reviewed by both

Lader (1976) and Ley (1977). The difficulty in establishing the most appropriate schedules is that information is hard to come by about the complex relationships between the pharmacokinetics, pharmacodynamics (whatever they are), and therapeutic effects. It would help if there were pharmacokinetic studies available on more drugs — it is amazing how many do not appear to have been studied this way. Perhaps all this would not be such a drawback were it not for the fact that tradition has long determined three or four times daily schedules and it seems this is a difficult habit to give up. It tends to prevent the sorts of clinical experiments necessary to establish the effects of simpler schedules on therapeutic effect and to prevent changes of clinical practice even when adequate information *is* available. For example, propranolol, when first introduced, was recommended to be given six-hourly though later studies have shown a twice daily dosage to be equally effective (and even once-daily dosage to be effective in the case of blood pressure reduction). Yet a majority of prescriptions for propranolol seem to specify three or four daily doses. Again, it is clear from clinical experience that trifluperazine can be given with full effect just once daily. And perhaps the most interesting recent demonstration has been that lithium carbonate, whether as Camcolit or as Priadel or Phasal, achieves the same serum levels for a given dose whether in divided doses or just once a day (Hullin, 1977).

One last point: although some 'unwanted effects' are clearly related to pharmacodynamic effects of the same order as the main effects (for example, extrapyramidal disturbances from phenothiazines), others appear to arise from different effects: for example, when amitriptyline is given in a one nightly dose there appears to be much less daytime sedation than with divided doses through the day. It seems likely that these latter effects relate to peak blood levels whilst the former effects are determined by the achievement of an adequate brain tissue concentration of a more steady kind necessary to produce the 'chronic' effects.

IV Conclusion

In conclusion then, as basic research begins to bring all sorts of pieces of information together into an increasingly coherent pattern clinicians are offered various opportunities both to pursue therapeutic efforts which avoid known drug dangers and move towards the use of drugs of simpler and safer nature and also to contribute to the business of filling in the gaps of th pattern of knowledge. They also have a need to try quite consciously to elaborate strategies for drug use which capitalise on known facts about the drugs and minimise known adverse effects. In trying to achieve these aims, however, we do seem to be faced with a very big problem: that of trying to reduce the lag between the establishment of knowledge and its practical implementation as standard. I should like to suggest that discussion in this session might, among other things of course, try to concern itself with this problem.

RESPONSE TO COMMENTARIES BY DR. BRIDGES AND DR. EAMES

David Grahame-Smith

I always feel rather embarrassed in front of a group of psychiatrists when trying to steer my way through my unashamed model of psychiatry. Dr. Bridges said a word or two about Sigmund Freud, and I have an interesting quote from Freud, who said: 'I have no inclination to keep the domain of the psychological floating as it were in the air without any organic foundation — let the biologists go as far as they can, and let us go as far as we can. Some day the two will meet.' Well, he was a neurologist before he became an analyst, and therefore knew there was such a thing as a brain. Although I have had long discussions with my philosopher friends in Oxford as to whether it is necessary to have a brain to be mad, I think we have to start off from there. This is in fact a very good starting point.

There is, presumably, something wrong with the brains of mad people, of depressed people, psychotic people, anxious people, and so on, and you have to assume that when you use a psychotropic drug it is affecting an endogenous molecule in the brain. The drug goes into the body, goes into the brain, attaches itself to some receptor site, for instance an enzyme or a membrane protein, and alters a biological process which then results in some improvement or alteration in the patient's condition — whether they get better, whether they get worse (and certainly all of us would agree that sometimes our patients get worse when we give them drugs). Normal people go psychotic sometimes when you give them certain drugs, such as LSD or other psychotogens. These drugs are affecting endogenous functions of the brain to produce their effect.

Now amongst the approaches I have described, and which Dr. Bridges and Dr. Eames spoke about, are studies of the effects of drugs in animals. These give an idea of the mode of their pharmacological action, or at least information about this. Then you have to go back to the patient and look to see if there is anything that suggests that the drugs are doing what you think they might be doing from your animal experiments. For instance, if you give neuroleptics to psychotic patients, you produce Parkinsonism, and we now know that

92

neuroleptic-induced Parkinsonism is due to blockade of dopamine receptors in the extrapyramidal nervous system, information largely gleaned from the study of the effect of neuroleptics on dopamine function in animals. From these observations has grown up the vast structure of the 'dopamine hypotheses' of schizophrenia. I think the dopamine hypotheses of schizophrenia will turn out to be wrong; that probably there is not a primary disturbance of dopamine function in schizophrenia. I say this purposely and intend to be controversial, because it is fashionable to talk about the dopamine hypotheses. People are riding on this roundabout, and there is a danger of being unable to see the wood for the trees. Let me explain: Dr. Bridges used the analogy of the old lady of Shropshire and digitalis and cardiac oedema. I want to give you a more modern example, the use of the 'Lasix plant'! As you well know, the extract of the 'Lasix plant' known as 'Lasix' is extremely effective in the treatment of oedema. Suppose you didn't know anything at all about heart failure, and you didn't even know that the heart was involved in heart failure (and I guess that four hundred years ago cardiac oedema was not known to be due to diseases of the heart). Suppose the old lady from Shropshire had given an extract of the Lasix plant to someone who had dropsy due to heart disease, and they had a diuresis. A clever pharmacologist then sits down, analyses this extract of the Lasix plant, and he finds it inhibits sodium reabsorption by the renal tubules — and you can't get more precise than that. It would then be said that the condition of dropsy is always due to renal disease, and that would be a perfectly reasonable conclusion to draw. In heart failure, dropsy is due *secondarily* to renal dysfunction and the diuretic acts on a secondary level. If in this case you trusted the action of the drug as indicating the *primary* abnormality in heart failure, one would not even be in the right organ.

Take neuroleptics and dopamine. Neuroleptics block dopamine. That may or may not be the reason that they are anti-psychotic. It seems likely that it has something to do with their anti-psychotic action, but it does not follow that there is a primary disturbance of dopamine function in patients with schizophrenia, because that disturbance in dopamine function that you are blocking may be secondary to something else that is going on in the brain, that has to feed through the systems relying upon dopamine for the psychotic behaviour to occur. You will then say to me: 'Well, what is the primary disturbance?' — and I would say I don't know, and I will admit that the fact that you have a lead into the problem through the pharmacological action of an anti-psychotic drug is better than nothing. You can at least work from there to find out what might be the matter, and I think that is a very important principle. I do think it is very important to stand back and be very critical about the implications of drug action.

Now the next thing, which I'm sure will turn you all off, is Figure 1 in my paper. It looks pretty horrible, but it is very important: it is this scheme that is at the core of all drug therapy. So it's complicated — actually I think it is a miracle that one can treat anyone with a drug and make them better — it is a miracle that you can manipulate internal molecular processes and cure illness or alleviate symptoms. It's even more a miracle because it's so complicated. I want just to lead you through the scheme because it is so important. On the left side are the details of what goes on when we give a drug. On the right side are the broad phases into which things can be split. Now I want to go into this because Dr. Eames said he didn't understand the term pharmacodynamics. My task is to explain what they are, because they are important.

First, the pharmaceutical phase, though. We depend upon the drug industry for that; we want good quality preparations with well defined properties so we know how much gets into the body over how long. That's generally not our job, except that if things go wrong, pharmaceutical problems are one of the things we have to think about, and things do go wrong from time to time. Not all preparations are well standardised and entirely predictable in their bioavailability.

Then we have the pharmacokinetic phase. This is fairly complicated, but it consists of the various things in the figure, and from a general point of view the drug plasma level tells us whether the drug is in the blood or not, and whether it's likely to get to the appropriate place.

Then we go to the pharmacodynamic phase. This takes in the pharmacological action of the drug at the site of the action. With psychotropic drugs the site of action is in the brain, but of course drugs act in lots and lots of places; in the case of tricyclic antidepressants, we have an effect on the heart, monoamine oxidase inhibitors act on the liver and inhibit amino-oxidase in the liver. A pharmacological effect is not synonymous with a therapeutic effect. Take the pharmacological effect of a tricyclic antidepressant to inhibit noradrenaline and 5-HT re-uptake at the synapse: that is pharmacologically proven, and that will occur in you or me whether we are depressed or not. That is different from the therapeutic effect, because you can produce a pharmacological effect and have no therapeutic effect at all if for some reason the depression will not respond to the pharmacological effect of the drug, even though the drug is producing its pharmacological effect. That is why this analysis is so important. In scientific terms you want to be able to define in the individual patient:

(a) Is the drug in the blood? — for if it's not in the blood it certainly won't produce any effect;

(b) Is it producing its pharmacological effect? — you want to know that because if it's not producing its pharmacological effect then you can be sure it won't be producing its therapeutic effect;

(c) As clinicians, you want to know whether it is producing its therapeutic effect. But as a clinical pharmacologist I want to break the process down into its component parts if possible, in each individual patient. That is impossible for psychotropic drugs because I can't get into the brain, but I

94

might be able to find ways of looking at various functions of the body — response of the blood pressure to tyramine; various platelet functions; various red cell functions, and so on, to show that at least somewhere the drug is having a pharmacological effect which should result in a therapeutic effect if indeed that particular condition is responsive to the pharmacological effect that this drug is producing. This is *not* a plea for plasma level measurement — measuring plasma levels in people taking, say, tricyclic antidepressants or neuroleptics is not what this is about. This is trying to analyse what is happening during psychotropic drug therapy. It is not a plug for doing plasma levels. I want to make that quite clear. We do, however, have to do plasma levels if we are going to analyse all these processes occurring with psychotropic drugs for administration, but that is at a research level. A careful analysis of this sort, coupled with clinical observations and animal experiments leads one to certain conclusions. I cannot be precise about all these, but it seems to me that we have been barking up the wrong tree for quite a long time with the tricyclic antidepressants in terms of their pharmacodynamic action. I think they may well act *acutely* by inhibiting monoamine re-uptake at the synaptic plate, but I begin to think that they then induce some adaptive change in the brain, which then becomes a secondary pharmacological effect, which in turn leads to the antidepressant effect of the drug. I'd like to go a little bit further and say that I think it quite possible that the longer term antipsychotic effects of the neuroleptics might easily be due to some adaptive change following on from dopamine blockade, because if you give an animal a neuroleptic such as chlorpromazine, and you give it not for a couple of days or, as most studies have been done, with giving one shot, but if you give it for a few months, all sorts of things happen to the biochemistry of dopamine and to its pharmacology within the brain. Things that you would never have thought of on the basis of the acute effect of the drug. I think this is going to be the way that neuropharmacological research is going to go — investigating psychotropic drugs and discovering more strange things about the incredible ability of brain tissue to adapt itself to the acute effects of drugs. You can show, after four weeks of treatment in a rat with chlorpromazine, incredible changes in the number of dopamine receptors that there are within the brain. The number increases enormously, teleogically in a sense, to overcome the blocking effect of chlorpromazine. This may be partly responsible for some of the movement disorders that you get in patients who are on long term chlorpromazine, and actually bedevils all post-mortem brain studies of schizophrenic patients. The problem here is that both in this country and America, pathologists have co-operated to provide brains from patients dying who have had schizophrenic illnesses. They are stored specially and categorised in this 'Brain Bank', and then bits are sent off around the world to people who want to do receptor binding studies, enzyme studies, levels of amines and so on. The problem is that most of these patients will have been receiving neuroleptic drugs for many years, so that if you find a change in the number of dopamine receptors, what is the meaning? There isn't any way round this at the moment, and it is an extremely difficult problem. Is the finding associated with the primary disease or is it an effect of the drug treatment?

I would now like to make some comments about the comments that have been made on my paper. I do disagree with Dr. Bridges about one thing, and maybe this will inject a bit of adrenalin into the situation.

He suggested that perhaps you could use antidepressants to diagnose depression. Well, carbamazepine is widely used in the treatment of neuralgic pain. Carbamazepine, if you look it up in Mims, or indeed in Goodman and Gilman, is an anticonvulsant, therefore is neuralgic pain epileptic? Until you know the intimate pharmacology of tricyclic antidepressants, I don't think you are in a position to use tricyclic antidepressants to diagnose depression; but if you want to say that this illness is an amitriptyline-responsive psychiatric syndrome, then that is all right. You give it and the patient gets better – but amitriptyline responsiveness doesn't necessarily equal depression. For instance, you can get pain in the chest from spasm of your oesophageal sphincter, which is very like angina, and trinitrin will relieve that, and a houseman of course will say that because the pain in the chest responds to trinitrin, it must be angina pectoris, but that is nonsense, because pain in the oesophagus can also respond to trinitrin.

The problem is that until you know all the things that a drug can do, it is difficult to use it in a diagnostic context. I would like to know whether you think that, because tricyclic antidepressants work in the treatment of enuresis, enuresis is therefore due to depression, or whether the tricyclics act on enuresis by some anticholinergic effect. There could be all sorts of reasons why they work in young children with enuresis. The other thing that I was surprised to hear you say was that you were worried that there was no objective evidence of psychiatric disease. Well, a neurosurgeon I don't think would worry that the earliest sign of a brain tumour was headache, for which there is not very good objective evidence. The patient comes and says 'I've got terrible headaches'. The neurosurgeon listens to the sort of headache that the patient has, and there may not be much else, and will decide on the basis of the history whether he should investigate that headache for the presence of a space-occupying lesion. I don't think one should worry that much, but after all this is the art of psychiatry. You often don't have very good objective evidence, you have to use diagnostic criteria other than the kind of objective physical evidence you get in general medicine.

On another point, however, I agree with Dr. Bridges. It is incredibly difficult to link the animal studies with what is going on in man. You have been kind enough to say some nice words about our studies on electro-convulsive shock. But all that might be a grand house of cards, though I hope it isn't. Just because we show that giving ECS to rats in a way similar to ECT in man produces pharmacological changes, we cannot be sure we are studying the relevant changes. At the moment, I cannot fit what an ECS does to the rat with what ECT does to man, and that is what the research is about, of course, to try to find some way to bridge that gap.

One possible way in which the gap might be bridged (and you have alluded to this) is through neuroendocrine studies. You quoted the studies of Carroll on the disorder of pituitary-hypothalamic control of ACTH secretion in patients with endogenous depression. That was a beautiful and classical neuroendocrine study, a classic of clinical science. The idea now is that something goes wrong in the brain of the endogenously depressed patient which affects not only the 'Mood' brain, but also the 'Neuroendocrine' brain. The neuroendocrine disturbance is not as it were secondary to the mood disturbance, but is part and parcel of a primary disturbance. A very, very important principle if it is true, that the neuroendocrine brain has gone wrong and the mood brain has gone wrong because something else has gone wrong in some primary way somewhere. Whether that turns out to be the case, of course, only further studies will tell, but one way of looking at ECS and seeing whether it is doing the same thing to man as it does to rats, is to do neuroendocrine challenge tests. In fifty years' time we may be doing such tests in psychiatrically ill patients to define the neurotransmitter function that has gone wrong in the brains of those patients. For instance, there is already evidence that in endogenously depressed patients there is a severely depressed response of growth hormone to either clonidine or apomorphine. Growth hormone in many of these patients will just not rise when the patient is in a depressed state, but then, as the patient gets better, the response comes back. These studies haven't reached the *full* light of day yet because they have not been properly evaluated.

I think that Dr. Bridges and Dr. Eames both made an important point about studying the patient who responds to the drug. That is a problem which has bedevilled other areas of medicine. One good example of which I can think is arthritis. If you don't define the type of arthritis and its severity, and so on, your clinical trials of anti-inflammatory agents don't mean a thing because you have such a lot of noise in your patient group, it blocks out those patients who do respond. The problem is that it is very difficult in one centre to accumulate patients with classic (and I use 'classic' to mean everybody would agree on the illness) psychiatric syndromes of the same type which do respond, without a doubt, to particular agents. You sit down and design your study of schizophrenia and say you want to study fifteen patients. Fifteen patients is nothing in the field of therapeutics. You want to study fifteen patients on whatever neuroleptic it might be. Once you say you want to study a patient with schizophrenia — there is no more schizophrenia! You can't find any anywhere. This is one of the great problems in clinical psychiatric research, which I can only see being overcome by multicentre arrangements. The problem about this is that you never have one person really getting a grip of what's going on, the study gets diffused all over the country, isn't very exciting, and usually leads to varying standards of diagnosis and treatment in various centres.

The other problem is ethics. The ethics of clinical trials and studies in psychiatry are fraught with difficulty, and it takes a very long time to do anything. One of the points that has been raised is how to introduce new knowledge more quickly into clinical practice. I think it just takes a very long time to do the necessary studies and evaluate them, and I think, frankly, it should (as long as a miracle treatment is delayed). In my opinion there are things done and fashions created which after quite a short time disappear, as they are found in practice not to be any good.

There has been some confusion about the terms 'neurotransmitters' and 'neuroregulators'. To me it depends on how big the synaptic gap is and how quick the post-synaptic response is. If the gap is fairly small, and the response is very quick, then it's a neurotransmitter. If the gap is very large and the response is rather slow and lasts a long time, then it's a neuromodulator. It is very interesting that in the extrapyramidal nervous system, when you look at the dopamine nerve endings and you look at the synapses, the gaps are small (a few Angstroms); the dopamine comes out, and you can show a very quick response. If you look in the forebrain at the dopamine nerve endings, there is nothing immediately around them. They are not up tight against the post-synaptic membrane. I guess in the extrapyramidal nervous system dopamine is a neurotransmitter producing its post-synaptic effect very quickly, and in the forebrain it is squirting out like an aerosol, tickling up everything that's in the area that has appropriate receptors on it, so that when the real neurotransmitter comes along, the neurone is ready to fire. There is a beautiful example: if you take a well-defined neuropeptide, and stick it down into the ventral tegmental area of the rat's brain, the rat gets very active, and has various stereo-typed movements which settle down after twenty minutes or so. Stop the infusion, and the rat now looks perfectly normal. If you wait twenty-four hours and then give a very, very small dose of amphetamine. What it has done is to change the function of the dopamine neurones which go from the ventral tegmental area to the forebrain. This change persists, so that the amphetamine now has a greater effect. That's what neuromodulation is — that kind of long-lasting change that relatively simple substances can bring about in neurones.

I have a certain sympathy with the cowboy approach that Dr. Eames proposes, that we need only bother with the drugs that produce the dramatic effects. Well, Mims would be composed of about a couple of pages if we did that. The fact is that if we look at the treatment of hypertension, this has improved enormously since the introduction of ganglion-blocking agents, which effected a miraculous change at the time — though we don't use them any more. Gradually over the years there have been many small improvements in antihypertensive drug therapy which added up have produced a considerable improvement in treatment. I think that small changes in an existing therapy are important. However, you don't make these advances by a study of fifteen patients on a drug or a placebo. You need fifteen hundred patients on the drug and fifteen hundred patients on the placebo, because if you're looking at tiny differences between two treatments, you need a lot of patients. If you want to see whether aspirin stops myocardial infarction, you need about two thousand five hundred people. If you want to see whether lowering moderate hypertension improves life span, so you don't get coronaries or strokes, you may need twenty thousand. Some people say if that's all drugs do, then it's not worth while using one. That may or may not be a valid point of view.

Practicalities of serum levels: I knew I would be taken to task about this. I agree with some of the things that have been said about practise. I don't think there is a place at present for advocating the routine use of plasma levels of tricyclic antidepressants or neuroleptics, but there are special cases where they might possibly be useful. The technology at the moment is very complicated and extremely expensive, and therefore impossible as a routine. But so, of course, was doing blood glucose many years ago, and also very difficult, but now it's very easy. The technology of measuring drugs is improving all the time, and one can assume that things soon will be very much easier, and it may in fact become a practicality. I don't know how you get the essential knowledge regarding the practical application of drug therapy into clinical practice more quickly. I've told you my own ideas about it: sometimes I think it's not a bad idea to go more slowly. Doctors and psychiatrists are not stupid. When they see a good thing, by and large they will pick it up, more quickly than slowly, because they want to help their patients.

By and large doctors are optimists and will try out things, so I don't think one should worry too much about time lags. The detailed neuropharmacological knowledge — well, that's jolly difficult. Practical psychiatrists have a complicated job to do a job that's difficult enough without thinking about rats and the effects of giving electroconvulsive shocks. I don't think that is really an essential part of practical psychiatrists' armamentarium at the present time, though, who knows, neuropharmacological knowledge might become as important to the psychiatrist as a detailed knowledge of the electrolyte balance is to the general physician. I think that's all I have to say.

References

Adamson, L, Curry, SH, Bridges, PK, Firestone, AF, Lavin, NI, Lewis, DM, Watson, RD, Xavier, CM and Anderson, JA (1973) Fluphenazine decanoate trial in chronic in-patient schizophrenics failing to absorb oral chlorpromazine. *Diseases of the Nervous System, 34,* 181–191

Andreasen, NC, Winokur, G (1979) Newer Experimental Methods for Classifying Depression. *Archives of General Psychiatry, 36,* 447–452

Asberg, M (1974) Individualisation of treatment with tricyclic compounds. *Medical Clinics of North America, 58,* 1083–1092

Asberg, M (1976) Treatment of depression with tricyclic drugs: Pharmacokinetic and pharmacodynamic aspects. *Pharmakopsychiatrie Neuro-Psychopharmakologie, 9,* 18–26

Asberg, M, Traskman, L and Thoren, P (1976) 5-HIAA in the cerebro-spinal fluid. A biochemical suicide predictor? *Archives of General Psychiatry, 33,* 1193–1197

Atsmon, A, Blum, I and Fischl, J (1972) Treatment of an acute attack of porphyria variegata with propranolol. *South African Medical Journal, 46,* 311–314

Blackwell, B (1973) Drug therapy: Patient compliance. *New England Journal of Medicine, 289,* 249–252

Blackwell, B (1976) Treatment Adherence. *British Journal of Psychiatry, 129,* 513–531

Bonham-Carter, S, Sandler, M, Goodwin, BL, Sepping, P, Bridges, PK (1978) Decreased urinary output of tyramine and its metabolites in depression. *British Journal of Psychiatry, 132,* 125–132

Boullin, DJ, Orr, MW and Peters, JR (1978) The platelet as a model for investigating the clinical efficacy of centrally acting drugs: relations between platelet aggregation and clinical condition in schizophenics treated with chlorpromazine. In: *Platelets: A Multidisciplinary Approach.* (Eds G de Gaetano and S Garattini) pp. 389–401. New York: Raven Press

Boullin, DJ, Knox, JM, Peters, JR, Orr, MW, Gelder, MG and Grahame-Smith DG (1978) Platelet aggregation and chlorpromazine therapy. *British Journal of Clinical Pharmacology, 6,* 538–540

Boullin, DJ, Woods, HF, Grimes, RPJ, Grahame-Smith, DG, Wiles, D, Gelder, MG and Kolakowska, T (1975) Increased platelet aggregation responses to 5-hydroxytryptamine in patients taking chlorpromazine. *British Journal of Clinical Pharmacology, 2,* 29–35

Bowers, Mg Jr and Rozitis, A (1974) Regional differences in homovanillic concentration after acute and chronic administration of antipsychotic drugs. *Journal of Pharmacy and Pharmacology, 26,* 743–745

Bridges, PK (1976) Depression by any other name. *Postgraduate Medical Journal, 52,* 130–135

Bridges, PK, Bartlett, JR (1977) Psychosurgery: Yesterday and Today. *British Journal of Psychiatry, 131,* 249–260. Leading Article *British Medical Journal* (1979) *2,* 513–514

Bulat, M (1977) On the cerebral origin of 5-hydroxyindoleacetic acid in the lumbar cerebrospinal fluid. *Brain Research, 122,* 388–391

Carroll, BJ, Curtis, GC (1976) Neuroendocrine identification of depressed patients. *Australian and New Zealand Journal of Psychiatry, 10,* 13–20

Carroll, BJ, Curtis, GC and Mendels, J (1976) Neuroendocrine regulation in depression I and II. *Archives of General Psychiatry, 33,* 1039–1044 and 1051–1058

Coppen, A (1977) Personal communication

Coppen, A (1978) Amitriptyline plasma concentration and clinical effect. A World Health Organisation Collaborative Study. *Lancet, i,* 63–66

Curry, SH (1974) *Drug Disposition and Pharmacokinetics.* Oxford: Blackwell

Curry, SH, Davis, JM and Janowsky, DS (1970) Factors affecting chlorpromazine plasma levels in psychiatric patients. *Archives of General Psychiatry, 22,* 209–215

de Alarcon, R and Carney, MWP (1969) Severe depressive mood changes following slow-release intramuscular fluphenazine injection. *British Medical Journal, 3,* 564–567

Evans, JPM, Grahame-Smith, DG, Green, AR and Tordoff, AFC (1976) Electroconvulsive shock increases the behavioural responses of rats to brain 5-hydroxytryptamine accumulation and central nervous system stimulant drugs. *British Journal of Pharmacology, 56,* 193–199

Forsman, A, Martensson, E, Nyberg, G and Ohman, R (1974) A gas-chromatographic method for determining haloperidol. *Naunyn-Schmiedeberg Archives of Pharmacology, 286,* 113–124

Friedhoff, AJ and Miller, J (Barcelona, 1979) The pineal gland as a model system for studying biological rhythms. *Proceedings of IInd World Congress of Biological Psychiatry*

Gaetano, G de and Garattini, S (1978) Platelets: a multidisciplinary approach. New York: Raven Press

Gallant, DM, Mielke, DH, Sprites, MA, Swanson, WC and Bost, R (1974) Penfluridol: an efficacious long-acting oral antipsychotic compound. *American Journal of Psychiatry, 131,* 699–702

Garver, DL, Davis, JM, Dekirmenjian, H, Jones, FD, Gasper, R and Haraszti, J (1976) Pharmacokinetics of red blood cell phenothiazine and clinical effects: acute dystonic. *Archives of General Psychiatry, 33,* 862–866

Garver, DL, Dekirmenjian, H, Davis, JM, Casper, R and Erikson, S (1977) Neuroleptic drug levels and therapeutic response: preliminary observations with red-cell bound butaperazine. *American Journal of Psychiatry, 134,* 304–307

Glassman, AH, Perel, JM, Shostak, M, Kantor, SJ and Fliess, JL (1977) Clinical implications in imipramine plasma levels for depressive illness. *Archives of General Psychiatry, 34,* 197–204

Gold, MS, Pottash, ALC, Davies, RK, Ryan, N, Sweeney, DR, Martin, DM (1979) Distinguishing unipolar and bipolar depression by thyrotropin release test. *Lancet, ii,* 411–412

Goodwin, FK, Post, RM and Sack, RL (1975) Clinical evidence for neurochemical adaptation to psychotropic drugs. In: *Neurobiological Mechanisms of Adaptation and Behaviour.* (Ed AJ Mandell). New York: Raven Press

Grahame-Smith, DG (1978) Pharmacological aspects of schizophrenia. *Biochemical Society Special Publications, 1,* 197–207

Grahame-Smith DG (1977a) Monitoring drug therapy: the use of cellular biochemical and pharmacological techniques. *Netherlands Journal of Medicine, 20,* 36–45

Grahame-Smith, DG and Green, AR (1977) The effect of electroconvulsive shock on brain monoamine function in the rat. In: *Depression.* Symposium Medica Hoechst

Gram, L, Reisby, N, Ibsen, I, Nagy, A, Dencker, SJ, Petersen, GO and Christiansen, J (1976) Plasma levels and the antidepressant effect of imipramine. *Clinical Pharmacology and Therapeutics, 19,* 318–324

Green, AR (1978) Repeated exposure of rats to the convulsant agent fluorothyl enhances 5-hydroxytryptamine and dopamine mediated behavioural responses. *British Journal of Pharmacology*

Green, AR and Grahame-Smith, DG (1974a) The role of dopamine in the hyperactivity syndrome produced by increased 5-hydroxytryptamine synthesis in rats. *Neuropharmacology, 13,* 949–959

Green, AR and Grahame-Smith, DG (1974b) TRH potentiates behavioural changes following increased brain 5-hydroxytryptamine accumulation in rats. *Nature, 251,* 524–526

Green, AR and Grahame-Smith, DG (1975) 5-hydroxytriptamine and other indoles in the central nervous system. In: *Handbook of Psychopharmacology,* Vol. 3, pp. 169–245. (Eds SD Iversen, LL Iversen and SH Synder). New York: Plenum Press

Green, AR and Grahame-Smith, DG (1976a) The effect of drugs on the processes regulating the functional activity of brain 5-hydroxytryptamine. *Nature, 260,* 487–491

Green, AR and Grahame-Smith, DG (1976b) (−)-propranolol inhibits the behavioural responses of rats to increased 5-HT in the central nervous system. *Nature,* 594–596

Green, AR, Heal, DJ, Grahame-Smith, DG and Kelly, PH (1976) The contrasting actions of TRH and cycloheximide in altering the effects of centrally actings drugs: evidence for the non-involvement of dopamine sensitive adenylate cyclase. *Neuropharmacology, 15,* 591–599

Greenblatt, DJ and Koch-Weser, J (1975) Clinical pharmacokinetics. *New England Journal of Medicine, 293,* 702–705

Heal, DJ, Green, AR, Boullin, DJ and Grahame-Smith, DG (1976) Single and repeated administration of neuroleptic drugs to rats: effects on striatal dopamine sensitive adenylate cyclase and locomotor activity produced by tranylcypromine and L-tryptophan or L-dopa. *Psychopharmacology, 49,* 287–300

Hirsch, SR, Gaind, R, Rohde, PD, Stevens, BC and Wing, JK (1973) Outpatient maintenance of chronic schizophrenic patients with long-acting fluphenazine. *British Medical Journal, 1,* 633–637

Hughes, J (1978) *Centrally Acting Peptides.* (Ed J Hughes). London: Macmillan

Hullin, RP (1977) Absorption of lithium from controlled-release preparations. *British Medical Journal, 1,* 1349

Iversen, LL (1973) Monoamines in the mammalian central nervous system and the action of antidepressant drugs. *Biochemical Society Special Publications, 1,* 81–96

Johnson, DAW (1975) Observations on the dose regime of fluphenazine decanoate in maintenance therapy of schizophrenia

Kendell, RE (1968) *The Classification of Depressive Illness.* Maudsley Monograph No 18 London: Oxford University Press

Kendell, RE (1976) The Classification of Depressions: A Review of Contempory Confusion. *British Journal of Psychiatry, 129,* 15–28

Kilch, LG, Andrews, G, Nielson, M and Bianchi, GN (1972) The Relationship of the Syndromes called Endogenous and Neurotic Depression. *British Journal of Psychiatry, 121,* 183–196

Klawans, HL and Rubovits, R (1974) Effect of cholinergic and anti-cholinergic agents on tardive dyskinesia. *Journal of Neurology, Neurosurgery and Psychiatry, 37,* 941–947

Kolakowska, T, Wiles, DH, McNeilly, AS and Gelder, MG (1975) Correlation between plasma levels of prolactin and chlorpromazine in psychiatric patients. *Psychological Medicine, 5,* 21–216

Kolakowska, T, Wiles, DH, Gelder, MG and McNeilly, AS (1976) Clinical significance of plasma chlorpromazine levels II. Plasma levels f the drug, some of its metabolites and prolactin in patients receiving long-term phenothiazine treatment. *Psychopharmacology Bulletin, 49,* 101–107

Kragh-Sφrensen, P, Eggert-Hansen, Chr, Baastrup, P Chr and Hvidberg, EF (1976b) Relationship between antidepressant effect and plasma level of nortriptyline: clinical studies. *Pharmacokosychiatrie Neuro-psycho-pharmacologie* (Stuttgart) *9,* 27–32

Lader, M (1976) Clinical Psychopharmacology. In: *Recent Advances in Psychiatry,* pp. 1–30. (Ed K Granville-Grossman). Edinburgh: Churchill Livingstone

Leff, JP and Wing, JK (1971) Trial of maintenance therapy in schizophrenia. *British Medical Journal, 3,* 599–604

Lewis, A (1971) 'Endogenous' and 'Exogenous': A useful Dichotomy? *Psychological Medicine, 1,* 191–196

Ley, P (1977) Psychological Studies of Doctor-Patient Communication. In: *Contributions to Medical Psychology,* Vol I. (Ed S Rachman). Pergamon Press

Machay, AVP, Healey, AF and Baker, J (1974) The relationship of plasma chlorpromazine to its 7-hydroxy and sulphoxide metabolites in a large population of schizophrenics. *British Journal of Clinical Pharmacology, 1,* 425–430

Martensson, E and Roos, BE (1974) Serum levels of thioridazine in psychiatric patients and healthy volunteers. European. *Journal of Clinical Pharmacology, 6,* 181–186

Matussek, N (1978) Neurodokrinologische Untersuchungen bie depressiven syndromen. *Der Nervenarzt, 49,* 569–575

Middlemiss, DN, Blakeborough, L and Leather, SR (1977) Direct evidence for an interaction of B-adrenergic blockers with the 5-HT receptor. *Nature, 267,* 289–290

Modigh, K (1975) Electroconvulsive shock and postsynaptic catecholomine effects: increased psychomotor stimulant action of apomorphine and clonidine in reserpine pretreated mice by repeated ECS. *Journal of Neural Transmission, 36,* 19–32

Modigh, K (1977) Personal communication

Moore, KE (1971) In: *Introduction to Psychopharmacology,* p. 117. (Eds RH Rech and KE Moore). New York: Raven Press

Orlov, P, Kasparian, G, Dimaxio, A and Cole, JO (1971) Withdrawal of antiparkinson drugs. *Archives of General Psychiatry, 25,* 410–412

Platt, Lord (1967) Medical Science: Master or Servant? *British Medical Journal, 4,* 439–444

Plotnikoff, NP, Prange, AJ, Breese, GR, Anderson, MS and Wilson, IC (1972) TRH: Enhancement of DOPA activity by a hypothalamic hormone. *Science, 178,* 417–418

Pollitt, J (1965) *Depression and its Treatment.* Heinemann: London

Pollitt, J, Young, J (1971) Anxiety State or Masked Depression? A study based on the action of monoamine oxidase inhibitors. *British Journal of Psychiatry, 119,* 143–149

Richards, AD (1964) Attitude and drug acceptance. *British Journal of Psychiatry, 110,* 46–52

Rivera-Calimlim, L, Castanida, L and Lasagna, L (1973) Effects of mode of management on plasma chlorpromazine in psychiatric patients. *Clinical Pharmacology and Therapeutics, 14,* 978–986

Rivera-Calimlim, L, Nasrallah, H, Strauss, J and Lasagna, L (1976) Clinical response and plasma levels: effect of dose, dosage schedules and drug interactions on plasma chlorpromazine levels. *American Journal of Psychiatry, 133,* 646–652

Roth, M, Gurney, C, Garside, RF and Kerr, TA (1972) Studies in Classification of Affective Disorders. *The British Journal of Psychiatry, 121,* 147–161

Sakalis, G, Curry, SH, Mould, GP and Lader, MH (1972) Physiological and clinical effects of chlorpromazine and their relationship to plasma level. *Clinical Pharmacology and Therapeutics, 13,* 931–946

Sakalis, G, Chan, TL, Gershon, S and Park, S (1974) The possible role of metabolites in therapeutic response to chlorpromazine treatment. *Psychopharmacologia (Berle) 32,* 279–284

Sayers, AC, Burki, HR, Ruch, W and Asper, H (1975) Neuroleptic induced hypersensitivity of striatal dopamine receptors in the rat as a model of tardive dyskinesia. Effects of clozapine, haloperidol, loxapine and chlorpromazine. *Psychopharmacologia (Berl), 41,* 97–104

Schildkraut, JJ (1969) Rationale of some approaches used in the biochemical studies of the affective disorders: the pharmacological bridge. In: *Psychochemical Research in Man.* (Eds AJ Mandell and MP Mandell), New York: Academic Press

Schildkraut, JJ, Orsulak, PJ, Schatzberg, AF, Gudeman, JE, Cole, JO, Rohde, WA and LaBrie, RA (1978) Toward a Biochemical Classification of Depressive Disorders. *Archives of General Psychiatry, 35,* 1427–1433

Schlesser, MA, Winokur, G, Sherman, BM (1979) Genetic Subtypes of Unipolar Primary Depressive Illness Distinguished by Hypothalamic-Pituitary-Adrenal Axis Activity. *Lancet, i,* 739–741

Shopsin, B, Wilk, S, Sathananthan, G, Gershon, S and Davis, K (1974) Catecholamines and affective disorders raised. A critical assessment. *Journal of Nervous and Mental Disease, 158,* 369–383

Singh, MM and Smith, JM (1973) Reversal of some therapeutic effects of an antipsychotic agent by an antiparkinsonian drug. *Journal of Nervous and Mental Disease, 157,* 50–58

Singh, MM and Lal, H (1978) *Dysfunctions of Cholinergic Processes in Schizophrenia.* Proceedings of the IInd World Congress of Biological Psychiatry. (Barcelona)

Snyder, SH, Banerjee, SP, Yamamura, HI and Greenburg, D (1974) Drugs, Neurotransmitters and Schizophrenia. *Science, 184,* 1243–1253

Steiner, M, Blum, I, Wijsenbeek, H and Atsmon, A (1972) Results of the treatment of psychoses with propranolol. The implications on the biochemical mechanisms of psychotic disorders. *Kupat-Holim Yearbook, 2,* 201–209

Van Praag, HM (1974) Towards a biochemical typology of depression. *Pharmakopsychiatria, 7,* 281–292

Van Praag, HM (1977) The significance of biochemical parameters in the diagnosis, treatment and prevention of depressive disorders. *Biological Psychiatry, 12,* 101–131

Vaughn, CE and Leff, JP (1976) The influence of family and social factors on the course of psychiatric illness: a comparison of schizophrenic and depressed neurotic patients. *British Journal of Psychiatry, 129,* 125–137

Walter, CJS (1971) Clinical significance of plasma imipramine levels. *Proceedings of the Royal Society of Medicine, 64,* 282–285

Wiesel, F-A, Alfredson, G, Likwornik, V and Sedvall, G (1975) A relation between drug concentrations in brain and striatal homovanillic acid levels in chlorpromazine treated rats. *Life Sciences, 16,* 1145–1156

Wiles, DH and Franklin, M (1977) Radioimmunoassay for fluphenazine in human plasma. *Clinica Chimica Acta* (submitted for publication)

Wiles, DH, Kolakowska, T, McNeilly, AS, Mandelbrote, BM and Gelder, MG (1976) Clinical significance of plasma chlorpromazine levels I. Plasma levels of the drug, some of its metabolites and prolactin during acute treatment. *Psychological Medicine, 6,* 407–415

Wing, JK, Cooper, JE and Sartorius, H (1974) The measurement and classification of psychiatric symptoms: an instruction manual for the PSE and Catego Programme. Cambridge: Cambridge University Press

Wood, RLl (1979) The Relationship of Cerebral Damage, Measured by CAT Scan to Quantative Intellectual Impairment. In: *Research in Psychology and Medicine,* Vol. I, pp. 339–346. (Ed Obourne, Gruneberg and Eiser)

Yorkston, NJ, Zaki, SA, Malik, MKV, Morrison, RC and Havard, CWH (1974) Propranolol in the control of schizophrenic symptoms. *British Medical Journal, 4,* 633–635

Yorkston, NJ, Zaki, SA, Themen, JFA and Havard, CWH (1976) Propranolol to control schizophrenic symptoms: 55 patients. In: *Neuropsychiatric effects of adrenergic beta-receptor blocking agent.* (Eds C Carlsson, J Engel and L Hansson). Munich-Berlin-Wien: Urban and Schwanzenberg

PERSONAL CONSTRUCT PSYCHOTHERAPY

Fay Fransella

The Theoretical Approach

In 1955, George Kelly published two volumes containing an alternative psychology. The theory is set out in the first volume, and the second volume consisted of a description of how the theory can be applied to explain the problems of, and provide help for, those in psychological distress. There are several suggestions to explain why the theory took twenty years to become established within the discipline of psychology as a viable alternative (see, for example, Davisson, 1978). But established it now is. What is currently developing is a realisation that it may have something important to offer as a framework within which to conduct psychotherapeutic and counselling endeavours.

One of the problems in attempting to describe the theory and the psychotherapeutic approach is that, like all other systems, it has its own language. However, it requires more than the learning of a language; it necessitates the development of a particular frame of mind with which to attempt the understanding of another person. I had not realised the importance of this latter requirement until I attempted to teach the approach to professional therapists trained in other approaches.

The theory's fundamental postulate and the eleven corollaries that elaborate it, together with the model of man Kelly presents, all stem directly from his philosophy of *constructive alternativism*. This states that 'all of our present interpretations of the universe are subject to revision or replacement'. Events are real and not just figments of the imagination, but they do not reveal themselves directly for us to see. Events are construed. In our attempts to understand and interpret as much of the life milling around us as possible, we develop an organised system of construction. By facing the world with our own personal set of such constructions we give it meaning and ourselves a sense of the continuity of personal experience. Kelly comments on the inventive nature of the person as follows:

Whatever nature may be, or howsoever the quest for truth will turn out in the end, the events we face today are subject to as great a variety of constructions as our wits will enable us to contrive. This is not to say that one construction is as good as any other, nor is it to deny that at some infinite point in time human vision will behold reality out to the utmost reaches of existence. But it does remind us that all our present perceptions are open to question and reconsideration, and it does broadly suggest that even the most obvious occurrences of everyday life might appear utterly transformed if we were inventive enough to construe them differently. (Kelly 1970)

Alternative approaches to psychotherapy from the construct theory viewpoint are thus alternative constructions of the nature of the person and of psychological disorder. Kelly decided that we each could profitably be viewed 'as if' we were scientists; scientists who go about attempting to gain increasing understanding and hence control over our environments. By construing events we are able to make predictions, to anticipate the occurrence of future events. Thus, we erect our hypotheses about a future event by having noted that, say, the sun rises and sets with monotonous regularity at the start and end of each DAY. We can therefore predict that tomorrow will be like today *in that* the sun will rise and set. We do not predict what the weather will be like tomorrow (unless we are amateur meterologists) nor what we will eat, nor whom we will meet. Our prediction in this case is precise.

The construing involved in interpersonal relations is, of course, far more complex. Some men are known to construe women as unpredictable drivers. They therefore predict that being behind a woman driver is a dangerous undertaking. To test this prediction the man has to behave – he has to carry out the act of driving behind a woman driver. For Kelly, behaviour is the experiment. It is by behaving that we test out the predictions derived from the hypotheses based on a previously established construction. In his article 'Behaviour is an Experiment' (Kelly, 1970a) Kelly says:

Instead of being a problem of threatening proportions, requiring the utmost explanation and control to keep man out of trouble, behaviour presents itself as man's principal instrument of inquiry. Without it his questions are academic and he gets nowhere. When it is prescribed for him he runs around in dogmatic circles. But when he uses it boldly to ask questions, a flood of unexpected answers rises to tax his utmost capacity to understand.

It is true that in most of psychology's inquiries some patently desirable behaviour is sought as an answer to the question posed. But the quest always proves to be elusive. In the restless and wonderful world of humanistic endeavour, behaviour, however it may once have been intended as the embodiment of a conclusive answer, inevitably transforms itself into a further question – a question so compellingly posed by its enactment that, willy

106

nilly, the actor finds that he has launched another experiment. Behaviour is indeed a question posed in such a way as to commit man to the role and obligations of an experimenter. (Kelly 1970a)

So the act of driving can be a man's test of the hypotheses that women drivers do odd things. If the woman drives impeccably, his prediction is invalidated. It is such invalidation of our construing that can bring about change. This man may say to himself that the sample was too small and that he must test his hypotheses again. He may say that the woman was having an 'off day' and that he was correct all the time. He may even reconstrue and consider the hypotheses that only *some* women are erratic drivers. On the other hand, he may attempt to 'make' the woman drive erratically. He may drive bumper to bumper, speed past her on the wrong side, or cut across her bows or hoot loudly and angrily. In all these latter cases he would be extorting validational evidence for a social prediction that had already proved itself a failure. This is how Kelly defines *hostility*. This man may have too much invested in this behavioural experiment to allow it to fail.

Construct systems are organised in a hierarchical fashion, so that the invalidation of a prediction at one level can have personally unacceptable implications at a more superordinate level. For this man, to accept that women are more than empty-headed sex objects might mean his having to question his own masculine superiority. His core construing of himself would be *threatened*. It is the awareness of impending change in construing or of the inadequacy of our system of constructs to cope with a present event that defines *emotion*. In psychotherapy such hostility is common — patients demonstrate that the therapist does not understand by designing behavioural experiments to show that their symptoms are still as bad as ever — perhaps having been threatened by the realisation that they may, indeed, soon be symptom free, therapists keep patients overlong in therapy to 'prove' they are successful therapists.

This driving example can be used to make two more theoretical points. In order for people to drive in relative safety on crowded roads with many other drivers there has to be some commonality of construing. Thus, even though each person has a construct system that is unique, similarities are said to exist when situations are construed in similar ways. Psychotherapy would be impossible if no similarity in construing existed between patient and therapist.

But similarity alone is not sufficient for understanding. Most drivers do not behave as the man in my example. Most attempt to predict what the drivers around them are going to do. Kelly argued that when we attempt to understand (construe) the construction processes of another, we are playing a social role in relation to that other person. For instance, when two people are conversing, the speaker is studying the effects his words have on the other. If the other begins to look blank, the speaker may interpret this as meaning he is going on too long — and will therefore stop. The other takes his turn at speaking and the position is

107

reversed. The behaviour of the two is now articulated — each interprets the reactions of the other and tests this prediction by behaving accordingly. It is only the attempt to construe the constructions of another that defines a role relationship, not the extent to which the interpretations are correct. This notion of role is central to an understanding of the psychotherapeutic process.

The Nature of Psychotherapy

Using the scientist model, one comes to see the person with a psychological problem as someone who is unable to test out their personal theories decisively and thus elaborate their construct systems, and their understanding of themselves and their interpersonal words. For instance, their construing may have become circular, so that they are endlessly testing and retesting the same hypotheses and appear unable to accept the implications of the data which they collect. Or they may have moved into the kind of chaos where constructions are so vague and loose that they cannot yield expectations clear enough to be tested.

Whatever the specific difficulty, the psychotherapist does not set out to 'sell' a particular construct system to the client as a predigested package. Rather he or she seeks to help the client tighten, reconstrue or test the validity of, the client's *own* construct system. If successful, that is if the client's system once again begins to move and elaborate, then the direction in which it goes and the issues it pursues are, in a very definite sense, no longer the psychotherapist's business.

Just as Kelly's view of the person stems directly from his philosophy of constructive alternativism, so it forms the base from which one approaches the person in psychotherapy. Kelly states that:

> We take the stand that there are always some alternative constructions available to choose among in dealing with the world. No one needs to paint himself into a corner; no one needs to be completely hemmed in by circumstances; no one needs to be a victim of his biography. (Kelly 1955)

We therefore have here a hopeful approach. But it in no way suggests that we each can always discover these alternatives for ourselves. We sometimes need another, or others, to point the way. Kelly saw this interaction between client and therapist as central for the clinical-psychological enterprise. Psychotherapy is a situation in which one person helped another to achieve:

> the psychological reconstruction of life. We even considered using the term *reconstruction* instead of *therapy*. If it had not been such a mouth-filling word we might have gone ahead with the idea. Perhaps later we may! (Kelly 1955)

The Psychotherapeutic Relationship

As construed by Kelly, the relationship between client and therapist is much more one of equals, each struggling with the same problem, than that of knower

108

and ignoramus. Kelly thought he saw the same struggles going on in psychotherapy as he saw going on between a PhD student and a supervisor. Both patient and student have selected the problem on which they wish to work; both may find that the initial question posed is not a very good one; both may find themselves 'stuck' during the course of the programme; both may look to their partner in the exercise and seek help in getting their construing disentangled so that they can get on the move again, and so forth.

Likewise, both therapist and supervisor accept what the patient and student bring in the first instance. Each pair works on this and tries to define the problem more clearly and in so doing perhaps even changes the question being asked. Therapist and supervisor each have experience in their particular fields which enable them to help their opposite number get out of difficulties.

The essence of the relationship is thus one of partnership. But one in which neither partner has the final answer — this they seek together. Since the relationship is couched in the metaphorical language of science, it may be helpful to let Kelly speak for himself:

> We have ruled out the notion of psychotherapy as the confrontation of the client with stark reality, whether it is put to him in the form of dogma, natural science, or the surges of his own feelings. Instead, we see him approaching reality in the same ways that all of us have to approach it if we are to get anywhere. The methods range all the way from those of the artist to those of the scientist. Like them both, and all the people in between, the client needs to assume that something can be created that is not already known or is not already there.
>
> In this undertaking the fortunate client has a partner, the psychotherapist. But the psychotherapist does not know the final answer either — they face the problem together. Under the circumstances there is nothing for them to do except for both to inquire and both to risk occasional mistakes. So that it can be a genuinely co-operative effort, each must try to understand what he himself is ready to try next. They formulate their hypotheses jointly. They even experiment jointly and upon each other. Together they take stock of outcomes and revise their common hunches. Neither is the boss, nor are they merely well-bred neighbours who keep their distance from unpleasant affairs. It is, as far as they are able to make it so, a partnership.
>
> The psychotherapy room is a protected laboratory where hypotheses can be formulated, test-tube sized experiments can be performed, field trials planned, and outcomes evaluated. Among other things, the interview can be regarded as itself an experiment in behaviour. The client says things to see what will happen. So does the therapist. Then they ask themselves and each other if the outcomes confirmed their expectations.
>
> Often a beginning therapist finds it helpful to close his cerebral dictionary and listen primarily to the sub-cortical sounds and themes that run through

his client's talk. Stop wondering what the words literally mean. Try to recall, instead, what it is they sound like. Disregard content for the moment; attend to theme. Remember that a client can abruptly change content — thus throwing a literal-minded therapist completely off the scent — but he rarely changes the theme so easily. Or think of these vocal sounds, not as words, but as pre-verbal outcries, impulsive sound gestures, stylized oral grimaces, or hopelessly mumbled questions.

But at other times the therapist will lend every effort to help the client find a word, the precise word, for a newly emerged idea. Such an exact labelling of elusive thoughts, is, at the proper time, crucial to making further inquiries and to the experimental testing of hypotheses. Particularly is this true when the team — client and therapist — is elaborating personal constructs. (Kelly 1969)

Psychological Disorder

From a personal construct standpoint, we behave in relation to how we construe the events confronting us, and so all the language to do with patients, symptoms, therapy and so forth is in terms of such constructions. Kelly defines psychological disorder as 'any personal construction which is used repeatedly in spite of consistent invalidation'. That is, the person is making poor predictions, the experiments are going wrong, the person is being a poor scientist. This person attempts to reconstrue and so achieve some validatory evidence for his construing. But he fails.

As discussed earlier, predictions about events are tested against reality by our behaving. The outcome of the experiment can be vital. When predictions are invalidated the person has to do something about this. One of the strategies open to us has already been mentioned. We can be hostile and make sure that our behaviour produces results that validate our construing. Or we can loosen our construing and make more tentative expectations about outcomes. If, in spite of varying our strategies for dealing with invalidation, we still continue to be proved wrong in our expectations, then we may so loosen the ties between our constructs in order to 'hedge our bets', that we become incapable of drawing the constructs together again. Bannister developed the theory of *serial invalidation* along these lines to account for the type of thought disorder found in some schizophrenics. He was at pains to point out that schizophrenic thought disorder was not, in his view, specific to schizophrenia but is more usefully viewed as one extreme of a continuum.

It should be noted that loosening and tightening are not of themselves pathological reactions, but are normal reactions to varying validational fortunes. What is being argued is that the thought-disordered schizophrenic has been driven to loosen *beyond the point* at which there are enough workable lines of implication between his constructs for him to retighten his

system. He has sawn off the psychological branch on which he was sitting.
(Bannister and Fransella 1980)

Bannister (1963, 1965) tested this hypotheses by serially invalidating a sample
of non-psychiatrically disturbed people. The experiments showed that
successively telling people they were correct caused them to tighten their
construing. However, telling people successively that they were wrong did not
cause them to loosen in the first instance. Rather, they first changed the *pattern*
of interrelationships between their constructs. Having done this, and with
invalidation applied to only one cluster of constructs at a time, loosening
occurred.

Bannister then went on to argue that one way to reduce thought disorder
might be to serially *validate* the person's expectations. Having isolated the
residual structure remaining to the schizophrenic, he was encouraged to 'see'
people in these terms. In this way, with protection against invalidation of this
rudimentary system, the person could begin to struggle back to thought order.
This research did not produce any startling 'cures' but did suggest that it was
possible for the schizophrenic to struggle back 'long and arduous though the
journey may be'.

Of course, invalidation happily rarely produces such devastating results.
More often the person who is unable to make the necessary psychological
adjustments becomes increasingly aware of the mess into which he is getting
himself. As he fails to reconstrue, his behaviour may become more and more
unusual both to himself and to others and, in the end, he may find a solution
— he may develop a symptom.

The Symptom

It is suggested that psychological symptoms may frequently be interpreted
as the rationale by which one's chaotic experiences are given a measure of
structure and meaning. (Kelly 1955)

There have been several accounts of the meanings symptoms have for a
patient and how these may be related to treatment outcome. For instance,
Wright (1970) discusses 'exploring the uniqueness of common complaints' and
says:

A symptom may be regarded as a part of a person's experience of himself
which he has singled out and circumscribed as in some way incongruous with
the rest of the experience of himself. (Wright 1970)

Within the illness model the patient may be seen as coming bearing an offering
— his symptom for removal. His symptom is diagnosed and he is offered
appropriate treatment. On the other hand, when focusing on the person as
construer, the emphasis is on exploring with him the paths along which his

111

construing of life has resulted in his present impasse.

Rowe (1971) showed how impossible it was for a depressed woman to improve since, for her, being depressed was 'good' and being well was 'bad'. Rowe (1978) elaborated this further in a descriptive study of a group of depressed women. She suggests that psychotherapy should be concerned with trying to understand the metaphors and myths that are an integral part of the patient's personal language system. For instance, she describes Rose for whom cleanliness was of vital importance. She needed rest, but was unable to remain quiet. During the course of psychotherapy it transpired she thought that it was only possible to face the Day of Judgment if one helped others and was clean. Since one never knows when that Day is coming, it is important always to be ready and clean. How could she possibly rest?

It has been argued (e.g. Fransella 1972) that some forms of behaviour, established for a long period of time, become so much part of a person's way of life, that symptomatic treatment is of little value unless the person is able to reconstrue. This applies equally to the alcoholic, the obese, the stutterer, the agoraphobic or the ticqueur. In several of these groups, a direct relationship between construing and change in the symptomatic behaviour has been demonstrated. Treating people with these disorders and, indeed, with **many** others, often results in therapeutic sessions soon moving far away from the presenting symptoms. This one would expect if people do indeed focus on a symptom simply as a means of making sense of the disturbing things that are happening to them.

Diagnosis

It is important to remember that the personal construct psychology viewpoint means that one accepts no dichotomy between mind and body, construing and behaviour, thinking and feeling. To say that one wishes to help a person reconstrue implies that one also wishes, and expects, changes in behaving, feeling and, possibly, in that totality called personality as well.

In personal construct psychotherapy, diagnosis is the planning stage of treatment. It concerns itself with the establishing of therapeutic hypotheses which guide the initial therapeutic sessions. The hypotheses will no doubt change as therapy progresses but initial diagnosis is essential, first to establish the pathways along which the person is free to move, and second to isolate those along which he or she may find it easiest to reconstrue and which, in turn, will lead to the most profitable new behavioural experiments.

Diagnosing is thus formulated in terms of the patient's own construct system. This means that diagnostic constructs are concerned with identifying aspects of the construing process that keep the person 'fixed' in his or her present state. Such constructs have to do with content of the construct system, dependency, the inability to start or complete a Creativity Cycle (loosening and tightening),

112

or a C-P-C cycle (circumspection, pre-emption and control), and much else besides. In construing the construct system of the patient, the therapist is attempting to subsume the patient's system within his or her own and to use the professional diagnostic constructs to provide a way of understanding why the undesirable behaviour continues and to give leads as to ways in which the person may be encouraged to view things from another standpoint.

Of equal importance to constructs relating to diagnosis are those to do with transition. Threat, for instance, is defined as 'the awareness of imminent comprehensive change in one's core structures'. It is argued that someone with a long-standing complaint, perhaps a stutterer, may well be threatened when faced with the real possibility that fluency is within his grasp. He has spent many years of life living the part of a stutterer. This is the most meaningful way he has of relating to people in the world around him — undesirable though it is. His therapy may well be extremely successful in a short space of time. He glimpses fluency as an alternative way of life. Yet he has no real experience of this — and the unknown can be truly alarming. When he arrives at his next therapeutic session, stuttering with gay abandon, the therapist may diagnose this as being the result of threat and explore this accordingly.

Likewise, too direct an approach to helping a person loosen his construing may result in anxiety; 'the recognition that the events with which one is confronted mostly lie outside the range of convenience of one's construct system'. Too many alternatives become apparent and no one can be tested out. With the resulting confusion little progress may be made.

The personal construct therapist is thus armed with a whole system of theoretical and professional constructs with which to make sense of another's psychological disorder. They are used as a basis from which clinical hypotheses can be formulated.

Aids to Diagnosis

Kelly offered two procedures for helping the clinician come to an understanding of the constructions of his client. The most widely used of the two procedures is the repertory grid, the other is the *self characterisation*.

The Self Characterisation

This is primarily designed to help the clinician arrive at testable clinical hypotheses about the construing of the patient. It forms part of the initial assessment and can be used in continuing process of diagnosis. It is an example of what Kelly calls 'the credulous approach'. 'If you do not know what is wrong with a person, ask him; he may tell you.' Here one is not interested in the truth or falsehood of a person's views, but in how that person views himself and his relation to others. The instruction for the self characterisation are an invitation to the person to 'tell' what is going on in his personal world.

I want you to write a character sketch of (e.g.) Harry Brown, just as if he were the principal character in a play. Write it as it might be written by a friend who knew him very *intimately* and very *sympathetically,* perhaps better than anyone ever really could know him. Be sure to write it in the third person. For example, start out by saying, 'Harry Brown is . . .'.

The instructions were worked out very carefully so as to give the person maximum room to manoeuvre and yet to minimize threat, and are fully described in Kelly (1955).

The following excerpts are from self characterisation written at the start of psychotherapy by a man suffering from a physical complaint which dated from his early adolescence. He found writing an excellent way of analysing himself as well as a way of communicating with the therapist.

Had I been asked not long ago to say what most characterised Roland I would have said his unresolved contradictions, his confidence in himself and his lack of confidence, the wish to draw attention to himself and his wish to be inconspicuous, his burning ambition and his unwillingness to do anything about it (the list could go on) or I could have said his puzzlement about the world. Even when I began to try and describe him I concentrated on his alienation from the world including himself. My first attempts began 'Roland is someone who, when writing his name, sees a stranger . . .' and 'Roland is a private person much pre-occupied with his own thoughts and reactions', and 'There is a photograph of Roland as a little boy taken at his birthday party. The other children look as if they are enjoying themselves. He looks puzzled.'

All these descriptions, and what would lead on from them, tell us something about Roland and if they went on to talk about his vomiting, his shyness, his fear of doing things in situations he doesn't understand, his compulsive smoking, his inability to use his abilities except in a very restricted way, they might provide some explanation of why he wants to change. But in one sense they don't tell us very much about who he feels he is and what he wants to be. (He would find it very difficult to express who he feels he is and what he wants to be, but he feels who he is and what he wants to be.) What they do tell us is something about the barriers in his life and some of the things he must learn to accept and overcome.

Now, I would say that what most characterises him is the phrase 'a grown-up child'. . .

In recent years he has grown-up and grown more childlike (when he was a child he felt very, very old). He is still growing in both directions, but he is thirty-one . . . time's winged chariot is hurrying near, and he hasn't got it right yet. He has to begin to make his world and he doesn't quite know how. *So now I would describe him as 'a grown-up child who doesn't know how to go on'.*

In this way he spelled out the nature of the therapeutic task as he sees it. It is to help him discover who he really is as well as just 'feels' he is; to help him tighten his construing (so that he could better understand and so predict himself and others), whilst still retaining the ability to fantasise and dream and be creative; and to help him get into action and so test out his true worth. It was such problems as these that he had not been able fully to sort out during his five years of Kleinian analysis.

Towards the end of therapy, he writes on the effect writing a self characterisation had just had on him.

> It focused on something which I suppose has been associated with panic — although not consciously associated — the feeling that I was going to have to change more drastically — in a sense either remain more or less the same or the change would have to be more drastic than I had thought. Writing the self characterisation focused my attention on *not* wanting to change. Not wanting to change as dramatically as I was feeling was necessary (in purely abstract terms), I'd lose 'me'. . .
>
> There was a 'me' I valued and liked and so on and it seemed it was going to have to go. So I tried to think what this 'me' that I was so concerned about was. And without actually being able to verbalise it very well, the 'me' I was frightened about losing was the 'child-me'. And that was to do with dreaming, day-dreaming, certain preoccupations with my own processes, perceptions and sort of playing with that . . .
>
> This then sort of brought me on to — brought out a contrast between the child and the adult and it seemed to me that if I can look at being sick in relation to this I could see being sick as a reasonable device . . .
>
> Seeing it in terms of being a very useful way of preventing myself from becoming an adult — it seems to be enormously successful.

The self characterisation is not simply a diagnostic tool indicating themes, anxieties, identity problems, loose or tight construing and so forth. But it can clearly be of value to a patient in his or her attempt to make sense of a problematic world.

The Repertory Grid

This technique started life as the Rep Test. Constructs were elicited from the person and then analysed in terms of content, tone, permeability, communicability and so forth. The grid format was then evolved by Kelly as a means of quantifying these aspects of the person's construct system. The many subsequent developments of the technique and examples of its wide applicability can be seen in Ryle (1975), Slater (1977), Fransella and Bannister (1977).

An example of the grid's use as a therapeutic tool can be given from the case just described. Apart from being asked to write a self characterisation for the

115

first session, the rep test was also administered to the patient. He named people important in his life to fit certain role titles (such as 'a person I admire', 'someone I dislike') plus his father, mother, wife and three aspects of the self. These were presented to him, three at a time and always including one 'self'. He was asked if there was any way in which two of the three people were alike and thereby different from the third. This is, in fact, the standard way of eliciting personal constructs.

These constructs were then laddered (Hinkle 1965). Each elicited construct is taken in turn and the person is asked by which pole of the construct he or she would prefer to be described. The person is then asked to state why they selected as they did, and to say what the advantages are of being described by one pole of the construct rather than the other. This process of asking 'why' is continued until the person is able to give no further reasons. For this man, some of the laddered constructs were *threatened by chaos* versus *can operate more effectively; floating* versus *can locate themselves; have possibilities for wholeness* versus *hollow; committed to one course of action for life* versus *have more possibilities open to them; wear masks* versus *without masks.*

The patient was then required to state how these constructs were related one to the other in a bi-polar implications grid format (Fransella 1972). The relationships between these constructs were then analysed in terms of the degree

FIGURE 1. Significant links with construct *successful — not yet successful* on 1st test occasion

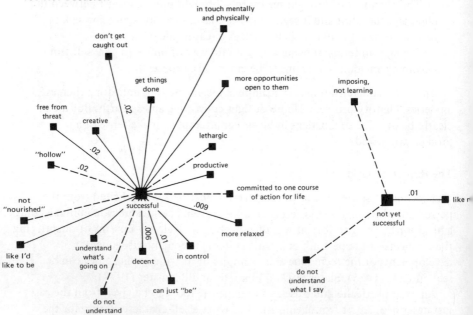

116

of matching or mismatching. The type of information this procedure provides can be seen in Figure 1, which shows only a few constructs which are significantly related to the self construct.

Like the self characterisation, the grid procedure is clearly part of the therapeutic procedure itself. People reconstrue as they are brought face to face with some unusual construct relationships or themes they see emerging or illogicalities of which they were previously unaware. This man had started to reconstrue during the laddering procedure. He was made aware of how 'claustrophobic' and rigid his dichotomisation of constructs into *masculine* and *not masculine* was — *masculine* things were 'bad' and *not masculine* (or feminine) were 'good'. This patient was also able to verbalise his sense of isolation and of a lack of identity when confronted with the construct relationships plotted in Figure 1. He said he felt exactly like that — 'out on a limb'.

FIGURE 2. Significant links with construct *successful — not yet successful* on 2nd test occasion

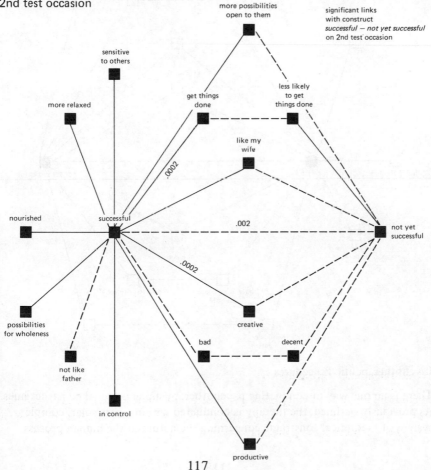

Grid methodology can also be used to plot change. Figures 2 and 3 show that one aim of psychotherapy was achieved. Some reconstruing had occurred in that he had linked *not yet successful* with other parts of his system. Being 'not yet successful' all his life, he had been able to remain the potential genius, the potential great artist, author, weaver of dreams. But at the same time he was getting older. He had never been able to risk failure or risk the invalidation of his potential and so never completed anything and never had a full-time job. There had been no commitment.

FIGURE 3. Significant links with construct *successful − not yet successful* on the 3rd test occasion

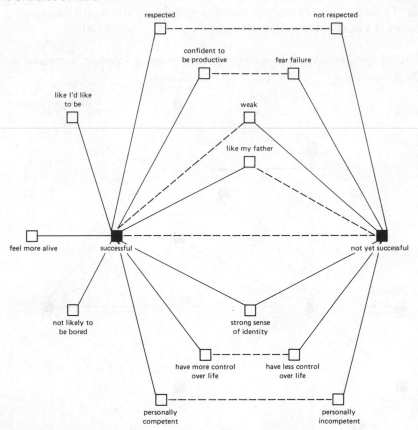

Psychotherapeutic Procedures

There is no one way of conducting psychotherapy along personal construct lines. As previously outlined, the therapy is conducted within a particular, complex system of theoretical constructs concerning the nature of the human process,

118

and particularly about the process of change. Since this system of therapeutic constructs is pitched at a very high level of abstraction, the personal construct therapist is able to call upon virtually any technique deemed likely to bring about some alternative construing in the patient. For instance, if the diagnosis is that the person has a system of constructs to do with personal relationships that is so 'tight' that movement is impossible, then some technique for 'loosening' that system might be employed — free association or guided fantasy for example; if the diagnosis is that the person operates a personal dualism and keeps emotional experience out of his life, then some procedure to bring him into contact with that side of himself might be used — such as some gestalt exercise.

Equally, with a person who finds it difficult to express himself verbally, a programme of systematic desensitisation as the basis for reconstruing could be useful. From a personal construct standpoint, this form of behaviour therapy would be introducing the person, systematically, to a previously avoided situation and *helping him construe it*. Implosion can be seen as having its effect by forcing the person to encounter a situation previously construed as 'impossible', likely to make me die', 'cause me to lose total control of myself' and the like.

This is not eclecticism. On the contrary, every course of action is directed by a highly explicit set of theoretical constructs. Where the approach is unusual is in having the theoretical constructs defined at a very high level of abstraction.

One practical consequence of this is that it changes the nature of psychotherapeutic research. One does not look to see whether therapy A is more effective than therapy B. One focuses instead on the *process* of psychological change. Given that a person's construct system functions at the present time in a certain way, one asks what is the best way of helping that person reconstrue and so enable him psychologically to 'get on the move again'. One starts matching techniques to aspects of psychological functioning and to certain individuals.

Kelly did, however, consider that some therapeutic procedures were particularly helpful in encouraging reconstruction.

Enactment

The clinical situation is viewed as a private laboratory where exploratory experiments can be conducted before being tried out in reality. Kelly had been impressed by the procedure of psychodrama described by Moreno. He felt that the method could be of use in giving the individual an opportunity of glimpsing what it would mean to try out a new approach to a problem. By enacting a role in the clinical sessions 'as if' you were someone else or 'as if' you were approaching a problem in a different way, new possibilities might be perceived. The woman who doubts her love of her husband, might be asked to enact the role of a person who really did not do so. What would be his reactions? How would she behave in the morning, in bed, in the garden, and so forth? What possibilities would not loving him open up for her?

Enactment is not just acting a part. It is an attempt to submerge oneself in a role so as to see how differently the world might look from that stance.

Controlled Elaboration

This is an essential feature of personal construct psychotherapy. The person's processes may well be psychologically channelled by the ways in which he anticipates events, but the anticipations are not serving him well. He needs to elaborate his system of constructs, but not in a haphazard manner. Controlled elaboration is aimed at helping the person tighten up the system of constructs, to produce self-consistency and possibly to attach some verbal labels to non-verbal constructs.

Since the way problems are construed is a major determinant of whether or not they can be solved, the task of the therapist is to help the patient formulate testable hypotheses. Intellectualisation is no good. At some point in time the patient has to be able and willing to go out into the world of reality and put his ideas to the test. Controlled elaboration helps him do this, whether it is in the form of verbalising pre-verbal constructs, sorting out inconsistencies or elaborating submerged poles of constructs.

Controlled elaboration has to be seen in contrast to two other forms of psychotherapeutic movement. There is the more superficial movement in which the patient has reconstrued himself and certain other features of his world but within his original system. This, however, may prove to be no more than a seesaw action — a 'slot-rattling' — in which the person is merely sliding himself up and down his original construct axes. At the other extreme there is the fundamental revision of constructs. This is the most difficult type of reconstruction to achieve and consists of changing some of the constructs in his old system for new ones. Behavioural change may not be as great with construct revision as with 'slot-rattling', but it is far more significant.

Fixed Role Therapy

There was only one particular technique Kelly describes arising from his theory to be used when something is needed to trigger off some psychological movement. Fixed role therapy embodies and illustrates many of the central ideas in personal construct psychotherapy. In the first instance, the patient is asked to write a self characterisation. The patient's therapist, in conjunction with another therapist, draws up a portrait of a person who is 'at ninety degrees' to the person in the self-characterisation. The aim is to portray a person who will suggest new dimensions along which life can be seen and not to encourage rattling from one end of existing dimensions to the other, which an exactly opposite sketch would encourage. For example, if a woman sees her relationships as about *dominance* versus *submission* then the fixed role sketch might describe a person who is fiercely *interested* in people but not, thereby, either dominant *or* submissive.

This sketch is shown to the patient and she is asked if she finds the person credible. If there are doubts, the sketch is altered until it is acceptable. The woman is then told that she should become this new person for the next week or so. She is to eat the kind of food she thinks this person would eat; wear the kind of clothes she would wear, respond to others as she would, dream the other's dreams. In fact, truly to be that other. She is being forced to experience herself and her behaviours in a different manner. Most important, she may be able to see that a person is self-inventing and that she is not necessarily trapped by her circumstances, by the body in which she lives or by her autobiography.

Details of fixed role therapy could be found in Kelly (1955), Bonarius (1970), Skene (1973) and Epting (1979). One study has been conducted to examine the efficacy of this approach to treatment together with rational emotive therapy and compared with no treatment (Krast and Trexler 1970). Both produced change. But it must be emphasised that fixed role therapy is only suggested by Kelly as a technique to be used with certain patients in certain circumstances. It is not synonymous with personal construct psychotherapy.

Group Psychotherapy

Although Kelly's theoretical approach to psychotherapy has been discussed mostly in the context of the individual, he did provide some guide-lines of how it can equally well be applied to the group. He describes six phases through which the psychotherapy group evolves. Starting with the establishment of mutual support, the group goes through stages of enactment within the group setting and on to the designing of experiments for each other to be experimented with outside the group setting. (See Kelly 1955.)

Conclusions

Personal construct psychotherapy takes as its starting point a personal acceptance by the therapist of the philosophy of constructive alternativism. This is a frame of mind in which the patient is seen as someone with his or her own unique way of viewing the world of reality. The therapist's job is to subsume this view of the world as far as possible within his or her own construct system. The more the therapist can stand in the shoes of the patient and see the world through the patient's eyes, the better able will the therapist be to help that patient reconstrue the world so as to get out of the dilemma in which she finds herself.

Personal construct psychotherapy involves the application of the theoretical constructs which form the psychology of personal constructs. This means that the therapist must have considerable knowledge of the theory in its entirety. Only then is she able to apply these constructs concerning the psychological workings of all of us to the patient's system.

Having applied these theoretical constructs to the patient's construct system, diagnoses can be made about the malfunctioning of that system as experienced by that person. The diagnoses having been made, specific techniques may be used to encourage helpful change. Diagnoses are only tentative and may change if proved wrong or be changed when the patient moves on to some other aspect of the problem.

Personal construct psychotherapy thus has at its disposal as many techniques as have been invented. With the procedures of other therapies becoming techniques, it is possible to start to examine, in a systematic manner, the type of technique that is best suited to particular types of construing. It then becomes of paramount importance to direct research to the study of the process of change in construing itself rather than to the efficacy of different types of therapy.

SOME NEWER PSYCHOTHERAPIES

Kerith Trick

Medicine, and to a lesser extent psychiatry has made enormous advances in the past fifty years. It has achieved this largely by studiously avoiding any consideration of what it is doing other than the setting of short term practical goals. Such goals have often been arrived at as a result of luck, serendipity, and a totally false theoretical basis. In this way great practical advances have been made unlike those more contemplative professions such as sociology which, having devoted considerable effort to render the obvious obscure and the self-evident untenable have on those occasions when they vacate their ivory towers for the real world accomplished only such major disasters as the town of Milton Keynes. Psychiatry has, however, become for many reasons an embattled profession and has thus been forced to re-examine some of its activities if only to defend itself against the attacks of those who regard mental illness as a myth invented by psychiatrists to keep themselves in business. One of the greatest areas of conflict is the field of psychotherapy. Here is an activity in which rich pickings can be made — particularly in North America and plenty of potential pickers can see no reason for a psychiatric closed shop to operate. The result has been an explosion of therapies. To go to a party in the USA without being in therapy leaves one far more exposed than if you had merely failed to do up your trousers properly.

How can one start to distinguish between the competing panaceas, is it to be Est or should one transcend by meditation, will it bio-energise you or should one create a positive struggle with Esalen? Perhaps a good Rogering would do the trick or would something more primal be the answer.

The term psychotherapy is now used to cover so many activities that it has become all things to all men and nothing to anyone.

Psychotherapy often sounds like the Samian Clay described by Galen: 'All who drink this remedy recover in a short time except those whom it does not help, who all die, and have no relief from any other medicine. Therefore it is obvious that it fails only in incurable cases.'

It is necessary to try and define the essential features of psychotherapy.

Raimy (1950) defined psychotherapy as 'an unidentified technique applied to unspecified problems with unpredictable outcomes. Practitioners of this technique require long and rigorous training'.

Winder (1957) defined the necessary characteristics of psychotherapy as follows:

1. There is an interpersonal relationship of a prolonged kind between two or more people.
2. One of the participants has had special experience and/or special training in the handling of human relationships.
3. One or more of the participants have entered the relationship because of a felt dissatisfaction with their emotional and/or interpersonal adjustment.
4. The methods used are of a psychological nature, i.e. involve such mechanisms as explanation, suggestion, persuasion, etc.
5. The procedure of the therapist is based upon some formal theory regarding mental disorder in general and the specific disorders of the patient in particular.
6. The aim of the process is the amelioration of the difficulties that cause the patient to seek the help of the therapist.

These criteria imply a number of assumptions that may or may not be correct.

1. The basic notion that the behaviour of an individual can be changed as the result of an act of communication.
2. That such changes are relatively permanent though the acts of communication are intermittent.
3. That such changes are desirable —
   (a) in the view of the therapist
   (b) and/or in the view of the client.

So far these characteristics are common to any form of learning and would apply equally to the activities of teacher or preacher as well as therapist. The essential aspect of therapy must be the relief of the distress experienced by the client. For the purpose of today's discussion we can therefore exclude those techniques that do not claim to treat emotional distress.

Winder's definition of psychotherapy at least allows comparison between the various forms currently on offer. Systems that do not satisfy those criteria may be excluded from consideration. While there is no way at present, and perhaps there never will be, of comparing the efficacy of different techniques, at least it may be possible to compare their characteristics and to see if any system has the merit of internal consistency.

In order to carry out a comparison it is necessary to construct 'models' of the various therapies. A model defines certain dimensions. The more relevant dimensions that can be arrived at the better the comparison can be. Anyone who studies copies of '*Which*' will be familiar with this technique — even in this instance it is impossible to recommend a 'Best Buy'. Perhaps 'Holiday Which' is a better example. You cannot compare a holiday in Italy with one in Greece, but at least you can know what you are letting yourself in for.

Dimensions that are appropriate in psychotherapy include:

1. Definition or 'diagnosis' of the state needing treatment.
2. Aetiology of that condition.
3. Relevance of the patient's behaviour.
4. Technique of treatment.
5. Prognosis.
6. Role of therapist and his qualifications.
7. Goals of treatment.

Let us now consider some of the more recent developments.

Rogerian Psychotherapy

Carl Rogers has exercised enormous influence on the development of psychotherapy. An academic originally trained as a Christian Minister, Rogers discovered his true interests as a counsellor.

Carl Rogers' (1964) model of man is that 'he does not simply have the characteristics of a machine, he is not simply a being in the grip of unconscious motives: he is a person in the process of creating himself, a person who creates meaning in life, a person who embodies a dimension of subjective freedom. He is a figure who, though he may be alone in a vastly complex universe is able in his inner life to transcend the material universe; he is able to have dimensions of his life which are not fully or adequately contained in a description of his conditioning or of his unconscious'.

Rogers regards 'diagnosis' as unimportant as 'any changes that occur during treatment are those brought about by the client himself'.

Aetiology

'The innermost core of man's nature is basically socialised, forward moving, rational, and realistic. The neurotic is one who has developed a distorted image of himself, one charged with masochistic self hatred.'

Patients' Behaviour

Behaviour as such is not of primary importance, it is the client's inner 'subjective state of mind' that is critical.

Prognosis will depend largely on the therapist's attitude, disposition, and behaviour.

125

Therapy

For Rogers 'the techniques of the various therapies are relatively unimportant except to the extent that they serve as channels for fulfilling one of the following conditions. These conditions are that the therapist has:

1. Empathy.
2. Warmth.
3. Genuineness.

The relationship between therapist and client is all important. The therapist creates a setting in which the client can become intensely aware of how he is evaluating himself. The therapist does not interpret or probe and is non-directive and non-authoritarian. He must be 'what he is' and there must be a congruence between him and the client — that is a matching of what he is experiencing, what he is conscious of and that which he conveys to the client. The therapist must have 'unconditional positive regard' for the client — regard not for what he does or says but for what lies within him.

The therapist acts rather as Cassius does for Brutus:

> 'Since you know you cannot see yourself
> so well as by reflection, I, your glass
> will modestly discover to yourself
> that of yourself which you yet know not of.'

By presenting to the client through the mirror of his 'unconditional positive regard' a new and desirable view of himself, the therapist helps him cast away his 'masochistic self hatred'.

Rogers has the merit of believing that the outcome and methods of psychotherapy can be tested along scientific lines. He carried out a massive study which failed to show any positive results. This may be due to his selecting schizophrenic patients as the subjects.

Existential Psychotherapy

In contrast to the optimistic view of human personality taken by Rogers, existential therapists tend to take a gloomy view of the human predicament.

Existentialism is the general title for a number of very different philosophies having only a rather tenuous connection with each other. The underlying theory goes back to Kierkegaard who in a series of books and essays proposed a view that saw human life as anguished and absurd, harrowing, and meaningless. Kierkergaard saw as the only solution to man's predicament, that man should accept 'faith' which for Kierkegaard meant a belief in a Christian God. Later existentialists such as Satre reject this aspect of the philosopy. They believe that man is trapped in existence, living in a totally arbitrary world in which one way of living is as 'good' or as 'bad' as another. Once an individual recognises this he is confronted with his 'dreadful freedom' — that is he is completely free to choose his own way of living in the world, there can be no guides, there is no way of escaping from making a choice, and having made a choice, no way of escaping from the consequences of that choice.

Obviously belief in such a philosophy almost excludes the notion of psychotherapy as a planned activity, and existential writers go to considerable lengths to avoid being tied down to any concrete methods of 'treatment'. E K Ledermann (1972) comes as near as he dare to doing so. He sees some forms of neurosis as being 'a moral phenomenon' — a manifestation of man's moral crisis. He quotes D R G McInnes' paper on undergraduate breakdowns, as showing that such neurotic problems present mainly as work and social difficulties, the sufferer experiencing a persistent feeling of pointlessness and futility.

Treatment relies on mobilising the moral resources of the patient by providing him with a target. The therapist assists the patient in his striving for freedom by confronting him with his situation and with the possibilities of self liberation. To do so the therapist chooses methods of treatment that put the patient face to face with his task.

The Qualification of the Therapist

Anyone can act in the role of therapist but a trained therapist will employ special techniques.

Methods

1. An initial interview in which the patient 'attains a view of his life' by telling the therapist his story from earliest childhood, relating his emotional development, and gaining insight into the factors and circumstances that prevented him from achieving his freedom.
2. Dream interpretation, reverie techniques, drawing and painting, and even drugs may be used to gain access to the patient's unconscious but interpretation differs from psychoanalytic interpretations.

While techniques are important they are not the essential element. The personal encounter between patient, therapist, and other patients is the vital factor.

Aim

The aim is not to correct social adjustment. The emphasis is not on the objective state of mind but on the subjective experience. The individual must attain 'authenticity' through 'transendence'.

Existentialists do not agree on the meaning of these terms. Bugental in his book 'The Search for Authenticity' defines an authentic person as 'a person is authentic in that degree to which his being in the world is unqualified in accord with the givenness of his own nature and of the world'.

'Transendence implies the complete confronting and incorporating of existential anxiety in all its forms. . . Transendence is complete awareness and full feelingful assent.'

It is hardly surprising then that assessment of existential psychotherapy cannot be judged by scientific methods. Statistics are inapplicable because each patient is a unique individual. There is no 'natural history' of the neurosis and hence 'relapses' are no measure of success or failure. Chronological time is unimportant, 'lived in' time is all that matters — each moment posing its own dilemmas which must be faced.

Gestalt Therapy

Claimed to be the second most prevelant form of therapy in the USA it was founded by Frederick Perls.

Definition

Neurosis is the result of distortions incurred in the warding off of forbidden trends. These trends are seen as needs of the total organism rather than as repressed fantasies. The organism is endowed with a drive to put itself together, of which conscious awareness is the active sign.

The person must be put in touch not with repressed memories but with current immediate organismic needs. Active awareness of the present is what promotes healing not the reflective and synoptic picture of one's entire life. Interpretation thus becomes an anti-therapeutic interruption.

Therapist

'A good therapist doesn't listen to the content of the bullshit the patient produces, but to the sound, to the music, to the hesitations. Verbal communication is usually a lie. The real communication is beyond words.' (Perls, 1969.)

Therapy

Takes place in concentrated workshop setting.

Dramatisation is the key. Instead of relating a conflict in words, the subject enacts it, alternately playing out as different parts.

There is no theory of transference.

No interest in group processes as such, and no theory of interpersonal relationships or of social psychology. Projection is seen as being the major form of disturbed communication.

Primal Therapy

Dr. Arthus Janov is a man of remarkable modesty. Having worked for some 17 years as a conventional 'insight therapist' he suddenly and by chance discovered the 'Primal Scream'.

One day on a hunch he invited a patient to call out 'Mummy, Daddy'. The patient did so getting more and more emotional until he gave a 'piercing, deathlike scream that rattled the walls of the office'. Following which the patient felt better and Primal Therapy was born.

According to Dr. Janov, Primal Therapy unlike any other treatment *cures* mental illness, thus there is only one valid approach to treating neuroses and psychoses and that is Primal Therapy.

Definition

Neurosis is a state of being, and its chief characteristic is tension.

Aetiology

'The substratum for all irrational behaviour is pain, no matter of what origin. One severe trauma or many accumulated smaller ones can produce neurosis. The neurosis is composed of both the defences the patient has erected, plus the tension created by the interplay of these and the "Pain".'

Behaviour

No behaviour is neurotic in and of itself.

The Therapist

'He who gets up off the floor first gets paid.' That is it is difficult at times to tell who is the patient and who is the therapist. There is no special magic about being a therapist.

Treatment

Every conceivable item that may arouse an 'old circuit' is utilised. Toys, teddy-bears, cribs, playpens, plastic nipples, and bottles for 'nursing'. 'Primal groups are unusual and almost ineffable.' Each person there is doing his own thing. Patients are encouraged to act out their feelings. The theory is the more one lets oneself 'go to pieces' the more together one gets.

Aim

To solve all the problems in the world.

Transactional Analysis

Eric Berns once wrote a book called 'Transactional Analysis in Psychotherapy' (1961) which sold about 10 copies. He re-wrote it in 1964 as 'Games People Play' and it was top of the best seller list for over a year. It also became the most popular form of therapy.

Definition

Within each person there are three ego states.

The Parent, the Adult, and the Child

The Parent has two main functions, first it enables the person to act effectively as the parent of actual children, secondly it allows the individual to act automatically to situations on the basis of 'that's how it has always been done'.

The Adult is necessary for survival, it processes data and computes probabilities. It also regulates the activities of Parent and Child and mediates objectively between them.

All three aspects of the personality have their own value and it is only when one or other of them disturbs the healthy balance that trouble ensues.

Therapy

Transactional Analysis is brief, to the point, and educational. There is no playing around. Good humour is the rule and the emphasis on verbal exchanges as members analyse each others' scripts and games.

Therapist

Someone trained in games analysis and able to comment on the 'healthiness' of particular games.

Goal

To give the Adult ego state – that is the mature, realistic, and ethical part, power over the harsh tyrannical Parent and the reckless impulsive Child.

Family Therapy

This involves a basic redefinition of the task of therapy. It is not concerned with the individual's inner subjective life but with the nature of relatedness.

A general statement of the theory is set out in George Bateson's 'Steps to an Ecology of the Mind' (New York 1972).

Definition/Diagnosis

Neurosis is an aberration within the family. The family merely happens to select one vulnerable member to express its pathology.

Therapy

The therapist studies the interaction of family members until he has clarified the rules governing their behaviour. He then intervenes, focusing on discreet behavioural inter-reactions.

Therapist

The therapist has to be actively involved in the family as he must provide the instructions and the energy to produce change in the system.

Goal

The aim is to break up feedback systems that perpetuate pathological communications and to replace them with a system that allows all members to develop their potential. In this review, I have left out a number of other forms of group and individual activities because they do not specifically lay claim to treat neuroses. Any therapeutic results are regarded as a bonus. Such activities are designed to enrich the life of the 'normal' individual. These include various forms of encounter and sensitivity groups, EST, transcendental meditation, and yoga. More importantly I have totally ignored behavioural methods of treatment, not because they are essentially different from other forms of psychotherapy but because they are being dealt with at length in other sessions.

The forms of therapy I have described run on a continuum from one extreme position in which verbalisation is regarded as the essence of treatment to the opposite end where verbalisation is regarded as anti-therapeutic and feeling is all. It may be that the central position, as so often is the case, holds out the best prospects for patients.

If at the end of this review one is left with no clear idea of the nature of psychotherapy then it might be helpful to quote a well known poem:

> 'Twas brillig, and the slithy toves
> Did gyre and gimble in the wabe;
> All mimsy were the borogroves,
> And the mome raths outgrabe
>
> 'Beware the Jabberwock, my son!
> The jaws that bite, the claws that catch!
> Beward the Jubjub bird, and shun
> The Frumious Bandersnatch!'
>
> —Lewis Carroll

The Jabberwock is alive and well and living in California.

RESPONSE TO DR. FRANSELLA'S AND DR. TRICK'S PAPERS

Kenneth Wright

I would like to say a few things which occurred to me while I was listening to Dr. Trick's paper. He mentioned some of the confusion which one feels when confronted with different systems of therapy, with their different languages, their different-ways of talking about patients and their life events. I sometimes feel that confusion, but as a practising psychotherapist, I suppose I have a more intense clinical experience to relate to what they say. What occurs to me is that in fact, when one is working with people in some depth, you do have to have a language of some kind to talk about the sort of processes which you can begin to observe going on. I think such languages do help to orientate one and undoubtedly they do help you to communicate with colleagues who happen to inhabit the same linguistic universe as oneself. If they do not, of course, that is where the problems begin. I think one of the drawbacks of such language systems is that they are in danger of becoming closed systems which can become closed to reality. This of course is a criticism which is often made of psychoanalysts, that their statements have become dogma and they are no longer describing reality but belief systems of the practitioner. It must have something to do with that kind of evolution that one finds so much fear of exchanging ideas between practitioners who have different language systems. I think at times one could say they are xenophobic, it is as if they belong to a different culture — 'we don't communicate with these other people, we only meet with our own kind'. I wondered how personal construct theory would talk about this phenomenon. I think it might have something to do with the fear of the invalidation of those constructs on which one's professional and perhaps personal security is based if you start exposing them to other people. I am quite sure in my own mind that the professional constructs that any of us hold are not solely determined by their scientific validity or by their respectability, but by much more personal aspects as well.

I had one further thought which related back to Dr. Fransella's paper which was that if we are going to get anywhere with this problem of different languages I think we probably have to have a language with which to talk about the different languages which constitute the different forms of therapy — I think what Gregory Bateson would call a 'meta-language'. You can't talk about a language in that language itself, you have got to have some other set of constructs to talk about them if you are going to be able to analyse them. I wonder whether personal construct theory might not begin to provide such a language for talking about other forms of psychotherapy. Dr. Fransella mentioned the high degree of abstraction of construct theory. I think it has to be an abstract language if one is to use it for talking about concepts. It has got to be contentless if it is going to be used to talk about the content of other psychotherapies. Of course it wasn't designed to do that, it was designed to make sense of the different construct systems (and the different languages) of different individuals, and the kind of forms they took.

I will try and string together a few of the thoughts about Dr. Fransella's paper, though they are rather fragmentary. Perhaps I should say I am a psychoanalyst and so what I am going to say will be strongly influenced by that. When I was listening to Dr. Fransella's paper one thing struck me which has struck me before when reading things about construct theory. What seems to me to be a kind of essential step in any type of psychotherapy is the problem of the patient who insists that *this* is reality, *this* is the way that things really are. We may feel that *isn't* the way things reallyare. We may in the grossest cases think that the patient is deluded and we may say to the patient 'this is a delusion', but I think in a kind of miniature form it is the same problem of delusion that we are confronted with very often, with other psychotherapy patients, where the patient insists that *this* is reality. For instance we might be confronted with a hypochondriacal patient, who insists that he has this pain and that there is something physically the matter with him inside. We may feel we have done all the necessary investigations and what is the matter inside is something to do with this person's feelings, something to do with his experience which is very deep within him. We might think of the person who insists that another person is 'such and such a way' or insists that people are always being nasty to him. We feel this may be a misconception, or the kind of thing that Dr. Fransella described as people 'setting-up' a situation — that they are actually engineering the reaction with the other person. I think this is a core kind of situation in psychotherapy that has to be dealt with. I think Kelly wrote about this rather nicely when he described the loosening up of relationship of the person's constructs to reality, so that they can begin to experience their world as something that is at least in some important respect subjective and not something which is entirely 'given out there'. I think at that point you can begin to get the patient moving. In psycho-analytic therapy one of the areas where this is most fought out is in the transferance. Transferance is not something that is 'given', transferance is a label that the therapist puts on to certain states of affairs. The

133

patient may be saying 'you are the most horrible man I've ever met, I hate your guts, why are you so nasty and why do you do this, that and the other'? While the therapist may feel 'I don't think I am quite as bad as that, really I think I have been pretty patient sitting here listening to all this'. I suppose that is one of the ways a therapist keeps going, being able to see this as transferance so that he can understand this kind of attribution which from the patient's point of view is a statement about reality. The therapist can begin to understand how this misappreciation can have arisen in terms of the patient's past experience, but this may still be a very long way from helping the patient to any kind of understanding. In psycho-analytic psychotherapy a lot of the working through of a patient's personal problems tends to take place in this area and without the capacity of the patient to come to this view subjectivity of the transference there is very little improvement that can occur.

I think I may have spoken long enough on some of these matters and I would like to come back to them during the course of the discussion. It is not my purpose to present another paper and at this point I will throw the discussion open to the meeting.

References

Bannister, D (1963) The genesis of schizophrenic thought disorder: a serial invalidation hypothesis. *Brit. J. Psychiat, 109*, 680–686

Bannister, D (1965) The genesis of schizophrenic thought disorder: re-test of the serial invalidation hypothesis. *Brit. J. Psychiat, 111*, 377–382

Bannister, D and Fransella, F (1980) Inquiring Man 2nd edition. London: Penguin Books (in press)

Bateson, G (1972) Steps to an Ecology of the Mind. New York: Chandler Pub

Bonarius, JCJ (1970) Fixed role therapy: a double paradox. *Brit. J. Med. Psychol., 43*, 213–219

Bugental JFJ (1965) *The Search for Authenticity.* London: Holt, Rinehard and Winston

Davisson, A (1978) George Kelly and the American mind (or why has he been obscure for so long in the USA and whence the new interest?) In: *Personal Construct Psychology 1977.* (Ed F Fransella). London: Academic Press

Epting, F (1979) *Personal Construct Psychotherapy.* New York: Wiley (in press)

Fransella, F (1972) *Personal Change and Reconstruction: research on a treatment of stuttering.* London: Academic Press

Fransella, F and Bannister, D (1977) *A Manual for Repertory Grid Technique.* London: Academic Press

Hinkle, DE (1965) *The change of personal constructs from the viewpoint of a theory of implications.* Unpub. PhD thesis, Ohio State University

Janov, A (1970) *The Primal Scream.* New York

Karst, TO and Trexler, LD (1970) Initial study using fixed role and rational-emotive therapy in treating public speaking anxiety. *J. consult. clin. Psychol., 34*, 360–366

Kelly, GA (1955) *The Psychology of Personal Construct.* Vols I and II. New York: Norton

Kelly, GA (1969) Personal construct theory and the psychotherapeutic interview. In: *Clinical Psychology and Personality: the selected papers of George Kelly.* (Ed B Maher). New York: Wiley

Kelly, GA (1970) A brief introduction to personal construct theory. In: *Perspectives in Personal Construct Theory.* (Ed D Bannister). London: Academic Press

Kelly, GA (1970a) Behaviour is an experiment. In: *Perspectives in Personal Construct Theory.* (Ed D Bannister). London: Academic Press

Lederman, EK (1972) Existential Neurosis. Butterworth

Perls, F (1969) Gestalt Therapy Verbatim. New York

Rogers, C (1964) Towards a science of personality. In: *Behaviourism and Phenomenology.* TW Swann. Chicago OP

Rowe, D (1971) Poor prognosis in a case of depression as predicted by the repertory grid. *Brit. J. Psychiat., 118,* 297–300

Rowe, D (1978) *The Experience of Depression.* London: Wiley

Ryle, A (1975) *Frames and Cages.* Sussex University Press

Skene, RA (1973) Construct shift in the treatment of a case of homosexuality. *Brit. J. Med. Psychol., 46,* 287–292

Slater, P (1977 (ed) The Measurement of Interpersonal Space by Grid Technique. Vol. 2. London: Wiley

Wright, KJT (1970) Exploring the uniqueness of common complaints. *Brit. J. Med. Psychol., 43,* 221–232

CURRENT TRENDS IN THE MEDICAL TREATMENT OF SCHIZOPHRENIA

Stephen Hirsch

1. Clinical Effects of Antipsychotic Medication

'The extensive literature of evaluative trials, constituting the most massive scientific overkill in all clinical pharmacology, has demonstrated the value of antipsychotic drugs in all forms of schizophrenia, at all ages, in all states of illness, and in all parts of the world. Alas, not in all patients.'

Leo Hollister (1978)

The point is well made, if not overstated, it is not possible to dispute the efficacy of antipsychotic medication in schizophrenia. However, it is necessary to try to eliminate the one misconception that keeps reappearing in advertisements and re-emerging in the minds of clinicians — that certain drugs are more effective for one syndrome while other drugs are more effective for another. More than 16 reports covering several large collaborative studies in the USA, each involving more than 250 patients, have failed to confirm a differential action of drugs on symptoms or syndromes, or identify subgroups of schizophrenics according to their response to different drugs (Hollister, 1974). In each case where differences emerged between drugs, for example that chlorpromazine was better for excited, disoriented, or hostile patients and fluphenazine better for paranoid or thought disordered ones, the differences were not confirmed in subsequent studies in patients treated with the putative drug. It has proved impossible to sort out any pattern of symptoms, signs, or demographic variables. or any combination of these which can be used to predict responses of an individual patient. At the same time, all clinicians know that there are differences between antipsychotic drugs; with the help of recent advances in biochemical pharmacology it is now possible to provide a rational basis for unravelling this paradox. In order to do so it may be helpful to draw distinctions between the effectiveness and potency of antipsychotic medication and to develop two new concepts; *the sedative and neuroleptic quotient.*

136

The *effectiveness* of antipsychotics (or neuroleptics)* is their ability to achieve the intended effect. We would like this to be the permanent elimination of all signs and symptoms of schizophrenia but we know that such medication is not wholly effective. The specific ability of neuroleptic medication to eliminate or diminish hallucinations, delusions, bizarre behaviour, and paranoid suspiciousness is its principal non-sedative antipsychotic effect. This antipsychotic action of neuroleptics is pharmacologically related to their ability to block dopamine transmission, particularly at post synaptic receptor sites within the mesolimbic system (Creese, Burt, Snyder, 1978).

Another specific effect of neuroleptics is their potent action in reducing psychotic anxiety, excitement, aggressiveness, and belligerence with relatively little hypnotic effect as compared with that resulting from traditional sedatives such as barbiturates, opiates, or anaesthetics when used to achieve the same control. This may be called the *specific antipsychotic sedative* action of neuroleptics and it is related to their affinity for alpha-noradrenergic receptors centrally and correlates highly with their potency in antagonising a lethal infusion of intravenous noradrenalin in rats. It can be distinguished from the un-specific sedative actions of neuroleptics which diminish hyper-arousal or excitement in anyone and is reflected in the strong hypnotic effects we see when neuroleptics are given to normal or nonpsychotic individuals.

Potency refers to the amount of drug (in mgm) required to achieve a desired effect (the ratio of dose/effect). For our purposes it is useful to think of potency in terms of the minimum dose required to achieve antipsychotic control of symptoms. Immediately we recognise that chlorpromazine and thioridazine are low in potency as compared to fluphenazine, haloperidol, or pimozide which have an effect on hallucinations or delusions with much smaller doses.

The potency of antipsychotics is related biochemically to their stereospecific (H^3) spiroperidol binding capacity in vitro $(r = 0.87)^\dagger$. Pharmacologically it correlates highly $(r = 0.92)$ with their ability to antagonise amphetamine induced stereotypy in rats — that is, their ability to block the effects of increased dopamine at the synapse (Creese, Burt and Snyder, 1976, 1978). The action of antipsychotics on specific symptoms emerges slowly over one to three weeks (or more) while the sedative effects of antipsychotics can become evident within twenty minutes if administered parenterally.

The *sedation quotient* of neuroleptics is their calming or sedative action relative to their specific antipsychotic effect; that is the degree of sedation that occurs when giving a sufficient dose to abate a thought disorder, hallucinations

---

* Though the term 'neuroleptic' strictly refers to pharmacological features of drugs with activity similar to chlorpromazine, the term has increasingly come to refer to drugs with a clinical antipsychotic action plus effects on the extra-pyramidal system.
† Spiroperidol has a powerful affinity for dopamine receptors and lower affinity for alpha-norepinephergic receptors. Almost all clinically effective antipsychotic drugs block the stereospecific binding of (H^3) spiroperidol at concentrations which correlate directly with clinical potency (Hollister, 1978).

or delusions. Chlorpromazine and thioridazine are strong alpha-norepinephrine blockers with high sedation ratios as compared with haloperidol or fluphenazine. Pharmacologically, the activity of a drug in antagonising alpha-norepinephrine (α NE) relative to its activity antagonising amphetamine (AM) induced stereotypy in the mouse is a measure of the sedation ratio (the ratio of α NE/AM antagonism) (Janssen et al, 1978). High potency drugs like trifluoperazine, fluphenazine, and pimozide have low sedation ratios. Thus drugs may be chosen because sedation is wanted or not, but the differences only refer to their properties at the lowest dose which produces an antipsychotic action — if high potency antipsychotic drugs are given in large doses they have powerful sedative effects. When initially introduced, high potency drugs like haloperidol or fluphenazine were only used at low doses (2 to 15 mgm daily) exhibiting their antipsychotic but not their sedative effect. Hence they were thought to have 'activating' properties when in fact they simply did not cause as much sedation. More recently we use the potent neuroleptics in high doses when specific antipsychotic sedation is required (20 to 90 mgm daily). In both cases tolerance to the hypnotic effects of neuroleptics develops in time, thus the differences between low potency neuroleptics and high potency ones disappear with the manipulation of dosage and as tolerance develops over time.

A similar story can be told about differences between drugs with respect to their *neuroleptic quotient,* or their tendency to cause extra-pyramidal symptoms for a given antipsychotic effect (EPSE/Antipsychotic Effect). While dopamine receptor blockade in the mesolimbic system is necessary for the therapeutic effect of the drug, dopamine receptor blockade in the nigrostriatal part of the brain results in extrapyramidal side effects (EPSE's). The differences between antipsychotics in their neuroleptic ratio is a function of their anticholinergic activity. Parkinsonian symptoms result when there is a decrease in dopaminergic activity in the nigrostriatum relative to acetylcholinergic activity. The unwanted dopamine blockade in this part of the brain which occurs with neuroleptic treatment can be compensated for by concomitant cholinergic blockade — thus drugs which have a strong anticholinergic activity automatically compensate for the dopamine blockade they produce in the extra-pyramidal system. The low potency neuroleptics, chlorpromazine and thioridazine have strong anticholinergic activity relative to the high potency ones. Thioridazine has the lowest neuroleptic ratio and the strongest anticholinergic effect of established antipsychotics, thus the lowest frequency of parkinsonian side effects; chlorpromazine is similar in potency but has less cholinergic activity. High potency haloperidol, trifluoperazine, and fluphenazine have high neuroleptic ratios because they have relatively low anticholinergic activity. While supplementary anticholinergic medication is more commonly required with drugs with a high neuroleptic quotient, this is less so when they are administered in very high doses when their anticholinergic activity is increased sufficiently to counter-balance their parkinsonian effects. This probably explains why acute dystonia and extrapyramidal side effects are if anything less common when haloperidol is given in very high doses, above 60 mgm per day.

It should be added that a certain degree of tolerance develops to the nigrostriatel activities of neuroleptics so that if the medication is begun with low doses and increased slowly EPSE's are less likely and less severe — moreover, their frequency diminishes with time as compensatory mechanisms take place reinstating the balance between dopaminergic and cholinergic activity (Hollister, 1978).

This thesis can be summarised as follows: the well tried neuroleptics are equal in their antipsychotic effect but differ in milligram potency. If drugs are compared at doses required to get the same basic antipsychotic effect, other differences are noted in terms of their sedative, parkinsonian, and other activities which can be expressed as a ratio of the severity of the side effect to the antipsychotic effect but because of the wide therapeutic range and tolerance to these drugs, dosage can be manipulated to enhance or diminish the secondary effect. Recent advances in biochemical neuropharmacology have identified the probable basis of different pharmacological activities of neuroleptics which explain these clinical effects. Table 1 summarises the clinical differences described:

TABLE 1 Potency, sedative and neuroleptic quotients in relation to a given antipsychotic effect

Drug	Potency	Sedative ratio	Neuroleptic ratio	Range of clinical daily dose
Haloperidol	++++	+	++++	2− 100 mgm
Trifluoperazine	++	+	+++	5− 60 mgm
Fluphenazine	++++	+	++++	15− 120 mgm*
Chlorpromazine	+	+++	++	75−2000 mgm
Thioridazine	+	++	+	75− 800 mgm**

Relative strength: High ++++, Low +
* One study used 1200 mgm/d (Quitkin et al, 1975)
** Upper limit set to avoid retinal pigmentation

Given the low toxicity and wide range of possible therapeutic dosages used in antipsychotic medication, for example, fluphenazine has been used in doses from 5 to 1200 mgm per day (Quitkin et al, 1975), it follows that one can manipulate dosage over time to enhance or diminish the sedative and neurological effects in relation to the antipsychotic action of the drug. Consequently these effects need not predominate when choosing medication; this highlights the importance of appreciating other differences between neuroleptics such as their effects on the heart, blood pressure, liver, and the epileptic threshold. These are well summarised in most textbooks of pharmacology and psychopharmacology (e.g. Hollister, 1978).

2. Whom to Treat

It is worth noting that not all schizophrenic patients require specific antipsychotic treatment. The asylum or the hospital can offer considerable relief from outside social and interpersonal pressures which precipitate schizophrenic symptoms (Hirsch, 1979) so that up to 25% of unselected acute admissions may recover without medication. Hence the success of mental hospitals with some patients before the days of physical treatment. While spontaneous remission is more likely to occur among the group traditionally recognised to have a good prognosis — first illness, acute onset, florid symptoms etc. — it is not possible to identify such patients with any accuracy. When comparing flupenthixol to placebo in acutely admitted patients, Johnstone et al (1978) found a significant improvement in all patients over the first two to three weeks; an advantage of active medication over placebo only emerged in the third week of treatment. If one is allowed to practice unhurried medicine, a period of at least one week's observation without antipsychotic treatment would identify those patients who begin to remit spontaneously and spare them the disadvantage and side effects of unnecessary medication. It should be remembered that despite 25 years of developments in the pharmacotherapy of schizophrenia the cure rate for the disorder has not changed since Kraeplin first described the condition. Bleuler (1974) carried out numerous studies of schizophrenia including 20 years' regular observation of over 200 patients and he states categorically that the proportion of benign psychoses with complete life-long recovery has not been altered by modern physical treatment (Bleuler, 1974). Given that the diagnoses are uncertain in a large proportion of cases there is much to say for taking one's time to assess patients before exhibiting medication.

The importance of environmental factors in determining the need for treatment applies equally to the schizophrenic who is obviously hospitalised in a stable unstressful environment. While some chronic in-patients require neuroleptic treatment for sedation and others require it to control florid symptoms, a considerable proportion (between 30% and 70%) are unchanged when medication is withdrawn (Prien and Klett, 1972) unless they are subsequently exposed to environmental threat (Hirsch, 1976). Given the danger of developing tardive dyskinesia and the positive protective environment of the hospital where treatment can be rapidly reinstated, most chronic in-patients should have the benefit of a trial off medication and others can be given the opportunity of a significant decrease of dosage. Even troublesome very disordered patients may benefit from such a trial.

3. Maintenance Treatment

The principal advance in patient care due to pharmacotherapeutics after the introduction of phenothiazines was the recognition of the third specific effect of neuroleptic medication – its prophylactic action in preventing the recurrence or recrudescence of schizophrenic symptoms. Davis (1975) reviewed 24 methodologically sound double-blind controlled studies of maintenance therapy covering chronic inpatients and outpatients. Among patients on active drugs only one study reported a relapse rate above 34%; the majority of placebo treated patients had relapse rates over 55%. Summing across studies, 698 patients out of 1068 who received placebo (65%) relapsed in contrast to 639 of 2127 patients on antipsychotics (30%); thus the prophylactic effect of neuroleptics had been established beyond question. The value of long acting depot injections for outpatient maintenance in schizophrenia has been confirmed in numerous studies including a double-blind placebo controlled trial (Hirsch et al, 1973). Though the value of oral maintenance treatment had been confirmed earlier (Leff and Wing, 1971), a strong view has grown up among clinicians, especially in the UK, that oral medication is not as successful as depot injections in preventing relapse. This is supported by the evidence from comparing relapse rates in patients before and after they were switched to long acting injections (Denham and Adamson, 1971; Johnson and Freeman, 1972). However, such studies included patients who were not successfully maintained on treatment prior to starting long acting injections. More recently a number of carefully conducted investigations have shown as much success with oral treatment over one or more years as earlier investigators had found with long acting medication. Moreover, the magnitude of the treatment effect as reflected by the difference in relapse rates between those on active medication – be it oral or by depot injection – and those on placebo is about the same (e.g. Hogarty et al, 1974).

Controlled studies directly comparing different oral neuroleptics against fluphenazine decanoate depot injections have recently found the same low relapse rates with oral neuroleptics such as pimozide (Falloon et al, 1978), penfluidol (Quitkin et al, 1978) or fluphenazine HC1 (Rifkin et al, 1972) as those observed on depot medications. In the latter two studies about 10% relapsed on active drug compared to 65% on placebo. While some patients may show more compliance than usual when taking tablets if they are in a trial, the numbers included are respectable enough to suggest that treatment by injection may not be necessary. Thus, these studies have established that oral maintenance treatment can be as effective as depot treatment.

Finally, it should be noted that like oral medication, the claim that different depot neuroleptics have different effects has not stood up to close scrutiny. Knights and colleagues (1979) were unable to find any meaningful differences between fluphenazine and flupenthixol in a study of 57 schizophrenics randomly assigned to one treatment or the other and followed for six months from the time they left hospital. Of those completing the trial 7% relapsed, 53% experienced depressive symptoms and 89% had extrapyramidal side effects (EPSE's). This study emphasises the high frequency of EPSE's during the first six months of treatment with depot neuroleptics. Prevalence rates reported by

141

other authors vary between 23% and 88% depending on how closely the signs are looked for. Side effects are more common in the first six months (Johnson, 1978). The symptoms can be abated by reducing the dose and increasing the frequency of injections using smaller doses. The value of anticholinergic medication after control of the acute symptoms is doubtful and has been called into question (see Johnson, 1978 and his references). The prevalence of parkinsonian symptoms from among patients on maintenance treatment is of the order of 20% but there is a constant interchange between those affected and those not. Discontinuation of anticholinergic medication led to an increase in parkinsonian symptoms of only 4% (McClelland, 1976). Other authors support the conclusion that such side effects are treated too soon for too long with too little clinical benefit after the first few days but with a possible increased risk of anticholinergic toxicity and tardive dyskinesia (Mindham, 1976; McClelland, 1976; Johnson, 1978).

4. When to Stop Treatment

Several studies of maintenance treatment have found that about 20% of patients withdrawn from treatment or switched to placebo do not relapse during the first one or two years (Leff and Wing, 1971; Hirsch et al, 1973; Hogarty et al, 1974). However, using a life table method of assessing the continued risk of relapse at any point in time Hogarty (1977) calculated that at three years following discharge the rate of relapse was still 3% per month or 2½ to 3 times greater than for patients on maintenance therapy. Nevertheless, there is a small proportion of patients who survive without relapse for quite a long time if medication is discontinued or they are treated with placebo from the time they leave hospital. Unfortunately there is no clinical or other measure to date that can predict who will survive when treatment is withdrawn except by trial and error. When discussing whom to treat I suggested that inpatients should be given a trial off treatment. Given the high risk of relapse as an outpatient off medication, we should be reluctant to allow patients with a previous illness to avoid maintenance treatment. When then can it be discontinued? Johnson (1976) withdrew treatment from 23 patients during the second year and 53% relapsed as compared with 12% who stayed on treatment (p < .01). During the third year of treatment 13 were discontinued and 69% relapsed compared with 15% on treatment. Hogarty et al (1976) withdrew patients from drugs who had been successfully maintained on treatment for the two previous years. Of 41 withdrawn, 27 (66%) relapsed during the succeeding year, which is no different from the mean relapse rate of 24 studies reviewed by Davis (1975). Relating to the initial period of maintenance treatment with antipsychotics, sociotherapy did not protect against relapse (Hogarty et al, 1976). Thus the risk of relapse following withdrawal from drugs does not abate for the first two to three years.

Maintenance therapy carries well known disadvantages including a high risk of parkinsonian side effects (Knights et al, 1979) tardive dyskinesia, and a more subtle parkinsonian syndrome with akinesia and bradykinesia which alters the patient's social presentation and causes depression-like distress (Rifkin et al, 1975). An alternative to discontinuing treatment is reducing the dosage. This has been tested in two large trials but unfortunately the patients, though chronic, were inpatients.

Cattey et al (1964) randomised patients to have either daily treatment as in the past, treatment Monday, Wednesday and Friday (58% reduction in dose), or to have placebo only. Within four months the relapse rates were 5%, 16%, and 45% respectively. Prien et al (1973) compared patients on a daily basis to patients on three, four, or five times a week regimens and found little difference in the relapse rate after 4 months, which was 1% and 6–8% respectively – the dose reduction being 19% to 43%. It is clear that dose reduction, or discontinuation of treatment in the first three years, at the very least carries an increased risk of relapse which, though less than on no treatment, must be balanced against other benefits.

6. Relative Contribution of Experiential and Pharmacological Factors on the Course of Schizophrenia

Davis (1976) combined patients from two clinical trials and found that the rank order correlation between drug treatment and placebo against improvement versus deterioration was $r_p = 0.60$, which meant that drugs explained only 36% of the variance of improvement – surprisingly little considering that more than 75% of the drug treated group improved and 50% of the placebo group deteriorated. In a study of outpatients from the time of discharge Vaughn and Leff (1976) replicated previous workers and found that the correlation between drug treatment and relapse was $r = 0.39$ explaining only 15% of the variance. However, their study was a prospective trial of the importance of hostile emotion and over-involvement (called high expressed emotion or HEE) by the key relative as measured at the time of patient's admission with schizophrenia. Of patients whose key relative rated high on EE 51% relapsed over nine months following discharge, but of those returning to live with a relative rated as low EE, only 14% relapsed. Moreover, the relapse rate of patients with a high EE relative was affected by the amount of time spent in the same room with the relative – 69% of those spending more than 35 hours per week relapsed in contrast with 28% of patients spending less than 35 hours per week. The correlation between going home to live with a high EE relative and relapsing was $r_p = 0.45$ and there was no relationship between whether the patient had maintenance treatment and whether the patient's relative was high or low on EE ($r_p = 0.01$). The presence of stressful life events has been shown to influence outcome in a way which suggests that medication raises the patient's threshold to life events (Leff, Hirsch et al, 1973) and a nixious environment at home

(Hirsch. 1976). These studies suggest that social experience plays a big role in provoking relapse but drugs modify its influence prophylactically in the well patient, and remedially in the ill patient.

A different aspect of the question is whether social and psychological treatments have a remedial effect independent of medication. May et al (1976) have carried out a massive controlled study of treatment with a five year follow-up. Psychotherapy was no better than milieu (control) treatment by itself; improvement with drug treatment with or without psychotherapy was significantly superior. A number of other studies have been conducted comparing social therapy or psychotherapy with or without drugs in chronic schizophrenics. Patients improved most with drugs and deteriorated most without drugs – at best social therapies had a slight, usually non-significant, influence (Greenblatt et al, 1965; Hogarty et al, 1974). The conclusion from such findings as these is that social and psychological therapies do not have the antipsychotic effectiveness of psychotropic drugs. But they do not help a patient find housing, get a job, or cope with social relationships as we might expect social treatment to do. It is perhaps disappointing that our social and psychological treatments as yet do not improve the patient's ability to cope with life's experiences and offer some protection against relapse such as drugs provide.

6. Radical Approaches to Current Treatment

We have reviewed some of the more recent concepts and developments with regard to conventional treatment of schizophrenia. It can be concluded that we have achieved considerable success in controlling the symptoms of schizophrenia so that patients can live outside hospital and have fewer episodes of florid illness. Though affected in a less severe degree the majority of patients with schizophrenia continue to carry disabilities as a result of their condition – we should be experiencing a growing restlesness at our inability to cure this malady. A talk about current trends would be incomplete without mentioning some of the bolder efforts currently being undertaken to deal with the drug resistant patient. I am skipping the account of very high dose treatment largely because these efforts have been unsuccessful (Quitkin et al, 1975; McClelland et al, 1976). Rather, I will turn my attention to unproven attempts at radical therapy still under investigation.

Propranolol

The potential antipsychotic activity of propranolol was discovered by Atsom and his colleagues in Israel (Atsom and Blum, 1970) and applied most extensively to schizophrenics by Yorkston who has carried out several open studies (Yorkston et al, 1974) and one double-blind trial in which propranolol or placebo was added to conventional treatment. Our interest in propranolol derives from several facts:

144

1. There is evidence that it acts on the medulla and hippocampus and it may not have a dopamine blocking effect like other antipsychotic drugs (Gruzelier, 1978).

2. It has interesting and different psychophysiological normalising effects not shared by other antipsychotic drugs (Gruzelier et al, 1979).

3. It has no extrapyramidal side effects (Yorkston et al, 1976)

4. There is an unproven impression that it improves demeanour and calms excitable patients and possibly affects other unspecifiable aspects of a schizophrenic's functioning in a way not observed with conventional medication.

The trials to date referred to above support, but do not conclusively prove, that propranolol has an antipsychotic effect. More recently (Yorkston et al, in press) we have shown a significant improvement in newly admitted acute patients randomly allocated to propranolol or chlorpromazine as their sole treatment. The rate and extent of change was not significantly different between treatments for 35 patients rated at six weeks or 27 patients rated at 12 weeks. There was no placebo control but the magnitude of the change on the BPRS schizophrenia subscales was about six points that of the order observed in most of the studies carried out in the USA (Overall et al, 1967). This study was hampered by the fact that medication was not increased once the initial signs of improvement were evident — thus the modal dose was 600 mg for propranolol and 300 mg for chlorpromazine at six weeks. Now, we would push the dose of propranolol until toxicity occurred then reduce it by 10% or 20%. A review of the literature suggests that patients should be offered at least 500 mgm chlorpromazine if they do not respond to lower doses (Klein and Davis, 1969). In a carefully conducted open study Sheppard (1979) has reported significant improvement in seven of eight patients treated with higher doses of propranolol.

Of greater interest is the d-isomer of propranolol — commercially propranolol is only available in the d/l racemic form. The d-isomer has much less beta blocking effect on blood pressure and heart rate so the dose can be increased rapidly to much higher levels making the drug feasible for clinical use. We have found that d-propranolol has the same psychophysiological properties as the racemate* and we are about to embark on a double blind comparison of d-propranolol to placebo in newly admitted patients to determine if d-propranolol has antischizophrenic properties.

Encouraged by the work of Cundall (personal communication) who reported good improvement in 9 out of 13 schizophrenics treated with d-propranolol in an open uncontrolled investigation we have carried out preliminary studies to get the measure of this drug. R Manchanda and I have treated and systematically monitored 7 patients with d-propranolol following admission and noted improvement in 5 of them.

Table 2 shows significant improvement of the BPRS schizophrenia subscores

*(Gruzelier et al 1979)

on patients treated in this open trial. Note that the mean dose of d-propranolol was 1100 mg per day as compared to 600 mg of d/l propranolol used in the previous trial.

TABLE 2 Open Trial – D-propranolol Schizophrenia Subscores – BPRS (Thought Dis.* + Non-Thought Dis.**)

	Before Treatment	One month Treatment	Dose mg
1	18	3	960
2	7	2	1600
3	9	6*** 7 days	800
4	15	2	1760
5	15	8	800
6	14	12**** 14 days	920
7	5	4	1040
X ± SE	11.9 ± 4.8	5.3 ± 3.6	1126 ± 390

*	Conceptual disorganisation, hallucinatory behaviour. Unusual thought content.
**	Blunted affect, emotional withdrawal, suspiciousness, grandiosity, mannerisms and posturing hostility and motor retardation.
***	7 days treatment.
****	Further improvement noticed at week 3.

Endorphins

Endorphins represent another area of recent discovery. These are psychoactive endogenous substances with morphine-like actions in the brain which can be found as part of a beta-lipoprotein produced in the pituitary. The possible role of abnormal or excessive endorphin production in the aetiology of schizophrenia was raised by Terenius et al in 1976 when they reported increased levels of endorphins in the CSF of patients with chronic schizophrenia. Subsequently Gunne, Lindstrom and Terenius reported reversal of hallucinations when four patients were infused with naloxone – a morphine/endorphin antagonist. In 1977 Kline and Lehmann et al reported that they produced transient amelioration of patients' psychotic symptoms after injection with beta endorphin. In 1978 Palmour and his associates in California found an abnormal lucine substituted beta endorphin in the serum and dialysates of schizophrenics.

Unfortunately subsequent investigations leave these initial findings in considerable doubt. Regarding the evidence that endorphin antagonists abolish schizophrenic symptoms an additional three studies involving a total of 50 cases also found a significant reduction of hallucinations following naloxone infusion but five other studies involving 51 patients including a replication by Gunne and his group who originally reported the antipsychotic effects of naloxone reported no effect. Emrich who has reported positive improvement in 40 of 50 cases studied concludes that the changes were small, lasted only hours, and could be due to alteration of what he calls 'stress factor' (Emrich et al, 1978).

Following up Kline's original study Berger used 20 mg of beta endorphin –

146

over twice the dose used by Kline – and found no dramatic improvement. The increased concentration of beta endorphin and related substances in the serum and CSF have not been substantiated either.

In contrast to this discouraging result, Verhoeven and others (Verhoeven et al, 1979) reported a double-blind crossover trial with des-try-gamma endorphin (DTGE), an endorphin non-opiate peptide with potent neuroleptic properties in animals similar to haloperidol. Employing a crossover design eight patients showed improvement in the first week and in four improvement was maintained for three months without further treatment. In all, 14 patients were studied, all responded to the drug but only four were well after the injections were discontinued. Another synthetic metenkephalin FK33–824 (Jorgensen et al, 1979) has also been shown to have neuroleptic activity. We have tried five patients on DTGE with absolutely no effect! Fortunately, we have since learned from our suppliers that the substance they supplied us was partially if not wholly inactive because of freeze drying for the purpose of shipment. The value of endorphins remains to be demonstrated.

Dialysis

Wagemaker and Cade (1977) have reported ten cases of chronic schizophrenia treated with dialysis of whom three recovered and are off treatment and five others are significantly improved. All patients had hallucinations or delusions and blunted affect and these symptoms responded to treatment. However, Port et al (1978) published a survey of 81 dialysis units contacted by questionnaire – 52 centres responded and reported experience with 53 patients dialysed for renal disease who have had a diagnosis of schizophrenia. Improvement of schizophrenic symptoms had only been noted in eight cases – 15% of those treated. Notwithstanding, we have treated two patients with renal dialysis each with more than ten years illness and persistent hallucinations and delusions as well as chronic apathy. Both needed constant observation at home or in hospital and both had had a trial of high dose neuroleptics and propranolol without effect. The first patient was dialysed twice weekly for eight weeks with no improvement. The second has shown a remarkable improvement in personality, liveliness, and drive as well as the disappearance of his hallucinations, ideas of reference, and delusions. His only persisting symptom is a delusional memory. When dialysis was reduced to once weekly for six weeks he deteriorated and when it was increased to twice weekly he rapidly improved. However he has now been withdrawn from dialysis at his own wish and has not deteriorated. A small dialysable molecule could play an aetiological role in schizophrenia in some patients.

Chances have it that none of these new treatments will prove to provide the breakthrough in the treatment of schizophrenia that we need. Nevertheless I believe that it behoves clinicians to continue to attempt to press forward the boundaries of their knowledge and therapeutic potency. The fact that there are over 3,000 references on the treatment of schizophrenia in the Index Medicus during the past three years is testimony to the fact that we have yet to find an effective remedy for this condition.

COMMENTARY ON CURRENT TRENDS IN THE MEDICAL TREATMENT OF SCHIZOPHRENIA

Douglas Bennett

Professor Hirsch's paper dictates the direction and content of my commentary. His starting point is his erudite and comprehensive review of present trends in the pharmacotherapy of schizophrenia. It is all too easy to be dazzled by his account of sedative and neuroleptic ratios or the estimation of the potency of anti-psychotic drugs in terms of their stereospecific (H^3) spiroperidol binding capacity in vitro. However, for all the talk of dopamine blockade and nigrostriatal action it is clear that patients treated with 'the putative drug of choice' do not respond more favourably than those randomly assigned to the drug. This situation is not so very different from that which I described 12 years ago, when I said of these medications that 'so far no study has shown unequivocal evidence for the superiority of any phenothiazine over chlorpromazine . . . the therapists choice often depends either on familiarity, the patients preference, or the wish to avoid undesirable side effects' (Bennett, 1967a). There is no room in pharmacotherapy for easy optimism. Leslie Iversen (1978) observed that 'the dopamine hypothesis may make the development of new drugs easier, since simple screening tests for anti-dopamine properties now exist'. However, new compounds discovered in this way will be likely to behave very similarly to those already in existence. Of course, there could be a breakthrough but we should not hope for too much, for to quote Iversen again 'it would certainly be naive to suppose that a metabolic defect could be regarded as "the cause" of schizophrenia'. Neurobiological research may help, however, to unravel the complexities of the situation. At least it seems that we can now select medications that will cause our patients less troublesome side effects.

At times Professor Hirsch seems to share some of these reservations. Thus he maintains that despite 25 years of development in the pharmacotherapy of schizophrenia the cure rate for this disorder has not changed since Kraepelin first described the condition. Of course, much depends on the concept of cure. Can one even talk of cure in schizophrenia? Certainly the prognosis in terms of

149

social adjustment for patients with schizophrenia has improved. Kraepelin (1919) thought that about 17% of in-patients treated at his Heidelberg Clinic were socially adjusted many years later. Mayer-Gross (1932) followed up 260 schizophrenic patients out of a total of 294 admitted to the same Heidelberg Clinic in 1912 and 1913. Sixteen years later, although there had been a high death rate, 35% had made 'social recoveries' outside hospital. Harris and his colleagues (1956) followed the course of 125 schizophrenia patients admitted to the Maudsley and Bethlem between 1945 and 1950 and found that 45% could be regarded as social recoveries five years later. A further 21% were socially disabled but living out of hospital. More recently a study of 111 patients first admitted to three British psychiatric hospitals in 1956 showed that 56% had recovered socially 5 years later while 34% were socially disabled but out of hospital (Brown et al, 1966). There has been improvement in the rate of social recovery if not of cure. This is unlikely to be attributable to medication alone since most of the change occurred before modern medications were introduced. It seems inadvisable to talk of cure when one is dealing with a poorly understood but incapacitating condition which will relapse in the presence of social stress or which, in the absence of sufficient social stimulation, may result in severe disablement. A combination of relief from precipitating and everyday stresses and active treatment usually results in the fairly rapid remission of acute symptoms but a liability to further attacks often remains and this vulnerability must be recognised as a form of 'invisible' chronic impairment (Wing, 1978). Now I do not wish to take up the cudgels on behalf of social treatment in opposition to medication. What I believe is that both play their part and it is a surprise to me that Professor Hirsch has not taken a broader view of treatment since he is extremely well informed on the subject. Certainly there is much more to the treatment and management of schizophrenia than the prescription of psychotropic medication. For as Professor Hirsch indicates, when drug treatments are compared with placebo they only explain 36% of the variance of improvement (Davis, 1976) or in the Vaughn and Leff (1976) study only 15% of the variance.

It is necessary to make a distinction between the use of medication or placebo and the effect of social factors in the acute and chronic stages of the disorder. Thus in Prien and Klett's (1972) study 30–70% of the chronic patients in hospital were unchanged when medication was withdrawn. Wing and Brown (1961) go further. In their study of female schizophrenics in three mental hospitals they show that the amount of medication prescribed in these hospitals, while varying widely, could not be related to the differences in the patients clinical and social state.

I commend Professor Hirsch's suggestion that in-patients should be given a trial off treatment as advocated by Caffey et al (1964) in view of the risks of continuous treatment. There are also risks of inadequate treatment. Oral medication may or may not be as effective as depot injections but research findings that suggest that it is take little account of other studies of patient compliance rates which have given figures (not only for those with psychiatric disorders) as low as 80% among in-patients and 40% among out-patients.

When we come to study acutely ill patients with schizophrenia treated at home or in out-patients we find in controlled studies that when the medication is withdrawn its removal leads to relapse in some cases. (Pasamanick et al, 1964; Gross et al, 1961). Even so we have to remember that some patients relapse on medication and some do not relapse when it is discontinued (Leff and Wing, 1971). In 1967 I expressed a belief that for the schizophrenic patient 'both drugs and family relations play their part in preventing or precipitating a relapse of the illness'. I added that 'their combined effect has never been investigated' (Bennett, 1967b). However, in 1976 Vaughn and Leff reported their findings and showed how medication reduced the chances of relapse for patients with schizophrenia in families that showed high expressed emotion. The outlook for such patients is improved by reducing contact with relatives and by the maintenance of phenothiazine therapy. What is important is that in some difficult family situations ataractic medication alone cannot prevent the relapse of schizophrenia. In other family situations medication does prevent relapse.

Professor Hirsch says that social treatment has little if any effect. I am not sure how he would regard the provision of a sheltered work-shop which ensures that the patient does not spend too much time doing nothing or the provision of lodgings which reduce contact with a home where there was high expressed emotion. Would he see this provision as socio-therapeutic? Would a family approach directed at reducing high expressed emotion fit into that category?

In his paper Professor Hirsch seems to equate sociotherapy with milieu therapy. He refers to May's 'massive control study' in which drugs were shown to be superior to milieu in the treatment of schizophrenia. Drugs as chemical substances are very much the same in London or California but hospital milieux can vary enormously. One must specify, as Brown et al (1966) and Wing and Brown (1970) have done, the detailed nature of the social situation in a way that can be replicated. What then of May's milieu? Milton Greenblatt in his introduction to May's book (1968) says that 'I think Dr. May's "milieu therapy" leans toward a former idea of a loose collection of "non-specific therapies", such as occupational therapy, group meetings, and the like, mostly supervised or dominated by non-medical personnel. In fact, as utilised in this study, it forms a base line or back drop against which the more "specific therapies" could demonstrate their potentialities'. This milieu is only a very limited kind of therapeutic organisation of the hospital environment. Certainly it does not test the full potential of milieu methods. May's own description of the milieu takes up one page of a 300 page book and describes mostly the buildings and the numbers of nursing staff. The programme is described in five lines. It 'included nursing care, hydrotherapy and occupational, recreational, and industrial therapy. The nursing staff held community-type ward meetings once a week with all the patients and a half-time social worker was assigned to provide case-work according to the patients' needs.' Of course May is not alone. People talk of the hospital environment as if there was one such thing. Hospital environments differ and so do wards in the same hospital (Brown et al, 1966). Some psychoanalysts such as Hartmann have gone further. He speaks of the 'average expectable environment'; not to be confused with the average expectable therapist of the average expectable patient.

The interaction between social environment and medication is complex. It is nowhere better illustrated than in the study by Lorna Wing (1956) in which the behavioural changes in patients treated with reserpine were rated and compared with ratings made by a social psychologist of the behaviour of untreated patients in the same disturbed female ward (Folkard, 1959). Ratings of the mental state of the patients taking reserpine showed a significant reduction in 'hostility'. Observations made by the social psychologist showed no significant difference between the experimental and control groups in regard to the number of patients involved in aggressive incidents. Surprisingly both groups improved. It was suggested that reserpine not only reduced aggression in patients receiving it but also in patients not receiving the drug whom the treated patients had previously provoked. These authors showed that subsequent changes in the social situation of the ward, caused by opening the ward doors or changing the staff could result in a similar alteration in the number of aggressive incidents. Ødegaard (1964) sampled the national figures for admission to all Norwegian mental hospitals in three 5-year periods: 1936/40, 1948/52 and 1955/59. He showed that the discharge rate between the first two quinquennia was greater than that between the second and third. Yet it was in the interval between the second and third quinquennia that treatment with reserpine and chlorpromazine had been introduced. When the discharge rates for individual hospitals were analysed they showed a marked negative correlation between the levels of discharge in 1948/52 and 1955/59. In other words Ødegaard believed that the pharmacotherapeutic drugs brought less benefit to patients in those hospitals with initially favourable therapeutic situations and a high discharge rate.

Medication is often a useful crutch in a difficult family situation or in a backward hospital. We are all well aware of the inadequate staffing of mental hospitals, but reading Professor Hirsch's paper I wondered whether the District General Hospital Unit too might not be deprived of beds and time and that this might also encourage a reliance on medication. This thought was reinforced by his remark that if only unhurried medicine were possible one might be able to observe a patient for a week before prescribing medication.

This brings me to some discussion of the effect of medication on the staff as well as on the patients who swallow it. Perhaps Rathod's (1958) study is the most interesting in this respect. Two groups of disturbed women patients in separate wards, three quarters of whom were schizophrenic, were observed over a period of three and a half years. Their behaviour and the incidence of disturbances on the ward were recorded. The control period during which drugs had not yet taken effect was followed by a period where one third of the patients were taking chlorpromazine. The behaviour of the patients on both wards was improved. In the third period almost half of the patients were on phenothiazines but there was no further improvement in their behaviour; instead, there was a slight deterioration. In the fourth period an active social programme of occupation and recreation together with staff discussions was introduced on both wards. At the same time the phenothiazine drugs were replaced for all except a few patients by placebo tablets. This was done without the knowledge of either patients or staff. The social programme was accepted enthusiastically in one ward and was virtually rejected in the other. Patient behaviour continued to improve — most markedly in the ward adopting the social programme. Not only were both wards as quiet as when tranquillisers were being given but further improvement in patient behaviour resulted from the social changes. In the last phase nurses in the best ward were told about the placebos and within a short time the ward showed signs of increased disturbance. I think it is important to remember that while drug treatment and social management alone are partially effective at different times and at different stages of the schizophrenic disorder they are much more efficacious when they are considered together. It is not my purpose to repeat my views on the social treatment of schizophrenia here (Bennett, 1978). Nor can I do more than draw your attention to the importance of psychological treatments which are not mentioned by Professor Hirsch but are well discussed by Gwynne Jones (1978) in Professor Wing's recent book on schizophrenia.

I come now, to the last section of Professor Hirsch's paper in which he states his belief that it behoves clinicians to press forward the boundaries of their knowledge and their potency. One cannot disagree with that. Yet this whole section causes me some ethical and scientific unease. I regard the search for a final chemical solution as inherently dangerous and extremely reactionary. I might say the same about the so called 'radical treatments'. As psychiatrists we still have to live down past excesses of therapeutic zeal. These include the induction of organic confusional states by multiple daily convulsions with ECT, the use of death defying insulin comas, the deliberate induction of extra-pyramidal symptoms with neuroleptics, not to mention the ill-considered use of pre-frontal leucotomy. Maurice Partridge in a follow-up study of leucotomy patients commented that bizarre diseases require bizarre treatments and in psychiatry they got them. In those days we did not need trials since we knew that we were doing good. I hope that we have learned something in the years between. Yet Professor Hirsch introduces us to the 'open trial' which seems to be an acceptable euphemism for an 'uncontrolled' trial. Endorphins are spoken of as an area of recent discovery. But it reminded me that at one time opium was frequently employed in the treatment of mental illness. Even dialysis has an historic analogy. Hack Tuke in his Dictionary of Psychological Medicine published in 1892 tells of a physician named Denis in Paris. In 1667 Denis employed the transfusion of blood in a young man who became sane. The blood was taken from a calf. On the following morning he was less insane. Encouraged by this success the remedy was repeated. The result was very satisfactory as to his mental condition but a high fever set in which ended fatally. It was admitted that the patient recovered his reason and had been obliged to visit the Professors of the medical school in Paris in order that they might see for themselves that he was sane. No wonder he became feverish said Tuke. I hope that we are not as easily convinced as the Professors of 1667 since that is no way to increase the boundaries of our knowledge. It is on our critical sense that the well being of our patients and future knowledge depends.

COMMENTARY ON CURRENT TRENDS IN THE MEDICAL TREATMENT OF SCHIZOPHRENIA

David Curson

My task was to produce a discussion paper in reply to Professor Stephen Hirsch's excellent review of current trends in the treatment of schizophrenia. I interpret that task as attempting to expand on particular areas of treatment and focus attention on certain issues I think the audience might consider relevant.

There is little to criticise in the factual content of pharmacological principles and mechanisms and the lucid summary of the drug trials which have been conducted. However, I do feel that we need to examine carefully a number of salient issues in the field of schizophrenia treatment.

In my view no discourse on the treatment of a psychiatric disorder can be complete without some reference to diagnostic and nosological issues. Schizophrenia is no exception. Some might feel it is a principal area of concern.

Professor Hirsch seems to allude to this problem in his opening remarks where he sets out to scotch some prevailing myths about syndromes and their responsiveness to chemotherapy. As one reads on there is an increasing awareness that treatment is being construed principally as treatment with psycho-active drugs and there is only a passing reference to other aspects of management.

I would propose that an understanding of treatment encompasses the concepts of definition and classification. In simple terms the clinician needs to be sure (and be sure that others are sure) of what he is attempting to treat before he knows whether the treatment prescribed is effective or not.

A number of assumptions are prevalent and perhaps they demand (if not cry out for) examination, e.g.:

(a) All clinicians share the same concept of schizophrenia.
(b) All clinicians are capable of identifying schizophrenia in a manner consistent with the methods adopted by researchers who test the forms of treatment in a scientific way.
(c) 'Positive' or 'Hard' symptoms of schizophrenia, e.g. delusions or

hallucinations are the ones that really matter and are the proper target of treatment (treatment itself being conceived by psychiatrists as drug treatment).

Definition Issues

The debate about the concept of schizophrenia continues and the relative contributions of symptoms (Schneider, K 1959; Strauss and Carpenter, 1973 and 1974; Carpenter, Bartko et al, 1976), behaviour (Wing, 1961), course (Bleuler, 1974), outcome (Strauss and Carpenter, 1972 and 1977) and possible etiology, be it psychological, biological, or sociological (Dunham, 1976; Eisenberg, 1977; Dohrenwend, 1975 and 1976; Claridge, 1972) have been investigated and reviewed by large numbers of workers. From Kraepelin (1899) and Bleuler (1911) to the present day the emphasis has been seen to shift from one aspect to another..

Kendall (1975) has argued for agreement on the criteria for the diagnosis of schizophrenia. He reminds us of the need for diagnostic categories as a basis for research and of the fundamental scientific requirement of replication by different workers. 'Repeatability is fundamental and this principle applies to the definition of the subject matter just as much as it does to the experimental procedures involved and the results obtained. If our diagnostic criteria are unreliable and vary unpredictably from place to place this requirement is obviously not being met.'

There appears to be a preoccupation over the minutiae of methodology whilst agreed diagnostic criteria have tended to be played down. It is interesting that Davis (1975) who is referred to frequently by Professor Hirsch never once mentions the problem of diagnosis but enters into an extensive critique of methodology. When this problem is then taken back to the clinician (conveniently defined as the person responsible for treating the vast majority of schizophrenics) we have evidence that diagnostic criteria are even more disorganised and culture-bound (W.H.O., 1973; Cooper et al, 1972). When discussing the implications of a diagnosis of schizophrenia Kendall (1975) again remarks that part of the problem lies in the different emphasis different psychiatrists place on the importance of a particular constellation of symptoms, a condition with a particular (usually a poor) prognosis, and a condition with a particular (and speculative) aetiology. It is worth reminding ourselves that, even today, there are psychiatrists, psychologists, social workers, and even psychiatric nurses who believe as a fundamental truth the speculations of Fromm Reichmann (1948) about 'refrigerator mothers', Bateson and his 'Double Bind' (1956), Lidz and his 'Skew' (1973), and Wynne and Singer who attributed schizophrenia to fragmented and amorphous styles of communication in the families (1963, 1965). Is it any wonder that clinicians of all disciplines are unable to agree over appropriate treatment?

Strauss and Carpenter (1974) investigated the role of symptoms and their relationship to outcome, using patients in the International Pilot Study of Schizophrenia. Their results showed that the symptom criteria of Langfeldt did not discriminate selectively a poor outcome category of schizophrenia thus challenging the major empirical basis for the view that symptom criteria alone could account for a poor outcome concept of the disorder. They proposed the 'confluence of factors hypothesis' which is more complex than a unitary concept of schizophrenia as a disorder. 'If a particular group of symptoms is of a debilitating nature or accompanied by other difficulties such as long-standing social disability, and if these symptoms have already persisted for a long period of time in a person, these processes together might then present a particular picture but although it can be given a name – for example schizophrenia – it might not represent a specific disease but a confluence of chronicity, certain symptoms, and social disability, all of which can also exist independently.'

The same authors (1973) had shown that Schneider's First Rank Symptoms (FRS) were highly discriminating but led to significant diagnostic errors if FRS were regarded as pathognomonic. Furthermore, FRS did not have a postdictive or predictive function as no relationship could be established between FRS and duration or outcome of illness. In a later offering Hawk and Carpenter (1975) reported on a five year follow-up of their first outcome study. Outcome at five years and two years correlated highly and three variables stood out as key predictors of outcome at both points in time: duration of hospitalisation prior to in-trial evaluation, social contacts (perhaps indirectly and anecdotally referred to by Bleuler (1974)), and work function. Using cluster analysis Carpenter, Bartko et al (1976) showed one large and three small sub-groups each readily distinguishable from the other. They had expressed dissatisfaction with traditional sub-types as being indistinguishable by symptoms and signs and so hoped that their newer sub-types or sub-groups, namely 'typical', 'flagrant', 'insightful', and 'hypochondriacal' might be shown to be significantly and differentially related to variables such as drug response, clinical course and outcome, biological and psychological abnormalities, and psychiatric illness in relatives. Though the meaningfulness of this particular sub-division of schizophrenia may never be enhanced as the authors' hope, it certainly reflects a laudable attempt at challenging current unsatisfactory nosology.

One approach to the problem of classification is the use of operational definitions (Hay and Forest, 1972; Forrest and Hay, 1973). Essentially they are not only concerned with what the patient displays but also what he does not display or displays in addition to the other phenomena. In a sense they are but a formal expression of what clinicians are believed to do during the diagnostic process, but the absence of uniformity has already been referred to earlier.

Feighner's (1972) criteria for the diagnosis of schizophrenia are outstanding examples amongst several of the use of operational definitions. Many would

157

agree, however, that they are too stringent for clinical practice and perhaps too dependent on clinical course.

Many clinicians continue to use non-operational diagnostic criteria. Bleuler's four A's — incongruity of affect, autism, ambivalence, and association — are undoubtedly far too loose. Nevertheless they remain deeply entrenched in psychiatric folklore on both sides of the Atlantic. Schneider's FRS are of course in vogue. Mellor (1970) demonstrated that 72% of 166 patients diagnosed as schizophrenic in an English Mental Hospital had one or more such symptoms. At first glance this is impressive but not only does it leave unanswered the question of the other 28%, it also poses further questions when one considers the detailed, indeed luxuriant, mental state examination that was performed on those patients.

When attempts are made to base psychiatric nosology on drug response even more problems are encountered. Almost all are relevant to drug treatment in schizophrenia. Murray and Murphy (1978) point out that when administration of a drug is followed by behavioural change one cannot assume that it has affected the patient's illness per se since it may have acted on some associated factor such as premorbid personality. Alternatively, a clinical change may occur through a drug affecting some secondary consequence of a disorder; for example some alcoholics improve on tricyclics not because the drug affects their dependence but because they have become depressed as a consequence of their alcoholism.

Distinguishing features of drug responding sub-groups have often been identified but replication attempts have usually failed. The reasons for this lack of replicability have included:

(i)   Inability to identify reliably psychiatric phenomena.
(ii) Ignorance of whether drugs employed were reaching their site of action in appropriate concentrations.
(iii) Lack of specificity of most psychiatric drugs.

The second obstacle to replicability is that investigators have rarely taken into account the variables intervening between the prescription of a drug and therapeutic response. Factors such as non-compliance, placebo response, drug metabolism, and biological sensitivity appear capable of accounting for a large proportion of the variation of individual drug responses.

I suspect that the academics are moving towards agreement but I fear that clinicians are picking up the crumbs from the table and from information stemming more from drug company lunches than authoritative articles in the journals and are perpetuating the myths and fantasies of past and present generations. Professor Hirsch's summary of current knowledge is, therefore, timely but begs as many questions as it answers.

Perhaps we ought to consider some solutions whilst remembering that to set out to change the ideologies of practising consultant psychiatrists is a formidable

158

task. Despite all that has been written symptoms have proved to be a useful foundation for diagnosis. However they need to be viewed in their proper perspective. They can only retain some semblance of validity if they are elicited during careful and thorough examinations of mental state. This demands time and a working knowledge of psychopathology which some clinicians frankly lack.

Having obtained them they should not be viewed as the condition itself but phenomena of that condition. Furthermore, using certain symptoms as a basis for diagnosis and also as targets for treatment are not one and the same activity. Surely we are all familiar with symptoms that are disabling but when those same symptoms have gone the person remains severely disabled. Patients are simply no longer diagnosable using the same criteria! I can plead for appropriate training for potential consultant psychiatrists based on internationally agreed criteria, but there needs to be an explicit statement on the lines of Van Praag (1975) 'Empirical studies have failed to reveal clear pathognomonic symptoms'. He goes on 'schizophrenia conforms to the aetiological aspecificity of psychiatric syndromes' and proposes the need for a three dimensional classification of schizophrenia based on symptomatic typology, aetiological typology, and typology according to course. Chronicity as a feature demands caution however. If the diagnosis is not made until it is chronic this is not so much a validation criterion as a tautology. Roth and Barnes (1979) for example are attempting to validate a modified classification of schizophrenia using the original study of Hirsch et al with its wealth of preliminary inclusion data (1973) and the seven-year follow-up study of the same drug trial (1979). It may be of interest in this respect that two of the original cohort in the MRC fluphenazine double blind study have been re-diagnosed by the responsible clinical teams as manic depressives. Whilst a third patient in the opinion of the writer and his colleagues has probably been wrongly re-diagnosed manic depressive when she is clearly schizophrenic using current research criteria based on detailed mental state examination, social behaviour, course, and response to treatment. That this phenomenon can occur in a teaching hospital of some repute merely serves to underline the enormous difficulties in reaching a diagnosis. If I add that few clinicians have the opportunity to spend four hours assessing only one patient then the problems of routine psychiatric practice are magnified.

Whom to Treat

I agree with the points made by Professor Hirsch in this particular section. However a corollary might be entitled 'Whom can we treat'? Not only has every clinician encountered the obviously schizophrenic individual who refuses to accept treatment or, when he does, subsequently fails to comply by not attending clinics or secreting medication. Even the research worker encounters such people or has to allow for such groups. In this respect and despite the powerful pharmacological arguments clinicians, and I suspect their responsible nursing staff do prefer depot injections (Groves and Mendel, 1975).

Unfortunately, it is a double-edge sword. In maximising compliance we are also maximising side-effects and the more severe and irreversible such as tardive dyskinesia are most worrying. We can find ourselves inducing a physical disability which prevents re-settlement because lay people see such involuntary movements as peculiar and characteristic of madness even though, by a stroke of irony, the drug is preventing the madness which lies dormant but concealed from the world. At least when the patient has the capacity to default they may be protecting themselves from the worst excesses of enthusiastic medicine. It is perhaps for this reason more than any other that we need to condemn the widespread use of depot neuroleptics for conditions other than the schizophrenias and even then only for the more serious forms.

Maintenance Treatment

There is no doubt that available neuroleptics in oral or depot forms decrease the need for re-admission into hospital. Unfortunately the high hopes that these drugs brought about have been somewhat disappointed. They have not made the management of these patients either easier or simpler (Hamilton, 1972).

These problems of management (as opposed to treatment) are reflected even in patient selection into well designed and conducted studies. Professor Hirsch's own study (Hirsch et al, 1973) is a useful example. The data from the MRC trial were used to estimate the proportion of schizophrenic patients who can be expected to produce management problems on long-acting fluphenazine over 15 months. During the nine months of the trial and six months follow-up, five to six patients (14% to 17%) relapsed. Of the original St. Olave's catchment area based sample, eight patients (10%) had been excluded for reasons reflecting unsuccessful management despite long-acting fluphenazine (e.g. irregular attendance, severe alcohol, or drug abuse). Moreover one of the drug treated group dropped out because of symptomatic relapse (2.5%) thus 20% of patients over nine months and 26% to 29% over 15 months presented problems of management despite long-acting fluphenazine. Even this figure does not take account of the unknown number of patients who may have begun fluphenazine injections but for various reasons did not remain on the drug long enough to be included in the original cohort of patients attending the clinic.

Interestingly, this figure approximates to the 34% defaulting rate found by Johnson and Freeman (1973) in the earliest investigation of the problem. When administrative supervision was restricted to a single master register and all injections were given by fully trained psychiatric nurses able to evaluate mental state and side-effects the defaulting rate fell to 14%. The higher figure was associated with injections given by non-psychiatrically trained nurses (District Nurses) working in a multiplicity of agencies including local authority clinics, GP's surgeries, hospitals and home units.

160

As Johnson points out in his review (1977) the principal reasons for drug defaulting show a close agreement throughout a variety of studies with 3% to 5% of subjects discontinuing because of side-effects, 2% to 7% losing contact with the psychiatric services, and 6% to 10% refusing injections. A further small group withdrew on medical advice. It is important to note that the failure of the regimen due to side-effects and schizophrenic drift is a constant stumbling block and the problem of patient refusal is maximal during the first six months. It would seem that depot injections reduce defaulting from 45% or more to 20% or less. Such a figure cannot be ignored and depot preparations do have the advantage that the defaulters can be identified.

I would suggest, therefore, that whilst acknowledging the potential hazards referred to earlier in this paper the practising clinician might view the apparent equivalent potencies of oral and depot preparations as no more than academic. If the goal of a consultant psychiatrist is to keep his out-patient schizophrenics in the community and in so doing ensure that they are as non-psychotic as possible I suspect the choice between oral and depot drugs on practical grounds is obvious.

Of course, other factors will influence that choice. Often they are unstated. Staff compliance, enthusiasm, persuasive ability, and just plain skill are vital, if non-specific, variables. The organisation of a clinic, its area served, the provision and continuity of care (e.g. a different SHO every six months), division of responsibilities, ideological bias of professionals and para-professionals, and a variety of social factors must all contribute to the ultimate success or failure of long-term management.

I suppose it comes down to what everybody already knows. Chronic schizophrenics outside an institution are much more difficult to treat than acute schizophrenics inside or outside hospital. Unfortunately, it is much more difficult to measure the effects of what we do (or say we do) than what we give. So we inevitably return to anecdotes and myths.

Radical Treatments

Propranolol has offered psychiatry an exciting new drug to try out on schizophrenic patients previously resistant to the usual neuroleptics. I would tentatively raise a number of points on this issue. Note that propranolol is still considered experimental and, in the light of my previous comments, has been tested on acute schizophrenic in-patients. Its applicability to the chronic out-patient population which causes so much of the worry remains a long way off. Furthermore, since propranolol is an oral preparation the problems of compliance will once again lead to difficulties.

As for the d-isomer of propranolol, I am surprised to see it mentioned since those familiar with this area of treatment have already written it off. Even more surprising is the evidence of apparent effectiveness during open uncontrolled trials since Professor Hirsch has already mentioned spontaneous remission rates in hospital. My own particular criticism of the symptom-orientated treatment approach is also relevant to this issue.

No current treatment paper in almost any field of psychiatry would be complete without some mention of the endorphins. I suspect they may become another major industry after the limbic system and the reticular activating system. Let us remind ourselves that their significance is speculative and inconclusive. I await further developments with eagerness.

Non-drug Treatments

Hardly any mention is given to this area of clinical interest and ongoing research. Formal psychotherapy has been abandoned by all but the most zealous though talking treatments have a place perhaps under different names, e.g. counselling, major role therapy (Hoggarty, Goldberg et al, 1974), especially when the recovering patient is struggling with his residual personal and social handicaps and they are more effective when combined with on-going maintenance drug therapy.

Behaviour therapy, or more specifically behaviour modification based on the principles of learning theory, is certainly worthy of mention. Hamilton (1972) devotes some space to it when he advocates that research into rehabilitation is a top priority. We understand neither what factors in the treatment are effective and therefore how to improve them nor what factors in the patients determine their response or lack of it to treatment. Though it seems likely that rehabilitation based on the principles of operant conditioning is likely to prove fruitful, there is some disillusionment because of the failure of newly acquired or shaped behaviours to generalise to different environmental settings.

For the most behaviourally disturbed schizophrenic patients, however, there is every justification to proceed along these lines. Not only can they not function in the world at large but more recently and, indeed alarmingly, some mental hospitals refuse to accommodate them. The more cynical but concerned clinicians are already suggesting that the Prison Service is treating more schizophrenics who need urgent treatment than the mental hospitals!

I wonder if there is not another reason for the apparent and relative lack of interest in behaviour modification? Could it be that, since such procedures on the most behaviourally disturbed have of necessity to be carried out in a hospital or other institutional setting, it is running against the tide of fashion. The first trickle of patients left the asylums in the late 1950s and became a flood in the 1960s and early 1970s. The doctrine of community care became official policy (DHSS, 1975) even though some of the problems of discharged chonic psychiatric patients were revealed by Brown et al over 20 years ago. They stated 'community care will not represent an advance in treatment if it means that a burden has merely been transferred from the hospital to the family'.

162

To advocate a reversal of that policy is in some circles heresy, but for the most behaviourally disordered it is already happening if and when appropriate placement can be found. Is it not time that we reviewed these policies again? Do not the families deserve more from us after all the difficulties they have endured? Is it so heretical to suggest that hospital for a carefully selected few might be beneficial not if used as an alternative to prison or social dereliction but as a proper place to carry out specific treatment regimes that might ultimately enable some of those disabled patients to live, rather than survive, in a non-institutional setting.

Conclusions

I am aware that I have meandered through some philosophical pastures. If it stimulates discussion so much the better. Might I suggest the audience considers at least some of the following points generated by the principal paper.

(1) The question (as yet unresolved) of diagnosis, classification, and possible international agreement applied initially to research and, more ambitiously perhaps, to clinical practice. Drug treatment might then become more meaningful to clinicians and even (who knows) the patients and their families.

(2) The role of drugs has been exaggerated. Where oral, but especially depot neuroleptics are used in long-term management, there is a need to reconsider patient selection, the potential for side-effects, and the proper administration of delivery systems.

(3) The need to incorporate some biological measures into drug trials to enable us to discover more about the role of pharmacokinetics in drug responsiveness.

(4) The role of non-drug aspects of management; in particular the more effective use of available resources in the community to deal with crippling social and personal handicaps and the consideration at least of in-patient resources specifically set up to change the most disabling behavioural handicaps that result from the conditions we crudely lump together as 'schizophrenia'.

(5) Even if the schizophrenic remains asymptomatic, very large numbers are left with a lot of handicaps. Do we ask the patient what he or she feels about life. They often present repeatedly with what we call neurotic symptoms or unacceptable behaviour. Are these manifestations of the putative illness or are the patients really telling us they can't cope or that they don't wish to live in the community?

(6) Do we ever ask the relatives what they think or feel? They sometimes complain using the language they may believe the doctors will understand and even respond to (e.g. they're hearing voices again) even when there is no evidence. What may actually upset the relatives is behaviour that is rarely the subject of enquiry and may appear to the professional as minor or

163

trivial. Refusing to engage in everyday conversation, cadging cigarettes from people who visit the home, and walking around with their flies open can cause severe and ongoing distress (as I have discovered during my own study). Do we ever enquire about such matters and would we be interested anyway?

(7) Is the core of schizophrenia characterised by an inability to live in a normal environment? By insisting that our schizophrenic patients live in the community and remain exposed and often over-aroused by relatively normal social stimuli are we caring or are we being cruel? Are we expecting many to do what they are no longer capable of doing and are we leading others, especially relatives, to expect us to do what we can't.

As a final, and I daresay, provocative comment perhaps we should stop pretending we are really 'treating' schizophrenia at all. We control some of its symptoms some of the time, we manage crises sometimes better than others and if we know about them, and we pay lip service to community care when clearly it (the community) doesn't care. The provision of services can never be sufficient to cope with a disorder of such varying complexity and with such catastrophic social consequences for the sufferer. It is interesting indeed that in one of the more recent reports from the International Pilot Study on Schizophrenia (Sartorius et al, 1977) better prognosis was associated with the least developed countries. Either we need to look again at the elaborate and expensive services we provide or consider re-defining 'developed' as it presently applies.

RESPONSE TO COMMENTARIES BY DR. BENNETT AND DR. CURSON

Stephen Hirsch

I am sorry that my paper has caused such unrest to Dr. Bennett in particular, as I can only guess that this is the problem of generations. I was a disciple at his feet and nurtured in the same stable of social psychiatry which he has occupied. I did not come to this meeting as an antagonist to the social issues that were raised, but I saw my purpose as bringing you up-to-date with recent trends in the more medical aspects of treatment, and I do not think that most of the criticisms of my paper made by Dr. Bennett or Dr. Curson fall into that category.

I was asked to review the treatment of schizophrenics and by coincidence, at the same time, I was asked to write a chapter for a text book that is coming out shortly. In so doing I became aware that perhaps the most recent trend in psychiatry in the last five years, has been the tremendous advance in our knowledge, appreciation and understanding of the mechanisms of the anti-psychotic effects of drugs. I had to think about this in a number of contexts. For example, over the past year I have had to defend the running of Double Blind Placebo Trials to Ethical Committees. In doing so, I had to elaborate principles many of which I tried to put down in my paper, which I think explained many of the paradoxical issues which you are faced with, such as the fact that if drugs have an effect, it is only limited.

I have also had to face up to the arguments like those faced by Dr. Bennett eleven years ago that drugs do not differ in their anti-psychotic effects. Yet you as psychiatrists know that drugs do differ in their general effects, for example the fact that if you give very large doses of drugs you do not get more side effects than if you give moderate doses; and so I tried to put this in the form of a simple pharmacological model and I have been able to simplify it even more so since writing this paper because I think that, despite all the queries, several simple paradoxes can be explained. In fact, there seems to be more agreement between Dr. Bennett and myself than he wants to admit. I agree that our potency in treatment, i.e. our ability to cure schizophrenics, is limited, and indeed I may be more concerned about this than Dr. Bennett. That is perhaps where the difference between us lies, for if you look at the actual cure rate of schizophrenic patients who have been treated, the evidence suggests that it has not improved. Dr. Bennett does not want to talk about the cure rate, he wants to talk about the social functioning of patients. My question is: is the social functioning of patients and the improvements and gains that we measure in the social functioning of patients a gain in treatment, or is it simply the fact that we have begun to overcome the untoward effects of the social attitudes that society applies to our patients and the treatments that psychiatrists have been applying to patients over the last seventy five years?

So much of our so-called rehabilitation has to do with getting patients out of hospital, yet we as doctors are the ones that put them in hospital. For example, look at India. If we look at the current number of psychiatric beds in England compared with the days of Kreplin and Mayer Gross and extrapolate (per head of population) to the number of beds they would have to have in India today, then we arrive at a figure of 1,200,000 psychiatric beds. In fact, they have about 20,000 beds in psychiatric hospitals and fewer in district general hospitals. So it seems to me we are just trying to get back to the position that many countries in the world have had the good fortune perhaps never to have reached. If we look at the developing countries the morbidity of schizophrenia is actually less than in the developed countries, so I think that, when considering Dr. Bennett's comments, we could simply be talking about his own problems and that of his generation which is over-coming the ill effects of the treatments that psychiatrists have been giving.

The next point that I wanted to make is that we should understand what we are doing pharmacologically with our drugs because I think we probably know more about putting patients back into the community and putting them into hostels than we do about the rational bases for the use of our drugs. Secondly, we should appreciate the limitations of our drug treatment, a point which I hope I managed to get across in my paper for I have tried to document what drugs do and do not do. Thirdly, I took a point of view which does depart very radically from that of Dr. Bennett, that because our treatments are so impotent, we have to concentrate — at least in the research field — on developing new treatments. In the introductory talk to the C.I.M.P. in Vienna two years ago Roy Hollister gave a talk about treatment today, and made the point that the development of new treatments by the drug industry is based on finding a compound which does the same thing as the drugs we already have. By and large, the drug industry is only multiplying the number of neuroleptic drugs which have the properties described in my paper. In this I disagree with Dr. Bennett, perhaps because I come from a different perspective and also a generation younger, and I have not seen the disasters of psychosurgery and insulin coma treatment. Nevertheless, if we look at general medicine and some of its advances we find that some of the early and important developments were undertaken with a degree of recklessness — even perhaps of fame-seeking, or what have you, that have paid long term dividends. If we consider heart surgery for example, when they started putting in aortic valves there was about an 85% mortality rate. When they started doing mitral valve surgery it was less dangerous perhaps a 25% or 30% mortality rate, but now in both cases the mortality rate is down below 5%, which means a lot of lives have been saved. If I had somebody with chronic schizophrenia staying in a hostel in the community and attending a day centre, I would prefer to see his life possibly risked with the hope that he could have a possible cure than condemn him to that type of existence for the rest of his life, but that is a moral question that you have to answer yourself. At least I do not hold with the ideas that have been expressed that it is a dangerous thing to be looking for radical new treatments. I think our sophistication in terms of treatment is much greater than it used to be. Hopefully, when we do come out with a statement that endorphines work or dialysis works or anything else works, people will much more rapidly insist on putting such statements to the test. Unfortunately there is resistance by people who sit on certain committees who do not allow Double Blind Placebo Controlled Trials for treatments like Propranolol, Dialysis and so forth, because they want to dismiss them. You must judge for yourselves where the ultra-conservatism lies.

Now I will take up some specific points if I may in the two commentaries. We talk of Social Recovery — Social Recovery has improved considerably, but recovery from what and to what? I leave you to consider this. What about the role of the sheltered workshop? Dr. Bennett extols the role of the sheltered workshop in the after-care of the patient who has to return to live with a relative who shows high expressed emotion. Well, I suppose I might regard this as sensible, but I would also have to say that it has never been submitted to a controlled trial. It has not even been subjected to the systematic open study which Dr. Bennett criticises. Yet if you are going to throw out open studies in new treatments then Dr. Bennett will have to desist from sending such people to such establishments as Day Centres. I think I make the point in my paper that social factors are as important in outcome as neuro-pharmacological treatments, and that the differences between relatives showing high or low expressed emotion, or that having more or less than 35 hours a week contact with the noxious relatives, is as powerful a determinant in outcome as whether you put them on drugs or not. When you look at the interaction between drugs and social treatments, the drugs do have a significant effect in altering the response of patients to social environments; whether the social environment be defined as the amount of contact the patient has with the relative with high expressed emotion or the frequency of traumatic life events. I suppose it is only fair that I should mention one controlled trial that Douglas Bennett did not mention, even if this is hitting a little bit below the belt; this is a study of rehabilitation in a Day Hospital. In his study patients were randomly allocated to have two years rehabilitation in a Day Hospital or not. The study was carried out by Professor

Wing, the Day Hospital was Dr. Bennett's. The study suggested that Day Hospital treatment had no effect whatsoever, so I have to ask Dr. Bennett, in the face of lack of open studies on the one hand and controlled studies on the other, why he continues to advocate social treatment? Why does he have such confidence in social treatment as to exclude and inhibit others from pushing forward the frontiers of science, or whatever you want to call it. It might be retrogressive at times but at least we are making an attempt to develop a successful treatment of schizophrenia.

Let us now consider Dr. Curson's paper. He has made a number of points about the importance of diagnosis and the lack of consistency between psychiatrists, and I must say that it is a great credit to our original study that he was only able to find three patients out of 81 whom he could diagnose differently after nearly seven years! Most studies show that psychiatrists have 25% of their diagnoses changed after that time, so I think that we did fairly well, but we both used the same criteria, which might account for it. What about the importance of diagnostic criteria? Well, I agree with Dr. Curson. I have made all these kinds of points myself in the past and I do not in any way wish to suggest that I would not make them now, but there are vast differences between the diagnostic criteria for diagnoses in different places at different times. Nevertheless, in reviewing the literature on the treatment of schizophrenia, it was absolutely remarkable to me, and in many ways an eye opener, that one found that the effectiveness of drug treatment, in those groups where it occurred, came through and averaged out in a consistent way over a large number of studies. In the paper before you I mention the review by Davis of maintenance treatment. In I think about sixteen of the 22 studies involving about 3,000 patients they found a consistent positive effect of medication whether they were looking at in-patients or out-patients. In nearly all they found evidence of an important therapeutic and antipsychotic effect in preventing a relapse and the re-emergence of symptoms in schizophrenia treated with some type of maintenance therapy, and that is in a wide number of environments covering at least two countries and with wide differences in diagnostic practice. Summing up 22 studies, 65% of the patients on placebo relapsed as compared with 35% on active medication, which is of the same order as Leff and Wing recorded in their study, and not so very different, considering the different periods of time looked at, as we found in my own study on long acting medication. Looking at it slightly differently, let us consider some 44 studies involving the use of chlorpromazine as compared with a placebo carried out over a number of years in the United States. Although they may have been using different criteria for diagnosis of schizophrenia most, but not all, used the B.P.R.S. as their rating scale. What we find is that in all the studies where the dose of chlorpromazine has been over 500 mg per day, there is an advantage of active drug over placebo. Once you get down to below 300 mg per day (CPZ equivalent) you still have some studies in which chlorpromazine is better than placebo but there are also quite a few in which there seems to be a minimal effect or no difference. It is just this variance in drug dose related effect that indicates the robustness of the treatment compared with the amount of variance that arises from diagnosis. So I do feel confident in making most of the statements that are made in my paper about the efficacy of drug treatment despite the logical and reasonable criticisms that have been made.

References

Atsom, A and Blum, I (1970) Treatment of acute porphyria variegata with propranolol. *Lancet, i*, 196–7

Bateson, G, Jackson, D, Haley, J and Weakland, J (1956) Towards a theory of schizophrenia. *Behavioural Science, 1*, 251–264

Bennett, DH (1967a) Social Therapy and Drug Treatment in Schizophrenia Chap 4. In: *New Aspects of the Mental Health Services.* (Ed H Freeman and J Farndale). London: Pergamon

Bennett, DH (1967b) The Management of Schizophrenia. *Bri. J. Hosp. Med., 1*, 589–593

Bennett, DH (1978) Social Forms of psychiatric treatment Chap 9. In: *Schizophrenia: Towards a new synthesis.* 211–231 (Ed JK Wing). London: Academic Press

Bleuler, E (1911) Dementia praecox oder die Gruppe der Schizophrenien. In: *Handbuck der Psychiatrie.* (Ed D Aschaffenburg). Leipzig and Vienna Deuticke

Bleuler, M (1974) The Long Term course of the schizophrenic psychoses. *Psychol. Medicine, 4*, 244–254

Brown, GW, Carstairs, GM and Topping, G (1958) Post-hospital adjustment of chronic mental patients. *Lancet, ii*, 685

Brown, GW, Bone, M, Dalison, D and Wing, JK (1966) *Schizophrenia and social care.* Oxford Uni. Press London

Caffey, E, Diamond, LS, Frank TV, Grasberger, J, Herman, L, Klett, J and Rothstein, C (1964) Discontinuation of reduction of chemotherapy in chronic schizophrenics. *J. Chronic Diseases, 17*, 347–358

Carpenter, WT, Bartko, JJ, Carpenter CL and Strauss, JS (1976) Another view of schizophrenic subtypes. *Arch. Gen. Psychiat., 33*, 508–516

Claridge, G (1972) The Schizophrenias as nervous subtypes. *Brit. J. Psychiat., 121*, 1–17

Cooper, JE, Kendall, RE, Gurland, BJ, Sharpe, L, Copeland, JRM and Simon, R (1972) Psychiatric diagnosis in New York and London. *Maudsley Monograph No 20.* London: Oxford Univ. Press

Creese, I. Burt, D, Snyder, S (1976) Dopamine receptors and average clinical dose. *Science 194*, 546

Creese, I. Burt, D and Snyder, S (1978) Biochemical action of neuroleptic drugs: Focus on the dopamine receptor. Chapter 2 in Iverson et al 1978 op. cit

D.H.S.S. (1975) *Better Services for the Mentally Ill.* H.M.S.O.

Davis, J (1975) Overview: Maintenance therapy in psychiatry: 1 Schizophrenia. *American Journal of Psychiatry, 132*, 1237–45

Davis, J (1976) Recent developments in the drug treatment of schizophrenia. *American Journal of Psychiatry, 133*, 208–14

Denham, J and Adamson, L (1971) The contribution of fluphenazine enanthate and decanoate in the prevention of readmission of schizophrenic patients. *Acta Psychiatrica Scanda., 47*, 420–30

Dohrenwend, BP (1975) Socio-cultural and Social Psychological factors in the genesis of mental disorders. *J. Health Soc. Behav., 16*, 365–392

Dohrenwend, BP (1976) Clues to the role of socio environmental factors. *Schizophrenia Bulletin, 2*, 440–444

Dunham, HW (1976) Society, culture and mental disorder. *Arch. Gen. Psychiat., 33*, 147–156

Eisenberg, L (1977) Psychiatry in society – a socio-biological synthesis. *N. Eng. J. Med., 296*, 903–910

Emrich, HM, Moller, H, Lapse, H, Meisel-Kosik, I, Dwinger, H, Oechsner, R, Kissling, W and von Serssen, D. A possible role of endorphins in psychiatric disorders — actions of naloxona in psychiatric patients. Paper presented at the 2nd World Congress of Biological Psychiatry, Bardelona. 31.8.78–6.9.78

Falloon, I, Watt, DC and Shepherd, M (1978) A comparative controlled trial of pimozide and fluphenazine decanoate in continuation therapy of schizophrenia. *Psychological Medicine, 8*, 59–70

Feighner, JP, Robins, E, Guze, SD, Woodruff, RA, Winokur, G and Munoz, R (1972) Diagnostic criteria for use in psychiatric research. *Arch. Gen. Psychiat., 26*, 57–63

Folkard, MS (1959) A sociological contribution to the understanding of aggression and its treatment. *Netherne Monograph (1)*

Forrest, AD and Hay, AJ (1973) The Schizophrenias: Operational definitions. *Brit. J. Med. Psychol., 46*, 337–346

Fromm-Reichmann, F (1948) Notes on the development of treatment of Schizophrenia by Psychoanalytic psychotherapy. *Psychiatry 11*, 263–273

Greenblatt, M, Solomon, M, Evans, AS and Brooks, GW (1965) *Drugs and social therapy in chronic schizophrenia.* Charles C Thomas, Springfield, Illinois

Gross, M, Hitchman, IL, Reeves, WP, Lawrence, J, Newell, PC and Clyde, DJ (1961) Objective evaluation of psychiatric patients under drug therapy: a symptom and adjustment index. *J. Nerv. Ment. Dis., 133*, 399–409

Groves, JE and Mendel, MR (1975) The long-acting Phenothiazines. *Arch. Gen. Psychiat., 32*, 893

Gruzelier, JH (1978) Propranolol acts to modulate autonomic orienting and habituation processes in schizophrenia. In: *Propranolol and Schizophrenia.* (Eds E Roberts and P Amacher) 99–118. New York: Alan R Liss Inc

Gruzelier, JH, Hirsch, SR, Weller, M and Murphy, C (1979) Influence of d or dl-propranolol and chlorpromazine on habituation of phasis electrodermal responses in schizophrenia. Accepted for publication, *Acta Psychiat.* Scand

Hamilton, M (1972) Treatment of Schizophrenia: some critical considerations. *Brit. J. Psychiat. Special Publication No 10*, 59–63 London

Harris, A, Linker, I, Norris, V and Shepherd, M (1956) Schizophrenia: a prognostic and social study. *Br. J. Prev. Soc. Med., 10*, 107–114

Hawk, AB, Carpenter, WT and Strauss, JS (1975) Diagnostic criteria and five year outcome in schizophrenia. *Arch. Gen. Psychiat, 32*, 343–347

Hay, AJ and Forrest, AD (1972) The diagnosis of schizophrenia and paranoid psychosis: an attempt at clarification. *Brit. J. Med. Psychol., 45*, 233–241

Hirsch, SR, Gaind, R, Rohde, PD, Stevens, S and Wing, JK (1973) Outpatient maintenance of chronic schizophrenic patients with long-acting fluphenazine; double-blind placebo trial. *British Medical Journal, i*, 633–37

Hirsch, SR (1976) Interacting social and bilogical factors determining prognosis in the rehabilitation and management of persons with schizophrenia. In: *Annual Review of the Schizophrenic Syndrome 1974–5.* (Ed R Cancro)

Hogarty, G, Goldberg, S, Schoder, N and Ulrich, R (1974) Drug and sociotherapy in the aftercare of schizophrenic patients. II. Two year relapse rates. *Archives Gen. Psychiat., 31*, 603–609

Hogarty, G, Ulrich, R, Mussare, F and Aristigueta, N (1976) Drug discontinuation among long-term successfully maintained schizophrenic outpatients. *Dis. Nervous Syst., 37*, 494–500

Hogarty, G and Ulrich, R (1977) Temporal effect of drug and placebo in delaying relapse in schizophrenic outpatients. *Archives Gen. Psychiat., 34*, 297–301

Hollister, L (1974) Clinical differences among phenothiazines in schizophrenics. In: *Advances in Biochemical Psychopharmacology, 9*, 667–73. World Health Organisation

Hollister, L (1978) 'Psychopharmacology'. Chapter 5 in *Schizophrenia, Science and Practice.* (Ed John Shershaw). Harvard University Press

Iversen, LL, Iversen, SD, Snyder, SH (1978) *Handbook of Psychopharmacology Vol 10. Neuroleptics and Schizophrenia.* New York and London: Plenum Press

Janssen, PAJ and Van Bever, WFM (1978) Structure-activity relationships of the butyrophenones and diphenylbutylpiperidines. Chapter 1 In: Inversen, Iversen and Snyder. Op. cit

Johnson, D and Freeman, H (1972) Long acting tranquillisers. *The Practitioner, 208*, 385–400

Johnson, D (1976) The duration of maintenance therapy in chronic schizophrenia. *Acta Scand., 33*, 298–301

Johnson, D (1978) The prevalence and treatment of drug induced extra-pyramidal symptoms. *Brit. J. Psychiat., 132*, 27–30

Johnson, DAW (1977) Practical considerations in the use of depot neuroleptics for the treatment of schizophrenia. *Brit. J. Hosp. Med.,* 546

Johnson, DAW and Freeman, H (1973) Drug defaulting by patients on long-acting Phenothiazines. *Psychol. Med., 3,* 115–119

Johnstone, EC, Crow, TJ, Frith, CD, Carney, MWP and Price, JS (1978) Mechanism of the antipsychotic effect in the treatment of acute schizophrenia. *Lancet, i,* 848–851

Jones, HG (1978) Psychological Aspects of Treatment of Inpatients. Chap 8 In: *Schizophrenia: towards a new synthesis.* (Ed JL Wing). London: Academic Press

Jorgensen, A, Fog, R, Veilis, B (1979) Synthetic enkephalin analogue in treatment of schizophrenia. *Lancet, i,* 935

Kendall, RE (1975) What are our criteria for a diagnosis of Schizophrenia? In: *On the origin of schizophrenic psychoses.* (Ed HM Van Praag). Amsterdam, De Erven Bohn, B.V.

Klein, DF and Davis, JM (1969) *Diagnosis and drug treatment of psychiatric disorders.* Williams and Wilkins, Baltimore

Kline, NS, Li, CH, Lehmann, HE, Lajtha, A, Laski, E and Cooper, T (1977) ρ-endorphin-induced Changes in Schizophrenia and Depressed Patients. *Arch. Gen. Psych., 34,* 1111–1113

Knights, A, Okasha, M, Salih, M and Hirsch, S (1979) Maintenance therapy in outpatient schizophrenics: a double-blind comparison of fluphenazine and flupenthixol decanoate. *Brit. J. Psychiat.* In Press

Kraepelin, E (1899) Zur Diagnose und Prognose der Dementia Praecox. *Allgemeine Zeitschrift fur Psychiatrie und psychisch-gerichtliche Medizin, 56,* 254

Kraepelin, E (1919) 'Dementia Praecox and Paraphrenia' (Trans RM Barclay from 8th edition of *'Psychiatrie'*. Barth, Leipzig). Edinburgh: Livingstone

Leff, J and Wing, JK (1971) Trial of maintenance therapy in schizophrenia. *Brit. Med. Journal, 3,* 599–604

Leff, J, Hirsch, SR, Rohde, P, Gaind, R and Stevens, B (1973) Life events and maintenance therapy in schizophrenic relapse. *Brit. J. Psychiat., 123,* 659–660

Lidz, T (1973) *Origin and treatment of schizophrenic disorders.* New York: Basic Book Inc

May, PRA (1968) *Treatment of Schizophrenia.* Science House, New York

May, PRA, Tumah, H, Yale, C, Potepan, P and Dixon, W (1976) Schizophrenia – a follow-up study of results of treatment. II. Hospital stay over two to five years. *Arch. of Gen. Psychiat., 33,* 481–486

McClelland, HA (1976) Discussion on assessment of drug induced extra-pyramidal reactions. *Brit. J. of Clin. Pharm., 2,* 401–403

McClelland, H, Farquharson, RG, Leybury, P, Furness, TA and Schuff, A (1976) Very high dose Fluphenazine Decanoate. *Arch. Gen. Psychiat., 33,* 1435–1442

Mellor, CS (1970) First rank symptoms of schizophrenia. 1. The frequency in schizophrenics on admission to hspital. 2. Differences between individual first rank symptoms. *Brit. J. Psychiat., 117,* 15–23

Meyer-Gross, W (1932) In: *Handbuch des Geisteskrankheiten* Band IX. (Ed O Bumke). Berlin: Springer

Mindham, RHS (1976) Assessment of drug induced extrapyramidal reactions and the drugs used for their control. *Brit. J. of Clin. Pharm., Suppl 2,* 395–400

Ødegaard, O (1964) Pattern of discharge from Norwegian psychiatric hospitals before and after the introduction of the psychotropic drug. *Amer. J. Psychiat., 120,* 772–778

Overall, JE, Hollister, LE and Dalal, SN (1967) Psychiatric drug research. *Arch. Gen. Psychiat., 16,* 152–161

171

Palmour, RM (1978) *Endorphins in mental illness.* (Eds E Usdin and WE Bunney Jr). London: Macmillan

Pasamanick, B, Scarpitti, FR, Lefton, M. Dinitz, S, Wernert, JJ and McPheeters, H (1964) Home versus hospital care for schizophrenics. *J. Am. Med. Ass., 187,* 177

Port, FK, Kroll, PD, Swartz, RD (1978) The effects of haemodialysis on schizophrenia: A survey of patients with renal failure. *Am. J. of Psychiat., 135,* 6, 743–44

Prien, RF and Klett, J (1972) An appraisal of the long term use of tranquillising medication with hospitalised chronic schizophrenics. *Schiz. bull, 5,* 64–73

Prien, RF, Gibbs, RD and Caffey, EM (1973) Intermittent pharmacotherapy in chronic schizophrenia. *Hosp. Comm. Psychiat., 24,* 317–322

Quitkin, F, Rifkin, A and Klein, DF (1975) Very high dosage vs standard dosage fluphenazine in schizophrenia. *Arch. Gen. Psychiat., 32,* 1276–81

Quitkin, F, Rifkin, A, Kane, J et al (1978) Long acting vs oral injectable antipsychotic drugs in schizophrenia. *Arch. Gen. Psychiat., 35,* 889–892

Rathod, NH (1958) Tranquillisers and the patients' environment. *Lancet, i,* 611

Rifkin, A, Quitkin, F, Rabiner, C and Klein, D (1972) Fluphenazine decanoate, fluphenazine hydrochloride given orally and placebo in remitted schizophrenics. *Arch. Gen. Psychiat., 34,* 43–7

Rifkin, A, Quitkin, F and Klein, DF (1975) Akinesia: A poorly recognised drug induced extrapyramidal disorder. *Arch. Gen. Psychiat., 32,* 672–674

Sartorius, N, Jablensky and Shapiro, R (1977) Two year follow-up of the patients included in the WHO International Pilot Study of Schizophrenia. *Psychol. Med., 7,* 529–541

Schneider, K (1959) *Clinical psychopathology.* (Trans MW Hamilton). New York: Grune and Stratton

Sheppard, GP (1979) High dose propranolol in schizophrenia. *Brit. J. Psychiat., 134,* 470–76

Strauss, JS and Carpenter, WT (1972) The prediction of outcome in Schizophrenia. 1. Characteristics of outcome. *Arch. Gen. Psychiat., 27,* 739–746

Strauss, JS and Carpenter, WT (1973) Are there pathognomic symptoms in Schizophrenia? *Arch. Gen. Psychiat., 28,* 847–852

Strauss, JS and Carpenter, WT (1974) Characteristic symptoms and outcome in Schizophrenia. *Arch. Gen. Psychiat., 30,* 429–434

Strauss, JS and Carpenter, WT (1977) Prediction of outcome in Schizophrenia. *Arch. Gen. Psychiat., 34,* 159

Terenius, L, Wahlstrom, A, Lindstrom, L and Widerlov, E (1976) Neurosciences, Letter 3, 157–162

Van Praag, HM (1975) Controversial questions concerning Shizophrenia. In: *On the origins of schizophrenic psychoses.* (Ed HM Van Praag). Amsterdam: De Erven Bohn, BV

Vaughn, C and Leff, J (1976) The influence of family and social factors on the course of psychiatric illness. *British J. Psychiat., 129,* 125–137

Verhoeven, WMA, van Praag, HM, van Ree, JM and de Wied, D (1979) Improvement of schizophrenic patients treated with Des-tyr-gamma-endorphin. *Arch. Gen. Psychiat., 36,* 294–302

WHO (1973) *Report of the International Pilot Study of Schizophrenia. Vol 1,* Geneva

Wagemaker, H and Cade, R (1977) The use of haemodialysis in chronic schizophrenia. *Amer. J. Psychiat., 134,* 6, 684–685

Wing, JK and Brown, GW (1961) Social treatment of chronic schizophrenia: a comparative survey of three mental hospitals. *J. Ment. Sci., 107,* 847–861

Wing, JK (1961) Simple and reliable sub-classification of Chronic Schizophrenia. *J. Ment. Psych., 107,* 862–875

Wing JK (1978) Clinical concepts of schizophrenia. Chap 1 In: *Schizophrenia: towards a new synthesis.* (Ed JK Wing). London: Academic Press

Wing, L (1956) The use of reserpine in chronic psychiatric patients: a controlled trial. *J. Ment. Sci, 102,* 530

Wynne, L and Singer, M (1963) Thought disorder and family relations of schizophrenics I and II. *Arch. Gen. Psychiat, 9,* 191–206

Wynne, L and Singer, M (1965) Thought disorder and family relations of schizophrenics III. *Arch. Gen. Psychiat., 12,* 187–212

Yorkston, NJ, Zaki, SA, Malik, MKU, Morrison, RC and Havard, CWH (1974) Propranolol in the control of schizophrenic symptoms. *Brit. Med. Journal, 4,* 633–35

Yorkston, NJ, Zaki, SA, Themen, JFA and Havard, CWH (1976) Safeguards in the treatment of schizophrenia with propranolol. *Postgrad. Med. Journal, 52,* Suppl 4, 175–80

CURRENT TRENDS IN THE TREATMENT OF DEPRESSION

Anthony Clare

Introduction

It is difficult to attempt a review of the current state of the treatment of depression without some reference, albeit a passing one, to the problems which surround the epidemiology of depression and the issue of its precise classification. It is now well recognised and, indeed, has been since the classic study by Shepherd and his colleagues (Shepherd et al, 1966), that the great majority of individuals who suffer from affective disturbances do not encounter psychiatrists and do not receive specialised psychiatric treatment. In Britain, between 90 and 95% of people who suffer from psychiatric ill-health are treated by their family doctors. The bulk of these suffer from conditions which are difficult to classify according to the International Classification of Diseases. Most cases in the community are characterised by 'such features as depression, anxiety, pre-occupation with health, irritability and insomnia' (Williams, 1978). As a consequence, various categories have been suggested to describe the conditions such as 'sub-clinical neurosis' (Taylor, Lord and Chave, 1964), 'dysthymia' (Foulds and Bedford, 1975) and 'nervous tension' (Wing 1976). Most of the work, however, relating to the classification and the treatment of depressive disorders is based on samples of patients drawn entirely or for the most part from hospital populations. For example, the Collaborative Program of Research into what is termed 'The Psychobiology of Depression' undertaken by the US National Institute of Mental Health is based entirely on out-patient and in-patient samples, though nowhere in the published papers on diagnostic criteria, personality attributes, familial perspectives and clinical presentation is there a reference to this serious limitation (NIMH).

Nor can these epidemiological findings be ignored when the natural history of depressive disorders comes to be considered. The findings from a number of general practice studies suggest that affective disorders presenting to the GP can

174

be split into two sub-groups: short-term disorders enjoying a good prognosis, and chronic disorders with a refractory course of at least three years (Kedward, 1967). Taken together, these findings strongly suggest the existence of a 'pool' of psychiatric morbidity in the community comprising a hard-core population of patients with chronic illness and a variable population of vulnerable individuals presenting relatively short-lived reactions (Cooper et al, 1969, and Harvey-Smith and Cooper, 1970). It has also been shown that the social component of these disorders is often at least as important as their clinical features so that it is necessary to employ a socio-medical framework to do them descriptive and aetiological justice and to undertake adequate evaluations of treatment (Sylph et al 1969, and Clare and Cairns, 1978).

Thus, it becomes clear that a paper which sets out to consider the efficacy of current treatments must take account of the fact that much of the published evidence on the subject relates to a small and highly atypical sub-sample of the overall population of patients concerned. The proportion of clinically treated depressive patients has been estimated between 11% (Nielsen et al, 1965) and 92% (Odegard, 1972), the first figure being based on the sum of all depressive illnesses and the latter figure only on so-called 'psychotic' depressions. Patient samples derived from hospital statistics are most certainly biased in the direction of serious, psychotic, suicidal, chronic and therapeutically — resistant illnesses and such a skewed distribution has very probably increased over the past decade given the fact that out-patient and general practice treatment of serious and psychotic depression with anti-depressant pharmacotherapy has become more popular (Helmchen, 1979). It thus becomes necessary in any discussion of treatment to distinguish between the various categories of patients involved, not merely in terms of their symptom profiles and clinical diagnoses but also with regard to whether they are treated within the primary care system or are referred onwards to specialised psychiatric facilities.

General Practice Treatment of Depression

At the present time, the general practitioner who decides to treat a depressed patient himself without recourse to a psychiatric opinion can offer the patient support, reassurance and advice with or without the concomitant prescription of a drug or he can call on the assistance of another member of the primary health team such as a social worker, health visitor, nurse or psychologist, always assuming that such personnel are available. Or he can do both.

Current trends in the use of psychotropic drugs in general practice reflect the growing awareness in the rate of such prescribing (Parish, 1971). In England during 1975, over 43 million prescriptions were written for such drugs (15.3% of all prescriptions), costing over £25 million (DHSS 1977). Not all these drugs are prescribed for psychiatric reasons (Williams, 1978) but it seems reasonable to assume that the great majority of them are. Yet there is surprisingly little in the

175

way of unequivocal research results to indicate the usefulness of such drugs in the treatment of depression in this setting. In this country, the General Practice Research Group has carried out some useful attempts to evaluate scientifically such drugs (Wheatley, 1972). As well as demonstrating the feasibility of scientifically valid clinical trials in the primary care setting, the main aim of the GPRG was 'to try and determine the most suitable drugs for the treatment of the type of case seen by the general practitioner' (Wheatley, 1972). The main therapeutic conclusion arising out of several years of work make sobering reading. The first emphasises the importance of therapeutic faith in the role of drugs on the part of the general practitioner, a conclusion which may well be of importance to the psychiatrist anxious to evaluate his own role in the treatment of depression. The second emphasises the fact that 'none of the new drugs that we have investigated has proved to be significantly better than the two standard drugs, namely chlordiazepoxide in anxiety and amitryptiline in depression'.

There is a tendency on the part of psychiatrists to criticise general practitioners on the grounds that the latter do not prescribe psychotropics appropriately. By this is usually meant the fact G.Ps. often use drugs in doses which appear to be therapeutically useless, and employ them in a somewhat incongruous fashion, that is to say, they use a tranquilliser, such as diazepam, for what appears to be a predominantly depressive condition, or an antidepressant, such as imipramime, for what seems to be an anxiety state. The problem with such criticism is that while it seems well-based when viewed against current psychiatric practice, it may well be less surely founded when matched against the realities of everyday primary health care. It is a sad fact that little is actually known about how exactly patients in general practice use drugs that are prescribed for them. Such studies of efficacy as undertaken are for the most part carried out in the form of carefully controlled double-blind scientific evaluations with random allocation of subjects and highly artificial and standardised form of drug taking spread over an equally arbitrary period of time, usually three to four weeks. In actual practice, on the other hand, general practice patients exhibit various degrees of drug compliance, appear to use such drugs in a highly idiosyncratic fashion and are almost invariably subject to simultaneous environmental changes, additional therapy, self-medication and fluctuating social supports. An outcome study looking at the efficacy of psychotropic drugs in the light of such variables has yet to be published although at least one is currently under way.

It is worth noting that minor emotional illnesses are notoriously subject to suggestion or reassurance and responsive to change. They are thus sensitive to placebo and display a high rate of spontaneous remission. Patients in general practice with minor emotional states display a placebo response rate of around 50% in various drug studies compared with active drug response rates of about 75%. Blackwell points out that it is more than likely that the busy general practitioner who makes a habit of ending each interview with a prescription will be gratified and rewarded by the response that many patients report. 'To often neither the patient nor the doctor pauses to examine the role played by inquiry, discussion and reassurance' (Blackwell, 1973).

However, any general practitioner tempted to respond to the current anxieties concerning the possible over-prescribing of psychotropic drugs invariably asks what else can he do, what alternative treatment can he offer. The strong association between the clinical symptoms of depressive disorders in general practice and various problems of social adjustment underlines the need for a greater attention to be directed at the social aspects of these disorders in treatment. There have been a number of studies of collaboration between general practitioners and social workers (Collins, 1965 and Corney and Briscoe, 1977 and Forman and Fairbairn, 1968). Such reports have consistently advocated the need for closer liaison between the general medical, psychiatric and social services. To date, however, there has been little in the way of evaluative studies. One such study (Cooper et al, 1975) did assess the possible therapeutic value of attaching a social worker to a metropolitan group practice in London in the management of chronic neurotic illness. The psychiatric and social status of a group of patients before treatment and after one year was compared with a control group treated more conventionally over the same period. The results indicate that the experimental service conferred significant benefit on the patient population. Fewer of the experimental group were referred to psychiatrists and this group received less psychotropic medication. Whereas the initial clinical and social features of the two groups were closely similar, the experimental group improved to a significantly greater extent during the follow-up year.

There have been very few controlled attempts to evaluate medicosocial intervention in the community and none to have demonstrated benefit, however small, to so notoriously resistant a group of patients as those suffering from chronic neurotic disorders. (Segal, 1972.) For these reasons alone, the results of the investigation by Cooper and his colleagues carry some general implications which extend well beyond the findings themselves, limited as they are by the extent of the follow-up. As the authors themselves point out, the most significant conclusion may well be 'the demonstration that evaluative research in the mental health field can be carried out in an extramural setting'. With the growth of health centres, large group practices and various forms of attachment schemes, a trend can be anticipated towards increasing participation in primary psychiatric care in primary health by social workers, psychiatric nurses and psychiatrists themselves.

Another trend in the management of depressive disorders in general practice concerns the possible utilisation of such personnel as the health visitor and the district nurse (Brook and Cooper, 1975). There appear to be strong arguments in favour of such development in which the primary health care team would come to be regarded more and more as the keystone of community psychiatry. (World

Health Organisation, 1973). However, the discovery of a significant amount of social difficulties among depressed patients in general practice does not inevitably imply that social work intervention should be mobilised in every case. Some social problems appear intractable, and others beyond the resources of society to deal with. At the present time, too little is known about how those problems which could be alleviated might be identified.

Recent research into the possible role of various stresses and so-called 'life events' has important implications for the treatment of depression. In one celebrated study of a random sample of women living in South London, a large class difference in the prevalance of depression was found (Brown and Harris, 1978). This difference was particularly noteworthy among women with young children living at home. Severe life-events and major long-term difficulties occurring in the year prior to onset appear to play an important aetiological role. However, although these aetiological agents were more common among working-class women, they only explained a small part of the social class difference. George Brown and his colleagues have argued that the difference is essentially due not to the greater frequency of events and difficulties but to the much greater likelihood of working-class women breaking down once these have occurred. This greater 'vulnerability' was shown to relate to four specific social factors – the lack of an intimate confiding relationship, the number of children living at home under the age of 14, the loss of a mother before the age of 11 and whether or not the woman was employed before onset.

The notion that stress in the form of life events provokes illness is attractive but it is not without its critics. The association between life events and disorders such as schizophrenia and severe depression is small and accounts for less than 10% of the variance involved. (Tennant and Bebbington, 1978.) It is worth noting in this respect that the association between life events and illness does not appear to be any stronger for psychotic than neurotic depression. (Andrews and Tennant, 1978.)

Doubts have also been expressed concerning the distinction between 'provoking agents' and vulnerability factors. As Tennant and Bebbington point out, an allegedly provoking agent such as 'marital difficulties' and a vulnerability factor such as 'low intimacy' appear to be confounding each other's role in depression although Brown and Harris argue that these factors are distinct and independent. (Tennant and Bebbington, 1978.)

Nevertheless, the concept of vulnerability to illness remains attractive and has given rise to the notion that certain factors, notably social support, may reduce vulnerability to depression and thereby exercise a protective function. Scott Henderson and his colleagues, in a study of psychiatric out-patients (Henderson, 1977), report that depressed patients, compared with controls, have fewer good friends, fewer contacts with people outside their own household, fewer attachment figures and less support from these figures. Such work merits replication all the more so in view of the claims which are made concerning its implications for the treatment and the prophylaxis of depression. For example (Brown and Harris, 1978) argue that in many cases of depression a combination of chemotherapy and psychotherapy 'needs supplementing with social changes, such as work or meaningful activity outside the home' and they press for a new perspective on the role of medical and social agencies in the treatment of the condition. Amongst the 'many reforms in our current social organisation' which are suggested as part of a programme to combat depression in the community are an increase in the number of nursery school places and in the number of part-time employment opportunities for women. At the present time, these views must remain speculative and hypothetical, awaiting as they do further validation by other research workers.

Out-patient Treatment of Depression

Trends in the out-patient treatment of depression include the evaluation of maintenance therapy involving antidepressants, comparisons of the efficacy of drugs and psychotherapy, the prophylactic and therapeutic role of lithium carbonate, the treatment of refractory depressive illnesses with combined antidepressants and the measurement of drug plasma levels as an aid to maximising therapeutic efficacy and minimising unwanted side-effects.

A number of studies (Imlah et al, 1965, Kay et al, 1970 and Seager and Bird, 1962) have been undertaken since the introduction of the tricyclic antidepressants aimed at assessing the possible benefits of continuation therapy after the disappearance of depressive symptoms. However, the earlier studies were either confounded by the fact that the original treatment had included E.C.T., the assessments of drug response were not blind and the number of patients followed up tended to be small. The first large-scale trial by Mindham and his colleagues (Mindham et al, 1973) involved 92 patients who had been successfully treated for a depressive episode with one or two antidepressants, namely, imipramine and amitriptyline. The patients were allocated by an essentially random procedure to one of two regimens of continuation therapy – namely, the same drug in a dosage of 75–150 mg daily or a placebo of identical appearance, for a period of six months. Both patient and psychiatrist were 'blind' to the actual allocation. By the end of the period of continuation therapy 11 (22%) of the patients on active treatment had relapsed compared with 21 (50%) of those receiving the placebo. Continuation therapy was of benefit both to those rated as severely ill and those not severely ill at the start of the period of initial treatment. It was also of benefit both to those treated entirely as out-patients and to those who were admitted as in-patients for part or all of their initial treatment. There was a non-significant trend suggesting that continuation therapy with amitriptyline appeared to be more effective than continuation therapy with imipramine but the numbers involved were small and the initial treatment was not allocated at random. The psychiatrist had a free

179

choice between amitriptyline and imipramine for the initial treatment and, as a consequence, the two series of patients may well have been dissimilar at the start or continuation therapy.

The reduction of relapse rate on continuation therapy reported in this study may well be an under-estimate. Some patients had only 75 mg per day which may be an ineffective dose (Blashki, et al, 1971) and medication-taking amongst out-patients can be unreliable (Willcox et al, 1965). Mindham and his colleagues, however, did raise the possibility that the superiority of amitriptyline over imipramine in preventing relapse might reflect a sedative action on anxiety rather than an antidepressant one. In a study of psychiatric out-patients attending at the Connecticut Mental Health Centre in New Haven and the Boston State Hospital, Paykel and his colleagues (Paykel et al, 1975) suggested that amitriptyline exerted heterogeneous effects. The most consistent effect was on guilt and anxiety and there was a relatively weak effect on depressed mood but other components of the depressive syndrome, such as pessimism, hopelessness, paranoid feelings with a depressive flavour, somatic complaints and insomnia were all improved. The effects on anxiety and insomnia would be consistent with sedation. However, patients on amitriptyline showed less fatigue and less loss of energy rather than the reverse. The authors concluded that the overall effects were too widespread to be readily attributable to any simple effect on a single target symptom and some 'more general antidepressant action' seems likely.

Both these studies demonstrate that patients on active maintenance antidepressant therapy are less likely to relapse than those who receive placebo. The American study had a somewhat unusual design. Patients were treated with amitriptyline for four weeks preliminary treatment, extended in doubtful cases to six weeks. Those showing at least 50% improvement on a depression rating scale were included in the study. At the commencement of maintenance treatment, on a randomised basis, one-half of the patients commenced once or twice weekly individual psychotherapy from social case-workers. Both they and the remaining half also saw a psychiatrist once monthly for assessment and prescribing. All patients continued to receive medication for a transitional phase of two more months. At this point, a further randomisation occurred with respect to drug treatment. Within each group, one-third of the patients continued on amitriptyline, one-third withdrew double-blind on to placebo and one-third withdrew overtly on to no medication. Treatment continued in these six treatment cells for a further six months to a total of eight maintenance months or nine months from the beginning of treatment. Dosage of amitriptyline was flexible in the range of 100 mg to 150 mg daily.

This study suggested that after eight months of maintenance treatment in those patients who have not experienced a major relapse further medication maintenance conveys little advantage. The incidence of major relapse was more than halved on maintenance amitriptyline. The study sample was, however, confined to female patients and limited to drug responders. However, for clinical practice this latter is appropriate since in non-responders the important question is one of the next choice for acute treatment rather than continuation of the same drug.

The patients in the New Haven Boston study were followed up for a further 12 months. This follow-up revealed that a substantial proportion of the original 150 patients continued to receive either antidepressant medication or minor tranquillisers. There was suggestive evidence that the patients who received benzodiazepines rather than tricyclic antidepressants had a higher probability of relapse and a lower probability of recovery (Weissman et al, 1978). Two possible explanations for this finding need to be considered; is the difference between the two medication groups due to patient selection or is it due to one drug being more effective than the other? The data reported in this follow-up report favoured the treatment difference rather than the patient difference hypothesis. It is salutary to note that only 30% of this sample drug responders did not seek any further treatment during this twelve month period of follow-up (Weissman and Kasl, 1976).

The efficacy of *tricyclic antidepressants* and various *psychotherapies,* in comparison with one another and in combination, has not been fully established in randomised clinical trials. However, the New Haven Boston study quoted above showed that while psychotherapy improved overall adjustment, work performance and communication and reduced friction and anxious rumination it did not prevent relapse nor alleviate symptoms (Weissman et al, 1974). It is worth remembering that 'psychotherapy' in the New Haven Boston study meant 'supportive contacts on a weekly basis over eight months' by trained psychiatric social workers 'with sufficient experience and personal qualification to insure the quality of treatment'. Therapy emphasised the 'here and now' rather than reflective discussions or the uncovering of early childhood material.

A similar form of psychotherapy and tricyclic antidepressants were compared with one another or in combination in the treatment of acute depressive episodes (Weissman et al, 1979). Treatment with drugs and psychotherapy alone were equally effective and both were better than non-scheduled treatment, the last being defined as attending a psychiatrist as and when the patient felt like it. The results of this study suggested that most of the acute illnesses did not recover spontaneously in the short run. However, this rather surprising finding may well have been due to the fact that a number of patients whose episodes of illness were more chronic than acute were actually included within the study.

The conclusion drawn by Paykel and his colleagues to the effect that supportive psychotherapy appears to have little to add to pharmacotherapy with regard to producing symptomatic relief seems a reasonable one (Paykel et al, 1975). The conclusion drawn by Weissman and her colleagues to the effect that psychotherapy helps improve social adjustment requires modification however. Social adjustments in the Boston New Haven study was not assessed blind and

181

included some highly subjective items. In addition, there is the possible objection that what the psychiatric social workers were actually providing was not psychotherapy in the strict sense of the word but social support and advice.

A quite different trend in current approaches to depression concerns the use of *lithium*. There is convincing evidence of the prophylactic efficacy of lithium in preventing recurrence of manic-depressive illnesses. One summary of published reports on the subject showed that only 63 relapses occurred in the 271 patients on placebo (Davis and Janowsky, 1974). Factors believed to be associated with a good response to lithium include a history of bipolar affective disorder in first-degree relatives (Mendlewicz et al, 1973), a low frequency of pre-treatment episodes, pyknic build and cyclothymic traits (Taylor and Abrams, 1975). Conversely, a history of schizophrenia, a preceding schizoaffective episode or a lack of recorded history of affective illness all predict a poor response to lithium (Dunner and Fieve, 1974).

A number of studies indicate that lithium is effective in certain unipolar depressions but to date the results appear inconclusive. One recent review concluded that the magnitude of improvement associated with lithium was at least as great in unipolar as in bipolar depression (Davis, 1976). Other workers, however, using different approaches, noted that patients diagnosed as bipolar respond more frequently to lithium than do those diagnosed as unipolar (Mendels, 1976 and Noyes et al, 1974). Bowden, 1978, is only the latest among a number of researchers who have pointed out the difficulties in applying the unipolar and bipolar depressive classification for optimal selection of lithium responsive cases. As a result, many studies have taken lithium responders and compared them with non-responders without primary attention to diagnostic categorisation. The clinical characteristics of responders include anergia, psychomotor retardation, slowed thoughts, fatigue and lack of spontaneity. It still remains to be shown which if any, conditions are best treated by a combination of lithium and antidepressants. However, Garfinkel and his colleagues in Toronto (Garfinkel et al, 1979) have suggested that there is a reduced C.N.S. tryptophan uptake in unipolar depressive patients which may explain the current inconsistencies surrounding the therapeutic efficacy of tryptophan in depression and they speculate that lithium, which increases brain trytophan uptake, if combined with trytophan might improve the antidepressant effects of the latter and bring about a better therapeutic response.

Lipsedge, 1976, has recently and succinctly reviewed the present status of *combined antidepressant therapy* for refractory depressive illnesses. The use of a tricyclic antidepressant, together with a MAOI, remains controversial. In one recent study, however, a retrospective study of phenelzine or tranylcypromine together with amitriptyline or trimipramine in patients of whom over half had also received concomitant E.C.T., showed marked improvement in mood in almost all the cases (Tyrer, 1974). However, it was not possible to distinguish the effect of E.C.T. from that of the combined drug treatment. Sethna, 1974, carried out a trial of combined antidepressants with 12 depressed patients who had failed to respond to tricyclic anti-depressants, MAOIs and E.C.T. The patients were given phenelzine 45 mg/day and amitriptyline 75 mg/nightly and were reassessed at the end of three and six weeks. The combined antidepressant therapy was significantly more effective than the previous therapy. Adverse reactions were reported to be no worse than to antidepressants used singly, although 'toxic psychokinetic reactions' were observed in two cases at 10 and 16 weeks respectively after starting the combined treatment. It has been suggested that such combined treatment is anxiety-reducing rather than antidepressant and support for this view has come from one study in which combined treatment produced a more significant reduction in the Hamilton Rating Scale scores for anxiety than in the score for depression (Tyrer, 1974).

Over the past decade, there has been increasing interest in the possible relevance of *plasma concentration of tricyclic antidepressant drugs* in explaining variations in therapeutic response and the incidence of side-effects. With repeated administration of tricyclic antidepressants, plasma concentrations rise until a plateau or steady-state level is achieved (Alexanderson and Sjoqvist, 1971). Side-effects to nortriptyline, one of the active metabolites of the tricyclic antidepressants, have been reported to occur more frequently at high plasma nortriptyline levels (Asberg, 1974). The correlation between side-effects and plasma levels appears to disappear with time which may be a result of the antidepressant effect of the drug (Asberg et al, 1970). Plasma nortriptyline levels have also been correlated with changes in visual accommodation (Asberg and Germanis, 1972) and with a reduced magnitude of myocardial contractility (Barnes and Braithwaite, 1978).

Findings relating therapeutic response and plasma levels appear paradoxical. Initially, the antidepressant effect of nortriptyline in endogenous depressed patients did appear to be related to the plasma concentration (Asberg et al, 1971). However, maximum antidepressant effects were found to occur within an intermediate plasma level range while concentrations both above and below this range produced a poor response. Kragh-Sorensen and his colleagues (Kragh-Sorensen et al, 1973) have suggested that the upper limit for nortriptyline's therapeutic action is in the region of 175 mg/l with a therapeutic range of 50–150 mg/l recommended in order to maximise the antidepressant effect. In the case of amitriptyline, however, the relationship between plasma concentrations and therapeutic response is more complex mainly because of its partial conversion to nortriptyline during treatment. Since both compounds have different pharmacodynamic actions, the combined antidepressant actions are difficult to separate. In a discussion of these findings, attention has been focused on the fact that amitriptyline as a tertiary amine inhibits the uptake of serotonin whereas nortriptyline as a secondary amine inhibits the re-uptake of noradrenaline (Coppen, 1974). With purely nortriptyline medication, only the noradrenergic system is influenced, whereas in amitriptyline medication both the noradrenergic and serotonergic system are influenced. In addition, the relationship between the tertiary amine and its demethylated metabolites, and thus the speed of metabolism, is of importance to this effect. An example of this is imipramine which is metabolised more quickly than amitriptyline. During imipramine treatment over a long time span, high plasma concentrations of desipramine will be found whereas only relatively low and possible unimportant levels of imipramine will be produced. In contrast, amitriptyline is demethylated more slowly so that approximately equal concentrations of amitriptyline and nortriptyline can be found in the plasma. In the first reported study of plasma concentrations, a strong positive correlation between plasma concentrations of the parent drug plus the metabolite nortriptyline and clinical response was obtained (Braithwaite et al, 1972). In a more recent study of 28 patients treated with a standard dose of 150 mg amitriptyline over six weeks (Montgomery, 1975), patients with combined plasma levels of nortriptyline and amitriptyline within the range 80–200 mg/l exhibited a much better clinical response than those with levels above and below this range. Patients with such a combined plasma level are likely to be within the recommended range for nortriptyline alone (50–150 mg/l). In a review of the subject of plasma concentrations of antidepressants, Barnes and Braithwaite, 1978, conclude tentatively that the most frequent cause of therapeutic failure with nortriptyline medication may well be the attainment of too *high* drug plasma levels whereas for amitriptyline lack of response may be because plasma levels are too *low*. The clinical significance of plasma levels of other tricyclic antidepressants has not yet been thoroughly evaluated but one report concerning plasma protriptyline levels (Whyte et al, 1976) is in line with the above findings, showing as it does that clinical response is positively correlated with an intermediate range of plasma pretriptyline.

In-patient Treatment of Depression

Many of the above trends in the treatment of depression affect in-patients. However, two psychiatric treatments almost variably used on an in-patient basis are E.C.T. and psychosurgery; albeit the out-patient administration of E.C.T. is not common. Over forty years since Cerletti applied the first electrodes there is still disagreement concerning the efficacy of E.C.T. There has been no dearth of studies, just of good ones. Most of the support for the efficacy of E.C.T. in depression is drawn from two main studies, one conducted by the MRC in 1965 (Medical Research Council), the other conducted by the Scandinavian researchers Ottosson and Cronholm in 1960 (Ottosson, 1960). The M.R.C. trial reported that E.C.T. when compared with amipramine, phenelzine and placebo was easily the quickest effective treatment in cases of severe depression. The Scandinavian study strongly supported the view that it is the convulsion and not the amount of electricity passed through the brain which appears to be the therapeutic factor.

Recently, two British trials of E.C.T. versus 'simulated' E.C.T. have been reported. The first found that real E.C.T. was no more effective than the simulated version in relieving depressive symptoms but was more effective in reducing anxiety (Lambourn and Gill, 1977). The second study found E.C.T. to be 'significantly superior' to simulated E.C.T. in the treatment of depressive illness but in this study the simulated treatment was restricted to just two applications followed by real E.C.T. in the control group. The authors felt that it was 'ethically unjustified to withhold for a complete course (usually six to eight applications) a treatment generally regarded to be effective and to submit patients to perhaps unnecessary general anaesthesia' (Freeman et al, 1978).

It is still not clear which kinds of affective illness respond best to E.C.T. The proportion of patients showing a good response to E.C.T. is usually reported as 70 to 80%. However, not all depressed patients are helped by E.C.T. and attempts to predict response have not been wholly successful. For example, of the 44 patients included in one British study who showed a good response to treatment, 9 would have been predicted by the researchers' own guidelines as having a poor response, while of 64 patients showing a poor response 8 would have been predicted to be good responders (Carney et al, 1965). Even among patients with the typical features of so-called 'endogenous' depression, there are still approximately 15–25% that fail to respond to E.C.T. It has been suggested that the response to E.C.T. is worse in patients who have been ill for a lengthy period and, indeed, recently it has been suggested that E.C.T. may only be effective when given within six months of the spontaneous end of the depression, that is, within six months of when the mood disturbance would have normally corrected itself (Kukopulos et al, 1977). It has also been suggested that delusionally depressed patients do not appear to respond well to tricyclic antidepressants, whereas they do respond to E.C.T. (Glassman et al, 1975), a finding that might indicate one clear sub-group for preferential E.C.T. A more recent report, however, questions the differential efficacy of E.C.T. in the deluded group and these investigators found that over 50% of deluded depressed patients did respond to tricyclics (Simpson et al, 1976).

The present view of E.C.T. is summed up by the conclusion of the APA Task Force on the subject (Electroconvulsive Therapy 1978). 'E.C.T. emerges as a very effective antidepressant treatment', the report declares on the basis of an impressive evaluation of the evidence over the past 40 years and it continues: 'It is sometimes difficult to decide whether E.C.T. or antidepressant medication is the best *initial* treatment for severe depressive illness since the antidepressants have also shown clear efficacy for many similar patients. However, there is some evidence that certain depressed patients will respond only to E.C.T. and not to antidepressant drugs.'

The position concerning the role of psychosurgery in the treatment of severe and/or intractable depression is less clear however. The literature does suggest that patients suffering from severe mood disturbances are most likely to benefit

(Bridges and Bartlett, 1977). Indeed, crippling phobias, ritualistic and compulsive behaviours and profound, intractable and suicidal depressions figure most prominently in the mental state reports of patients referred for surgery. Evaluating the effects of surgery, however, is greatly dependent on the reliability, validity and comprehensiveness of the data as they are presented in the literature. One recent review (Valenstein, 1977), covering 153 articles published between 1971 and 1976, offers little room for complacency. The majority of reports lacked any objective assessment and relied totally on clinical acumen and subjective impression. Indeed, only 70 of the 153 mentioned tests at all. Five of the 70 mentioned unspecified 'psychometric evaluation' while a further 16 reported using intelligence tests. Frequently, they were declarations to the effect that after psychosurgery there were no or minimal changes in intellectual ability. 90% of the 153 articles were adjudged by the reviewer to be of low scientific value, a judgement which, if applied to an animal study, would make it unlikely that it would be accepted for publication by any respected experimental journal.

Nevertheless, it is worth noting that a multi-professional group reporting to the U.S. National Commission for the Protection of Human Subjects of Biomedical and Behavioural Research, after a most thorough review of the published work and an evaluation of several studies specially undertaken for it, found in favour of the use of psychosurgical procedures under properly supervised conditions (Report and Recommendations, 1977). Psychosurgical trends in the treatment of depression include the positioning of stereotactic lesions in the anterior part of the cingulum and the medical quadrant of the frontal lobe, and in the subcaudate area, the so-called 'limbic leucotomy'. There is disagreement concerning the precise number of seriously depressed patients for whom such surgery is indicated. One contemporary psychiatric enthusiast admits they may be 'very few' but believes that modern psychosurgery offers a reasonable prognosis to these patients who otherwise continue to suffer severe and even potentially fatal illnesses (Bridges, 1978).

Other trends in the current treatment of depression include attempts to clarify classification on the basis of responses to therapy. Wirz-Justice and his colleagues at the Basel University Psychiatric Hospital have observed that approximately 10% of their depressive patients after a therapeutic sleep deprivation demonstrated a lightening of depression, not, as is usual, on the first day, but on the morning of the second day; that is, after rebound sleep (Wirz-Justice et al, 1976). They assume that this is due to a mainly serotonergic dysfunction in the day-one responders and a mainly noradrenergic dysfunction in the two-day responders. A preliminary testing of this hypothesis suggested that day-one responders did indeed react better to clomipramine, which inhibits serotonin uptake, whereas day-two responders react better to maprotiline, which inhibits noradrenaline uptake. A similar line of reasoning concerns the view of Kupfer and his colleagues that those depressive patients successfully reacted therapeutically to amitriptyline, who after a single dose of amitriptyline medication demonstrated a reduction of the RMM sleep of more than 10% during the following night's sleep.

There is interest, too, in the possibility that a therapeutically ineffective material concentration of antidepressant in the blood, and thus a lack of effectiveness, can develop in the course of treatment. This loss has been attributed to an iron deficiency developing in the course of treatment, to a change in the secretion of stomach fluids, or to the process of enzyme induction (Helmchen, 1979). Helmchen also raises the possibility that this loss of effectiveness of antidepressant medication with a constant effective material concentration in the blood might be 'an expression of the development of tolerance' (Helmchen, 1979).

Still to be clarified is the way in which chronic depressive disorders develop, the relative importance of psychosocial, psychological and biological factors and the optimum treatment. Most of the major trends in contemporary treatment of depression are more in the nature of being steps along the way rather than final stages and the next decade will be a productive one if it should manage to improve our overall understanding of what is involved in psychiatry's most ubiquitous condition.

COMMENTARY ON CURRENT TRENDS IN THE TREATMENT OF DEPRESSION

Roger McAuley

A comprehensive review of the treatment of such a wide and diverse disorder as depression is by any standards an enormous undertaking. This is quite clearly and ably illustrated in Clare's paper. In the main his review demonstrates that in spite of the fact that the aetiology, definition, and classification of depressive disorders is so widely discussed and disputed, it is apparent that physical methods of treatment are so far the only ones clearly to be effective. It is important to note, however, that their role is more likely to be one of shortening the course of, rather than actually curing the depressive disorder. It is interesting to note the paucity of psychotherapeutic studies related to this area. As yet, it is unclear what part psychotherapeutic methods of treatment have to play. Following the publication of the Social Origins of Depression (by Brown and Harris, 1978) it would seem that the time is ripe for further attention to the psychotherapeutic treatment of depression.

This paper sets out to examine three separate areas relating to the psychotherapeutic treatment of depression. Firstly, some general issues which relate to the application of psychotherapeutic treatments in general. Secondly, a review of some major psychotherapeutic studies already published and thirdly an evaluation of the role of behaviour therapy. Overall, the objective is to complement rather than criticise or detract from the review by Clare.

Some Aspects of Psychotherapeutic Research

In the second edition of the Handbook of Psychotherapy and Behaviour Change, Bergin and Lambert (1978) introduce new notes of optimism about the effectiveness of psychotherapeutic treatments. They support the view that our efforts should be directed not towards whether such treatments are effective but rather to when and under what conditions they are effective. The last ten years have seen an improvement in the experimental design of many psychotherapeutic

188

studies — see for example the Temple Study reported by Sloane et al (1975) in which two treatments of neurotic disorders were investigated. The new experience emanating from such research, some of which is discussed below, has not been specifically applied to the treatment of depression. Some of the most important issues which such research has been concerned with include the concept of spontaneous remission and the cost and measurement of treatment effectiveness.

To be of value any psychotherapeutic treatments of depression must demonstrate that more cases improve following therapy than would be expected by spontaneous remission alone. Unfortunately this is not as simple as might initially seem. It is generally recognised that many depressed persons tend to improve over time. However, labelling this process spontaneous remission is unproductive since it tends to detract from the process of improvement itself. The large majority of depressed persons will improve for some reasons, which may include among others, biochemical or social ones. A clear understanding of the qualitative and quantitative processes of improvement may hopefully provide us with some clues as to why persons improve and thus lead to more effective treatment strategies. At a broad level Brown and Harris (1978) suggest that the lack of an intimate and confiding relationship confers some degree of vulnerability to depressive episodes. Attempting to change such relationship problems by therapeutic means may in the long term protect depressed persons from further depressive episodes. Further, the possible utility of work in this area is also reflected in the research into the factors and processes which influence the outcome of bereavement — see (Parkes, 1972).

Even if we do accept the concept of spontaneous remission there are difficulties in deciding its actual rate. It has been suggested that somewhere in the region of two-thirds of neurotic patients improve regardless of psychotherapy. However, any careful analysis of the rates of improvement should reveal that these will depend on the sample of patients studied (in terms of their levels of disturbance) and also on the type of measurements used. Very global measures will often reveal a much higher improvement rate than will very specific measures of, for example, social functioning. Perhaps in treatment research this whole issue of spontaneous remission would be better avoided by ensuring that groups of carefully matched subjects who are exposed to different treatments (and which should include a no-treatment group as well) are studied.

Even when it is demonstrated that some psychotherapeutic treatments are effective in the management of depression we must endeavour to ensure that they are cheaper and at least as effective as other treatments. Marks (1978) draws attention to the fact that in spite of the side effects associated with drug treatments these remain cheaper and relatively more effective than their psychotherapeutic counterparts. However, care must be taken prior to reaching any premature conclusions. The long-term as well as the short-term effects of the relevant treatment techniques must be considered. It is possible that some forms of psychotherapeutic techniques, while they may not help in the short term, may go some way to stimulating an improved long-term prognosis, for example, training in appropriate interpersonal social skills may help to protect a socially inept person from failing and becoming depressed in the future. The work of Weissman et al (1974) suggests that social casework may have effects on social functioning which are not demonstrable until some months after initial therapy. It remains to be demonstrated whether or not the effort and cost of psychotherapeutic treatments is worthwhile.

Increasingly over the past few years discerning behaviour therapists have become increasingly dissatisfied with their own traditional types of measurements of treatment effectiveness (see Ciminero et al, 1977). They have come to recognise that the measurement not only of actual behaviour change but also for example of attitudinal and cognitive changes may be important in understanding the treatment effectiveness. In a positive sense this has resulted in some movement away from the limits which a particular theory tends to place upon measurement. This general problem can be seen repeatedly in much of the treatment research into depression. Very often the major dependant variables are based upon the researcher's theoretical notions about the disorder. For instance, those who view depression as primarily an affective disorder might be most impressed by changes such as an improvement in mood and sleep and reduction in crying. Those who view cognitive changes as of paramount importance (see for example Beck, 1976) will develop measurements that focus on the person's thoughts and self-esteem. Similar criticisms can be made of persons supporting the reinforcement or learned helplessness theories of depression. Generally it would seem that multilevel assessments, looking at the individual over a wide level of functioning (including perhaps measures of affective state, cognitions and social functioning) should be employed as long as the aetiology of depression remains in doubt. To some degree this notion is supported in the work reported by Brown and Harris (1978) that suggested that life events may play just as significant a part in the more severe types of depression, as in those milder ones which are commonly thought of as more reactive in type. It is possible that evaluations which take into account the multiple levels of patient functioning even when used in drug trials, may lead to an understanding of the psychological processes involved in improvement. Perhaps indirectly these may lead to new psychotherapeutic techniques.

Major Psychotherapeutic Studies in Depression

It is amazing just how little research there has been into psychotherapeutic treatments of depression. A brief perusal of the reference list in Clare's paper indicates quite clearly that the majority of research has been orientated towards drug treatments. In fact there are only a few psychotherapeutic studies which have been sufficiently well experimentally controlled to warrant attention.

These studies which are focused on comparisons of psychotherapeutic versus drug treatments have been carefully reviewed and discussed by Hollon and Beck (1978). The most important of these are summarised in their Table 1 and briefly discussed below.

In a study of the treatment of depressed out-patients Daneman (1961) found that imipramine was vastly superior to placebo drug plus psychoanalytically orientated psychotherapy. However, the patients were treated by a single therapist (the author) who was also involved in the symptom ratings of subjects in both groups. A further source of difficulty in this study lies in the fact that it is impossible to tease out the effects of the psychotherapy due to the fact that it was always used in combination either with an antidepressant or with a placebo. Covi et al (1974) in the first of a series of NIMH supported studies used a more sophisticated experimental design. This involved a factorial design with three types of drug treatment (imipramine, diazepam and placebo) and two types of psychotherapy (high amount of contact and low amount of contact). In spite of the findings that imipramine was found to be superior and that psychotherapy was reported as ineffective there are a number of criticisms which can be made of this research. Firstly, 47% of the sample of patients initially screened failed to complete the study. Secondly, while a number of measurements were used these focused almost exclusively on symptoms and mood. No attempt was made to examine other areas of patient functioning. Again in this study the effects of psychotherapy alone were not studied. In the second of the NIMH studies Friedman (1975) reported the effects of four different combinations of therapy in a group of depressed married persons. These included an antidepressant plus conjoint marital therapy, antidepressant plus short contact individual therapy, placebo plus conjoint marital therapy and placebo plus short contact individual therapy. The measurements used included ones related to symptoms and to marital adjustments. The results of the study suggested that the antidepressant produced rapid relief and the marital therapy produced some improvement, though only on marital adjustment. However, the significance of the findings is ambiguous because of the method used in compiling the results. Cell by cell comparisons were not conducted. Rather, the number of improvements on the measured 203 variables were reported for the antidepressant versus placebo patients and for the marital versus short contact patients. The possibility of random sampling errors between the four treatment cells were not ruled out. Further the probability that a number of the 203 variables would show change by chance alone was not accounted for. Again in this study the effects of the psychotherapy alone (the findings of which are general only to married persons) were not examined. The last of the NIMH supported studies reported by Klerman et al (1974) and Weissman et al (1974) focused on the prevention of relapse in patients who had already responded well to antidepressant therapy. The therapies which were thus maintenance in type, included three levels of drugs (amitryptyline, placebo and no pill) and two levels of psychotherapy

191

(supportive weekly casework by an experienced social worker and weekly minimal contact for assessment of medication only). Measurements included those relating to symptoms as well as social adjustment. This study is perhaps the best in design of those mentioned so far. Its results which are summarised in the Table were clearly presented. Perhaps the one major criticism of this research is that the subjects who were selected on the basis of their previous good response to antidepressant medication helped bias the results in favour of drugs. However, in spite of this, there are hints that the supportive psychotherapy had some beneficial effects after six to eight months. The full significance of this finding is not yet clear. The last study discussed here is perhaps the most interesting and most controversial. Rush et al (1977) compared the effects of the cognitive therapy developed by Beck (1976) against those of imipramine. While this study is relatively small the results are startling. At twelve weeks after beginning therapy the cognitive therapy group were significantly better than the group treated with impramine although this latter group also improved significantly. The excitement which might follow upon these findings is not wholly justified. Firstly, the antidepressant drug used was terminated at the eleventh week of treatment. In view of the importance that drugs would appear to have in the maintenance of remission, this strategy has almost certainly had the effect of inflating the apparent effectiveness of the cognitive therapy. Secondly, as Marks (1978) points out the success in the cognitive group was achieved at the expense of 350% more therapist time than was devoted to the drug group. When one views the fact that there were no significant differences between the two groups at six months follow up one wonders whether such effort is really warranted. Lastly, these researchers used a higher dosage of antidepressant than was the case in the four other studies reported in the Table. Attention has recently been drawn to the fact that high dosages of antidepressants may in fact be anti-therapeutic. It is possible that the high dosage levels may to some degree have been masking the true effectiveness of the antidepressant used.

Recently there have been several studies that have explored the use of a variety of behavioural techniques (see Lewinsohn et al, 1974 and Fuchs and Rehm, 1977). These studies are not discussed here mainly because they have focused their attention on mildly depressed college students. It is at this moment difficult to assess whether or not the findings of these studies can be generalised to the population with which most psychiatrists are commonly involved. In summary it is impossible to draw any firm conclusions on the effects of any of the variety of forms of psychotherapy explored in the studies mentioned above. The reasons in the main, relate to methodological problems in study design. On the other hand the findings of some of the studies do suggest that further explorations are essential.

Behaviour Therapy and the Treatment of Depression

Strangely the amount of attention that behaviour therapists have devoted to depression has been somewhat limited. The majority of work in the past ten years has been devoted to reports of single case studies and to speculative theorising about the aetiology of depression. There are really only three research workers who have been involved in careful systematic research. Lewinsohn and his colleagues in Oregon (see Lewinsohn, 1974) have been examining and attempting to treat depressive behaviour from a reinforcement or operant standpoint while Seligman (see Seligman, 1975) has been exploring the concept of helplessness as it relates to depression. Lastly there is the work of Beck (see Beck, 1976) which has focused on exploring the treating of cognitive abnormalities in depressives. This section is devoted mainly to the work of these researchers.

The Work of Lewinsohn

Lewinsohn holds that depression is often due to an individual's low rate of response contingent on positive reinforcement. He suggests that positive reinforcers may be unavailable or that few events are reinforcing and/or the person lacks the social skills to elicit reinforcement. Among the most interesting parts of this research are those devoted to the depressive's interactions. Lewinsohn (1974) has demonstrated that the depressive has fewer people in his interactional field, elicits less behaviour from his peers, emits fewer positive reinforcements, and that he has a longer response latency in conversations than is normal. These findings are akin to lowered assertiveness — a feature that has been stressed by Wolpe (1971) and Seligman (1975). Lastly, Lewinsohn (1974) holds that the depressive's mood disturbance is secondary (rather than primary) to the reduction in positive reinforcement. However, as will become clear, his research does not completely support this latter viewpoint.

Two treatment strategies have been developed out of this research and successfully applied to mildly depressed subjects. The first involves encouraging the depressive to engage in reinforcing activities. The activities are individually selected for each patient on the basis of their effect on mood as judged after the completion of an inventory — the Pleasant Events Schedule. Basically this inventory selects those events that have been enjoyed in the past and are now most positively correlated with a pleasant mood. In some instances the treatment sessions are made contingent upon completion of such assignments. The second treatment strategy involves the training (or re-training) in appropriate interactional skills. For this purpose subjects are treated in groups. Here they are taught to observe and pinpoint behaviour problems, to define goals and initiate plans for behaviour change, and lastly to examine and carry out this change both within and without the group setting. The value of Lewinsohn's research requires to be qualified. His work has focused exclusively on the typography of depressed behaviour and does not attend much to the actual antecedents of depression. In particular what brings about the failure to engage in pleasant or reinforcing activities and what is the significance of the social skills deficits in the long term?

193

This author suspects that many of these deficits exist only as part of the depressive state. Little attention has been given to covert behaviour such as the individual's appraisal of his circumstances. Authorities such as Bandura (1977) have increasingly over the recent years come to recognise the importance of examining in whatever way possible the individual's private world. Lastly and importantly, most of Lewinsohn's work has been conducted on mildly depressed college students. While this does not in any way invalidate his research it does raise the question of how his findings generalise to 'ordinary' psychiatric populations.

Seligman's Theory of Depression

During the past twelve years Seligman and his colleagues (see Seligman, 1975) have been exploring the effects of non-contingent (unrelated) aversive events on behaviour. Initially this research was conducted on animals. Following the application of several non-contingent shocks it was found that the animals exhibited motivational and learning deficits that generalised to a variety of experimental situations. Similar findings have been reported for human subjects in a variety of laboratory situations though this latter research has been much more inconclusive. After studying these motivational deficits it was suggested that the most likely cause was that the animal or person had learnt that his environment was uncontrollable and thus he ceased to act on his own behalf. In other words the locus of control had shifted in the subject's experience from an internal to an external one – he had become helpless. Seligman has suggested that such a phenomenon may help to explain some depressive disorders and especially those which are reactive in type. The parallels between helplessness and depression are in some instances remarkably similar. They include motivational deficits, difficulty in learning, lowered aggression, somatic symptoms and the fact that both disorders tend to dissipate over time.

This model of depression has not been associated with any particular treatment technique. While techniques such as the re-establishment of engagement in reinforcing activities and social skills training may all have relevance the major difficulty with the helpless subject is one of response initiation. It would seem that reversal of helplessness must involve direct force or pressure or some technique that circumvents the helplessness cognitive set. In this latter instance the paradoxical injunction (which is a strategy used by family therapists) may prove helpful. In an attempt to solve such problems as response initiation Seligman (see Abramson et al, 1979) has had to re-examine the whole concept of helplessness. Interestingly in a reappraisal of the helplessness on the basis of attribution theory he makes some interesting but as yet untried suggestions. Basically these include techniques which are rather similar to those used by cognitive theorists, for example see Beck (1976). There is no doubt that helplessness is a feature of some depressed patients. However, caution must be exercised prior to drawing any conclusions on the basis of Seligman's theory. The majority of human research has been conducted on college students and as yet there is no answer as to how helplessness in a specific circumstance generalises into a depressive disorder, i.e. helplessness over a wide variety of situations. A last point which has been noted by Becker (1974) is that most of the parallels between helplessness and depression seem most germane to severe endogenous depression rather than to the reactive type.

Beck's Theory of Depression

'The essence of Beck's Theory is that the root of depression is a negative cognitive set. The depressed person is seen as having a negative view of himself in the world and of the future. The depressed affective state is secondary to these negative cognitions. Depressive episodes may be externally precipitated and it is the individual's perception and appraisal of the event which is depression inducing.' — Blaney (1977).

Specific treatment techniques have grown around Beck's Theory. He recommends that the techniques are most useful after the low point of the depressive illness has been reached. The therapy is conducted in several well defined stages. Initially the patient is shown how cognitions such as 'I'm a failure' can shape behaviour and emotion. Following this he is taught how to pinpoint cognitions and track their relationship to behaviour and emotion. In the third stage the patient is taught to apply logic and reality to these cognitions. Usually this involves seeking out varieties of explanations for negative happenings rather than attributing them to negative personal attributes. Finally the patient is encouraged to extend and continue to use the techniques in the future. The effectiveness of this type of therapy (see Rush et al, 1977) was discussed in the last section of this paper.

Interestingly the theory and techniques discussed by Beck and his colleagues are in many ways remarkably similar to those of Behaviour Therapists interested in a self-control model of depression. In fact the only major difference in the models is one involving terminology. Unfortunately the self-control work is very much in its infancy and there are only a few studies in which the ideas were used in a therapeutic manner. For instance Fuchs and Rehm (1977) applied the techniques successfully to a small group of depressed persons. Since the patients were only mildly depressed and the follow up period was only six weeks it is difficult to draw any useful conclusions from this study.

The major part of Beck's work has focused attention on the cognitive problems of depressed patients. Other researchers have attempted to explore how depressive states might be induced by manipulation of a person's beliefs or cognitions. This work which has been summarised by Blaney (1977), lends some credence to the notion that depression may have a cognitive source. Of all the behavioural theories of depression Beck's is perhaps the most persuasive

195

mainly because its development and associated treatment techniques have evolved out of situations involving 'real psychiatric patients'.

Other Behavioural Theories and Treatments of Depression

The remaining part of this section is devoted to other aspects of behavioural theories and treatments of depression which have been discussed in literature but which have not generated much related research. Included are the significance of loss of reinforcement as a precipitant of depression and factors that might maintain depressions such as avoidance behaviours, faulty self-control mechanisms and direct rewards for depressive behaviour.

1. Depression and loss of reinforcement: Loss of a spouse or limb or job are all events which may be associated with a loss of a wide range of positive reinforcers for ongoing behaviour. The role of such events in the onset of depression is quite obvious. In many depressed patients the importance of loss of reinforcement may be subtle and more difficult than this to establish. While many behaviour therapists have speculated about this the research work of Brown and his colleagues (see Brown and Harris, 1978) is most important to the understanding of how life events of a loss type can precipitate depression. In particular they draw attention to the importance of the individual's appraisal of the significance of the loss.

The treatment techniques that have grown around this viewpoint of depression for the most part involve therapists attempting to encourage the patient to engage in activities involving the lost reinforcers or where this is not possible (for example, after loss of a spouse) setting tasks involving other potentially reinforcing activities. To some degree this has already been discussed in the section devoted to Lewinsohn's work. One interesting way of re-establishing reinforcement using a time-projection technique has been reported by Lazarus (1968). Under light hypnosis a depressed girl was asked to imagine herself increasingly becoming involved in activities which she had enjoyed prior to a recently broken romance. The girl improved dramatically after two sessions. Finally McLean et al (1973) drew attention to the value of training persons who live in the patient's interactional field to reinforce constructive task oriented behaviour.

2. Depression and Avoidance Behaviours: In some depressive disorders and particularly in the case of grief reactions, avoidance behaviours such as denial of illness may be prominent. Functionally such behaviours may serve to protect the person from the painful consequences of the loss. Unfortunately this set of circumstances also serves to encapsulate the depressive disorder and thus prevent its resolution. Resolution may be effected by desensitising techniques. In some cases with the assistance of drugs the process can be made less painful — see McAuley and Quinn (1975).

3. Reinforcement of Depression: Liberman and Raskin (1971) describe how

196

depressive behaviour can be learnt directly as a result of reinforcement. In some persons depressive behaviour may be used (in a deviant sense) as a method of gaining attention or approval. This situation is most likely to occur in persons whose social competence is in the first place rather poor. It is particularly important to recognise this form of depression since it may require different treatment approaches than hitherto described. Depressive behaviour will need to be extinguished and this may be achieved by ensuring that the behaviour goes unrewarded and by training the patient in more appropriate interactional skills. In summary the behavioural work with depression has provided us with some exciting ideas and techniques. However it is difficult to evaluate at this point the utility of these when applied to the average routine clinical practice. There is at the moment a definite need to extend research work into both theory and treatment. Only after this may we be able to evaluate the place that behaviour therapy or any of the other forms of psychotherapy discussed in this paper, has in the treatment of depression.

COMMENTARY ON CURRENT TRENDS IN THE TREATMENT OF DEPRESSION

Hugh Ferguson

Dr. Clare has reviewed this topic boldly and writes with his customary clarity and slashing insight.

It should have been a pleasure to make comment and elaboration of this excellent paper, but, to use one of Dr. Clare's own words, it proved too sobering. Ironically, this man of wit and humour, who entertains as he elucidates, contrived to sadden. His very clarity exposes the limited progress being made, despite great effort, in treating psychiatric disorders.

One has heard the indictment that psychiatry has become the 'treatment of the treatable' and it had seemed that our ability to treat depression was one of the cornerstones of the psychiatrists' rather shaky edifice of healing. Being humble about the chronic schizophrenic or the sociopath seemed fair: with limited resources of manpower, money and time, helping the depressed, the acutely psychotic or anxious could at least justify our professional status and competence.

Dr. Clare in his preamble and discussion of depression in society immediately confines us to skills in treating only 1 in 10 of those who seek help for depression and rightly directs us to question the findings of clinical research based on this proportionately small and skewed population. He reminds us, in a most comprehensive review of treatment, that even with those we do treat, we have not achieved a reliable way of classifying, analysing, or judging treatment responses.

His paper, which I feel should be the main basis for my digressions can be somewhat artificially divided into two parts.

To precis what one could call the first half of his paper, he comments on the nosological confusion especially in minor illness most often treated by the general practitioner; on the types of short-lived or low grade illness in the community; and on the role of social pathology. He stresses the value of Primary Care Team co-operation and the role of social change. The issues of placebo effect, by drug, and reassurance, are dealt with, as are life-change events and factors of vulnerability.

Running through this section of his paper is the dominant theme of minor mixed anxiety/depressive states which, as Shepherd (1974) and Marks (1974) separately outlined, is most likely to form a larger percentage of psychiatric morbidity in general practice than in out-patient and in-patient psychiatric settings. Despite this, there is a definite trend in psychiatric practice for patients to be seen at a younger age or at an earlier stage in the depressive course and for clinical features to be of a milder 'neurotic' pattern. Our concepts and responses might not indeed, as Dr. Clare suggests, be so superior to the general practitioners'.

In essence, his paper focuses attention on neurotic depression, with all the problems of blurred definition and nosology.

Dr. Clare has wisely avoided an elaboration of the confusion surrounding the classification of depressive disorders with its plethora of dichotomies and cluster analyses, but to complement his paper some further elaboration of neurotic depression seems valid.

Kendall (1974) has reminded us that sophisticated techniques have failed to resolve our confusion and that a Type A — Severe and Type B — Mild Division, as originally suggested by Lewis (1934), could be said to have survived well.

There is an enlarging ground-swell of opinion that the milder depressive categories represent a residual category after the major depressive states have been excluded. As Kiloh, Andrews et al (1972) said, neurotic depression is made by exclusion of endogenous depression and is likely to be heterogeneous. 'Its existence as a separate entity as an artefact.'

One hundred neurotic depressives were studied prospectively by Akiskal, Bitar et al (1978) and 60% were found later to have no rigorously defined depressive state. The next logical focus of attention on this most limited classificatory exercise is:—

Secondary Depression

The concept of secondary depression was an outcome of researchers' needs to find a homogeneous group of depressions. Woodruff, Murphy et al (1967) divided depression into two mutually exclusive groups by natural history:—
Primary — a depressive syndrome occurring with no prior history of any other psychiatric disorder.
Secondary — a depressive syndrome with some non-depressive antecedent disorder, particularly anxiety states, personality disorders and alcoholism. The prognosis of the 'less pure' secondary states would more closely match that of the antecedent disorder.

However arbitrary and despite its defects, the primary-secondary dichotomy is emerging as one of the most useful in current practice. Both the similarities and the differences between primary and secondary are intriguing. Andreasen and Winnokur (1977) recognised certain distinguishing familial characteristics, but found primary and secondary depressives to be surprisingly similar in symptomatology, onset and duration of symptoms, gender ratio, and treatment response, i.e. its predictive value was questionable.

The Akiskal study did, however, claim some distinction on non-symptomatological grounds. Thus:

Primary Depression

1. No previous, non-affective disorder
2. Signs as prominent as symptoms, i.e. more objective
3. Perceived as a definite break in personality
4. Course – more episodic than chronic
5. Prognosis – generally good
6. Family history – if present, highly specific
7. Hypomanic complications with antidepressant medication
8. Emerging physiological markers, i.e. increased urinary H.M.P.G.
   shortened R.E.M. latency
   changes in cortisol secretion

Secondary Depression

1. Pre-existing non-affective disorder
2. More prominently loaded with symptoms, i.e. more subjective
3. Perceived as an exaggeration of usual complaints
4. Course – more chronic than episodic
5. Prognosis – depends on underlying disorder
6. Very rare incidence of family history
7. No pharmacological hypomania
8. No biological markers yet detected

Secondary depression, which Winnokur equates with neurotic depression, could be said to represent, at least in part, a deterioration in mood by the awareness of having an underlying disorder and its consequent stresses – a form of demoralisation – although such concepts are being touched upon in Dr. McAuley's paper. To remind us, however, that such depressions are not necessarily trivial Weissman, Prusoff et al (1977) recognised that many secondary depressives were severely agitated, had endogenous-like features, and stressed the risks of diagnosis by depressive rating scales which could result in the entire spectrum of psychiatric disorders being artificially clustered together.

Despite this incidence of severity which often directs such depressives to our clinics, the general practitioner, as has been stated and re-stated, is the most likely source of treatment and, as Goldberg and Blackwell (1970) claimed, most cases of psychiatric morbidity in general practice are affective disturbances of

200

which some two-thirds will have cleared in the six month followup.

The pool of psychiatric morbidity to which Dr. Clare refers running a more protracted course must contain many who could be described as secondary depressives. These clinical states by nature of their underlying pathology will be more dramatic with more complaints of rage, phobias, somatic disturbances, and more parasuicide.

It seems reasonable to conceive secondary depression as an illness superimposed on a more chronic one — compare sub-acute bacterial endocarditis and rheumatic fever — the complication demanding the more immediate attention. Many complaints presented to the general practitioner and indeed the psychiatrist will be depressive-like decompensations provoking early attack on depressive symptoms with various drugs. Thus it will be the depressive aspects of psychiatric morbidity which will attract attention and skew the statistics of psychiatric classification in general population studies towards depression. In our state of knowledge and resources the early attack seems inevitably based on pharmacology.

But why such an increase in antidepressant preparations? Increased awareness? — yes. Increased expectations from patients? — of course. But in 1966 90% of the total antidepressant market was covered by four drug companies with their five preparations covering the majority. In 1975 ten companies were competing for the same proportion of the market with a total number of preparations jumping from 14 to 21. There has, therefore, to be increased pressure from drug companies who have, as yet, we are told, to produce an antidepressant significantly superior to its fellows.

Placebo Responses

We are faced with the paradox of increasing knowledge about the spectrum of depressive states, both primary and secondary, and their responses to medication and a contrasting awareness of the potency of placebo responses in medicine in general and in minor psychiatric disturbances in particular.

Our confidence in ourselves as therapists is constantly being challenged by accusations that by treating a natural response to a life situation with drugs we are labelling too many as ill. This is a particular worry in the area of the so-called neurotic depressions which do respond to antidepressant medication with a placebo response of near 50%. Yet, as stated, many of these so labelled depressives have disturbances severe enough to create risks of suicide or produce such biological changes that the concept of illness becomes valid. It is an unanswerable question at this time.

By using potent drugs — with obvious side effects — this placebo effect is surely enhanced. Thus, there could be an increase in (Beecher, 1955) the calculated 35% of the population described as placebo responders. These people have few, if any, real distinguishing characteristics with a possible tendency

201

perhaps to conformity and acquiescence. The warnings of delay in response to antidepressants which we give, the immediacy of their potent side effects, our sense of conviction of their worth and, above all, the severity of the symptoms all add to the potency of placebo. Thus, those with low grade undramatic anxiety/depressive complaints have a poorer placebo response, especially when depressive decompensation is not a marked feature.

The end result is that general practitioners in particular, but psychiatrists and out-patient clinics too, all faced with the high frequency of neurotic and minor or secondary affective disorders, are participating in what Dr. Clare has quoted elsewhere as 'the relentless march of the psychotropic drug juggernaut'.

All this pressures us to explore the psychosocial dimension in minor or indeed major psychiatric disability, and Dr. Clare does well to emphasise the strategies of the general practitioner in his role as member of the primary care team.

Life Events

He has described the work of Brown on the factor of vulnerability in depression and separated this from stress precipitation. The concept of vulnerability is a fascinating if problematical one.

The difficulties in methodology of study of life events has led to doubt about reliability and resultant conflicting evidence. Most of the studies have been retrospective and Jenkins and Hurst (1979) have stressed the importance of faulty recall for events more than six months in the past.

Patients' accounts perhaps depressively exaggerate the import of an event and there has been in the past poor concordance with data from relatives but more controlled studies are now giving evidence that depressives have indeed a larger number of negative events or exits in the recent past (Brown, Harris et al, 1973) and (Thompson and Hendrie, 1972).

It has been demonstrated (Paykel, 1979) that there is the highest incidence of exits in suicide attempters, followed by depressives, but the lowest rates of the three cohorts occur in schizophrenia.

Brown, Harris et al (1973) work does lend weight to the belief that negative life events have a FORMATIVE role in depression even if the extent of this role is uncertain. His vulnerability factors include distant loss, although one notes that the vulnerability factors mentioned by him (i.e. having young children, lacking employment, lacking a confidante, and with a loss of the mother before 11 years) all applied to the 8% incidence of depression in his community group, i.e. who have not sought treatment. The low social class incidence possibly was a factor in terms of more limited access to medical treatment unless the relatively minor nature of the depression was the determinant.

On balance, these vulnerability factors relate mainly to stresses of social type or lack of social support — with early loss affecting the largely developmental

202

phases of personality formation.

The areas of coping devices and treatment access are so multifactorial in depression that definition is extremely difficult but Dr. Clare's way of addressing us to the problem of nosology and psychosocial parameters is indeed provocative.

In the 'second half' of his paper he concentrates on physical treatments, most particularly, the tricyclics, lithium, E.C.T., and psychosurgery. His review was much more comprehensive than his brief precis suggests. He highlighted:

1. The value of continuing drug therapy, particularly in adequate dosage; he suggested that if no relapse had occurred after eight months further continuation was of doubtful value.
2. Plasma tricyclic levels are relevant to both side effects and treatment response.
3. The relationships between secondary and tertiary amine drugs are studied with a reminder of the relative selectivity for secondary amines blocking uptake of noradrenaline, tertiary amines the blocking of serotonin uptake.

Discussion of plasma steady-state levels is made both of the drug and its active metabolites and mention is made of a possible curvilinear relationship in secondary amines in treatment, i.e. too high a level is counter-therapeutic, whilst in tertiary amines linear relationships are most likely with risks of ineffectively low dosage and low plasma levels.

Despite the finding by general practitioners that no drug was found to be superior to amitriptyline the need to find predictive factors for drug response is as high as ever.

Predictive Factors

Predictive studies rely on the assumption that one can identify pretreatment differences between poor and good responders, i.e. the conditions necessary for clinical change. In other words, assessment and prediction are inherently interdependent.

Indices of prediction may be *clinical* — and on this we are more reliant — or *biochemical*. Biological indices are slowly emerging especially for primary illness. Clinical studies have to show large and significant effects of a drug compared with another, or placebo, and different predictors for those receiving or not receiving the treatment drug being studied. All the aforementioned problems in classification, be they unitary, dichotomous, or cluster analyses bedevil such studies as Dr. Clare pointed out early in his paper.

Prediction by Age and Gender

Raskin, Schulterbrandt et al (1970) found imipramine to be more effective in patients over 40 years — female patients under 40 faring better on placebo. In keeping with this is the tendency for depression in older people to have more severe or psychotic features.

Gender is a much more complex parameter — a reminder of the heterogeneity of depression.

The 1965 M.R.C. study reported a better male response to imipramine, but women if given T3 in addition showed significantly enhanced responses, Prange and Wilson (1972). The work was confirmed by Wheatley (1972) and Coppen, Whybrow et al (1972), the Coppen study comparing imipramine and L-tryptophan

The current inference regarding the thyroid states in depression is that high cortisol levels blunt the pituitary response to thyrotrophin releasing factor with thus lower than normal levels of T.R.H.

A further study by Raskin (1974) differentiated imipramine responses from other antidepressants. Older females did well on imipramine only, older males on other medications also. Younger females again did poorly on imipramine and well on placebo with released hostility being the cause of poor responses.

Naturally, discussion of depression in women would have to include the role handicaps and vulnerability issues referred to elsewhere.

Pre-Morbid Personality

As a predictor, such pre-illness factors are established in bipolar and severe unipolar depression with increased incidence of stable or cyclothymic personalities and relatively good treatment responses unless delusions are present.

The neurotic/secondary groupings would have a loading of pre-morbid emotional turbulence or chronic personality disorder related to low self-esteem and exaggerated reactions to psychological let-down, over-dependency, helplessness, pessimism, and overuse of projection and dramatisation. Such factors predict variable and often poor drug treatment response.

Differential responses were studied by Kupfer, Picket et al (1976) who separated unipolar depressives into tricyclic responders whose pre-illness personalities were loaded with obsessionality or anxiety whilst lithium responders had cyclothymic personalities.

Genetic and Family Predictors

The response of a patient to a particular drug is likely to be similar to that of a first degree relative who becomes depressed. Twin studies have proved inconclusive.

Acetylation of M.A.O.I. has been studied (Pare and Mack, 1971) with slow inactivation by acetyl transferase occurring in 60% of the population — resulting in enhanced drug efficiency. Fast acetylators, the remaining population, will have poorer responses and higher side effects.

On balance, in every depressive episode our practice of taking family medical histories, drug responses of family members, and fast drug responses in patients is fully warranted.

Clinical Symptom Predictors have not proved reliably useful.

The usefulness of imipramine in retarded depressives without anxiety or delusional malperceptions or marked hostility in the case of young females is established. The usefulness of amitriptyline, especially in older age groups in endogenous states with anxiety is established. Mianserin appears to have similar values with reduced anticholinergic side effects.

One reasonably consistent finding has been the poor response in severe depressive delusional states that worsen unless phenothiazines are given in addition or more usually unless E.C.T. is used (Glassman, Kantor et al, 1975).

Using the Newcastle scale for depression (Rao and Coppen, 1979) confirmed this poor response in those with high scores reflecting delusional depression using amitriptyline. Predictably poor results to those with low scores in the neurotic range were found. This is further confirmation that antidepressant medications are effective mainly in the middle ranges of unipolar depressive illness.

Prediction by Classification has already been discussed briefly. Pervading most of the literature in depressive treatment is the theme that diagnostic classifications do not predict treatment responses well. Only in the primary bipolar and severe unipolar depression has some consistency emerged.

Biochemical Prediction of Antidepressant Response

Such research is at a tentative stage. Interest in the suppression of the pituitary adrenal response by dexamethasone is based on the fact that some depressives, especially severe forms, escape such suppression. (Brown, Johnston et al, 1979) added weight to the premise that such escape from dexamethasone suppression is a marker for good tricyclic responses.

Measurements of urinary 3-methoxy 4-hydroxyphenylglycol (M.H.P.G.) have suggested biological sub-types of primary depression with suggestions (Beckman and Goodwin, 1975) that amitriptyline responders had high pre-treatment levels and imipramine responders low M.H.P.G. levels. In complement, patients with low levels of 5 H.I.A.A. responded to amitriptyline and high 5 H.I.A.A. levels predicted response to imipramine — further confirmation that amitriptyline is less likely than imipramine to be converted into a secondary noradrenaline blocking metabolite.

The injection of dextroamphetamine improved certain depressives especially if severely disturbed — and such patients had a more favourable response to imipramine in keeping with the findings of low M.H.P.G. responders to imipramine.

On balance, of all predictor studies, the clinical ones remain the more useful concerning choice of drug, despite the obvious confusion. Useful examples are the clinical characteristics of lithium responders, the disadvantages of imipramine in hostile young females, and the usefulness of additional neuroleptics with depressive delusional illnesses.

205

An attempted resume of newer antidepressants, such as maprotiline and mianserin would be inevitably lengthy and anyway premature since plasma steady-state levels of such drugs and their active metabolites still have to be reliably studied.

To conclude, one would like to return to Dr. Clare's paper, which has covered so widely and so well such a range of topics. No attempt has been made here to emulate such a feat. The intention was merely to complement Dr. Clare's paper in a few areas and to enhance further what one hopes will be an enjoyable session.

RESPONSE TO COMMENTARIES BY DR. McAULEY
AND DR. FERGUSON

Anthony Clare

The two discussion papers complement rather than contradict anything that appeared in my paper. I told Dr. McAuley before this that, when I got his paper and looked through his references, it filled me with great dismay to see there is a whole area in current trends in the treatment of depression that has escaped my supposedly eagle eye. When I read the results of his review, particularly the psychotherapy of depression, I then realised that, for all that appears, there is really very little we know about it, as he has demonstrated himself, which is salutary and perhaps rather sad.

The problem in this area — in fact I had some misgivings about tackling it at all — is, for a start, the term 'depression' itself. This raises questions of a single symptom right the way through to a fairly classic and recognisable syndrome cluster. The population studied can range from community samples, the general practice populations, psychiatric out-patient populations to the in-patient populations.

Thus each time a paper appears, one looks to see how the sample has been defined or selected and whether the treatment is in a medical setting or non-medical setting, before ever beginning to look at the kinds of treatments that are being explored. So it is, in my experience, that before one gets to assess many of these respectable studies; respectable in the sense of ones that are quoted, and these respectable studies are often wanting in some of the basic requirements of decent research.

I would like to pick up one or two points that highlight the discussion. I think that it is salutary to note that in Weissman's study in Newhaven, a study which selected good responders to drugs to begin with and looked at psychotherapy with and without drugs in a very complex and very well designed way, only 30% of good drug responders did not seek further treatment during the twelve month follow-up period. So we are dealing with a condition that, even in the best groups, has a tendency to relapse, and the tendency for people

207

to say that there is no cure for depression, only symptom relief or methods of shortening illness periods may have something to it. (Lithium, however, is a substance that cures rather than treats if, by cure, you mean that as long as you take the drug you remain mentally healthy.)

The next point I would like to make is the issue of psychotherapy which interests me as I work in General Practice and work very closely with Social Workers. I always wonder when I see studies of this as to what exactly it means. It is also interesting to see the coyness with which those who use the term describe the actual content of what they do. However, the Temple University, Pennsylvania, study spelt out exactly what they did — they taped a number of interviews, and they selected their psychotherapists carefully. Sloane, indeed, to get round the accusation that he was using psychotherapists who were insufficiently trained, took psychotherapists who had at least twenty years' analytical training. When this data was presented to the Maudsley Hospital, of course, one analyst there said that these psychotherapists were old fashioned! In the Weissman study, on the other hand, it is very difficult to know what psychotherapy is. In fact, I'd call it 'social support', provided by a Social Worker and that it is 'here and now' therapy and is not in fact exploratory or carried out according to any formal psychodynamic theory — yet it is called psychotherapy. The same term, as you know of course, is applied to widely different exploratory psychological techniques.

The issue, too, of drug dosage in trials of depression is an important one, the whole thorny question being the extent to which failure to respond is due to either too high or too low dosage. It was also interesting for me to know how much of drug research work was done with mildly depressed college students, and there again, this is a warning about some of the newer studies, in particular cognitive and behavioural therapies as well as psychotherapy.

Just before I came to this Conference, there was an E.C.T. Conference in Leicester. It was interesting to see the extent to which a conference provoked disagreement masquerading as harmony, which may say something about us professional people. There was a bunch of scientologists protesting outside the door under fire, and the disagreements within seemed to be tempered by the fact that there were disagreements without. For my money, the evidence for the usefulness of E.C.T. in severe depression seems to be unchallengeable, yet figures now coming from the States and presumably, when the College's own study gets under way, from here show that E.C.T. is rapidly falling in terms of its use. Indeed, it may be that the Royal College will crown its achievements by reporting on the use and efficacy of E.C.T. at just about the time when E.C.T. is no longer used!

My final point is about the need for research into that big pool of psychosocial morbidity in General Practice. It is quite interesting, perhaps even alarming, to note that, after fifteen or twenty years of the psychopharmachological revolution, with General Practitioners bombarded with criticisms about their use of psychotropic drugs and an escalating drug bill, there are no studies, indeed not a single descriptive study about the efficacy of prescribing such drugs in general practice.

Most drug trials done in general practice are classical drug trials – you take two groups of patients and you give them certain drugs at a specific time. The drugs are given regularly and you rate them at the beginning and you rate them at the end. In general practice, of course, it is not like that. Patients, believe it or not, are free and what they actually do with their drugs ranges from, as you know, flushing them down lavatories, there to sedate the fishes in the North Sea, to ingesting them in rather large and irresponsible quantities, as you know from the Accident Wards of many of our general hospitals. Although there are some studies on the escalation of drug prescribing and the amounts of drug prescribing, there are no studies on how the GP actually goes about response, the actual response, the actual dose, the outcome, the intervening social factors and yet we are talking about, in fact, a multi-million pound industry.

And so to finish, because this is about current trends and the treatment of depression, one of the things I think, particularly about the treatment of depression, is that we've actually got to discover the way that drugs are actually used, not only because of my interest in General Practice research but because you, as hospital prescribers, are crucially important and are actually influencing GP's expectations about the drugs he uses, not to mention patient expectations. In other words, you greatly influence patients that you may never see. Your descriptions of depression, your descriptions of treatment, your descriptions of outcome, all based on hospital populations, greatly influence general practitioners and, in turn, greatly influence patients. We know that a large proportion of those prescribed potent anti-depressant drugs are on them for at least six months. We do not know how the patients that go on using them in general practice differ from the patients who use them and then discontinue using them when they feel better.

Is the group who stay on psychotropics a 'disease' group, and are those who just take them if they need them a 'normal' group, or do you increase the number of people in the 'disease' group merely by increasing your overall prescribing? Evidence from drug studies, and certainly our own, supports the view that those GP's who prescribe highest have most patients on long-term psychotropics. The second thing, of course, which must be borne in mind is that today, at any rate, a significant number of people use drugs in a highly idiosyncratic and individual type of way and apart from the public disquiet about drugs, there is no doubt that patients do find drugs helpful. A significant proportion of patients use them for very short times with apparent benefit. They take them in almost a stimulus relief pattern as indicated rather than as prescribed. So one current trend concerns a study that is under way at the moment which involves assessment of GP's and their expectations concerning why they prescribe and what they do prescribe, and their patients' expectations of drug use, their actual drug use, their response to drugs and the possible relevant factors concerned in their response.

Well, that brings us to the end of my discussion on these papers. It would seem that, if you take them together, they really complement each other. Dr. Ferguson has looked at the classifications of depression, an area which I stayed clear of as frankly I have never understood the difference between the six different names by which various people classify depression although, in clinical practice, I still look for and occasionally find classical endogenous features and I still look instinctively for certain reactive factors. I have considerable admiration for Dr. Ferguson in tackling it in a manner which certainly provided considerable clarification for me. No doubt some of you may feel classification is crucial, and may raise it, in which case, if you do, I will have no hesitation in handing the questions over to Dr. Ferguson to deal with.

References

Abramson, LY, Seligman, MEP and Teasdale, JD (1979) Learned Helplessness in Humans: Critique and Reformulation. *Journal of Abnormal Psychology.* (In Press)

Akiskal, HS, Bitar, AH, Puzantian, VR, Rosenthal, TL and Walker, PW (1978) The Nosological Status of Neurotic Depression. *Archives of General Psychiatry, 35,* 756–766

Alexanderson, B and Sjoqvist, F (1971) Individual Differences in the Pharmacokinetics of Mono Methylated Tricyclic Antidepressants: Role of genetic and environmental factors and clinical importance. *Annals of the New York Academy of Science, 179,* 739–751

Andreasen, NC and Winnokur, G Familiar Factors in Affective Disorders. A.P.A. Meeting, 1977

Andrews, G and Tennant, C (1978) Life Events Stress and Mental Illness. Editorial. *Psychological Medicine, 8,* 545–549

Asberg, M (1974). Plasma Nortriptyline Levels – Relationship to Clinical Effects. *Clinical Pharmacology and Therapeutics, 16,* 215–229

Asberg, M, Cronholm, N, Sjoqvist, F and Tuck, D (1970) Correlation of Subjective Side-Effects with Plasma Concentrations of Nortriptyline. *British Medical Journal, 4,* 18–21

Asberg, M and Germanis, M (1972) Opthalmological Effects of Nortriptyline Relationship to Plasma Level. *Pharmacology, 7,* 349–356

Asberg, M, Cronholm, N, Sjoqvist, F and Tuck, D (1971) Relationship between Plasma Level and Therapeutic Effect of Nortriptyline. *British Medical Journal, 3,* 331–334

Bandura, A (1977) Self Efficacy: Toward a Unifying Theory of Behavioural Change. *Psychological Review, 84,* 191–215

Barnes, T and Braithwaite, R (1978) Drug Treatment in Depression. In: *Current Themes in Psychiatry* (Eds Gaind, RN and Hudson, BL) Macmillan, London

Beck, AT (1976) *Cognitive Therapy and the Emotional Disorders.* New York: International Universities Press

Becker, J (1974) *Depression: Theory and Research.* Washington: Winston

Beckmann, H and Goodwin, FK Antidepressant Response to Tricyclics and Urinary MHP6 in Unipolar Patients. *Archives of General Psychiatry, 32,* 17–21 (1975)

Beecher, HK (1955) The Powerful Placebo. *J. Amer. Med. Ass.,* 1602

Bergin, AE and Lambert, MJ (1978) The Evaluation of Therapeutic Outcome. In: *Handbook of Psychotherapy and Behaviour Change.* (Eds SL Garfield and AE Bergin). New York: Wiley

Blackwell, B (1973) Psychotropic Drugs in use today: the Role of Diazepam in Medical Practice. *Journal of the American Medical Association, 225,* 1737

Blaney, PH (1977) Contemporary Theories of Depression: Critique and Comparison. *Journal of Abnormal Psychology, 86,* 203–223

Blashki, TG, Mowbray, R and Davies, B (1971) Amitriptyline and Amylobarbitone in General Practice. *British Medical Journal, 1*, 133–138

Bowden, CL (1978) Lithium-responsive Depression. *Comprehensive Psychiatry, 19*, 227–231

Braithwaite, RA, Goulding, R, Theano, G, Bailey, J and Coppen, A (1972) Plasma Concentrations of Amitriptyline and Clinical Response. *Lancet, i*, 1297

Bridges, PK (1978) A Contemporary View of Psychosurgery. In: *Current Themes in Psychiatry*, Vol 1 (Eds RN Gaind and DL Hudson). London: Macmillan

Bridges, PK and Bartlett, JR (1977) Review Article: Psychosurgery: Yesterday and Today. *British Journal of Psychiatry, 131*, 249–260

Brook, P and Cooper, B (1975) Community Mental Health Care: Primary Team and Specialist Services. *Journal of the Royal College of General Practitioners, 25*, 151, 93–110

Brown, AB, Johnston, R and Mayfield, D (1979) The 24-Hour Dexamethasone Suppression Test in a Clinical Setting. *American Journal of Psychiatry, 136*, 4B, 543–547

Brown, GW, Harris, TO and Peto, J (1973) Life Events and Psychiatric Disorder. *Psychiatric Medicine, 3*, 159–176

Brown, GW and Harris, T (1978) *Social Origins of Depression*. London: Tavistock

Carney, MWP, Roth, M and Garside, RF (1965) The Diagnosis of Depressive Syndromes and the Prediction of ECT Responses. *British Journal of Psychiatry, 111*, 659

Ciminero, AR, Calhoun, KS and Adams, HE (1977) *Handbook of Behavioural Assessment*. New York: Wiley

Clare, AW and Cairns, VE (1978) Design, Development and Use of a Standardised Interview to Assess Social Maladjustment and Dysfunction in Community Studies. *Psychological Medicine, 8*, 589–604

Collins, J (1965) *Social Casework in a General Medical Practice*. London: Pitman

Cooper, B, Fry, J and Kalton, G (1969) A Longitudinal Study of Psychiatric Morbidity in a General Practice Population. *British Journal of Preventative Social Medicine, 23*, 210–217

Cooper, B, Harwin, BG, Depla, C and Shepherd, M (1975) Mental Health Care in the Community: An Evaluative Study. *Psychological Medicine, 5*, 4, 372

Coppen, A, Whybrow, PC, Noguera, R, Maggs, R and Prange, AJ (1972) The Comparative Antidepressant Value of L-Tryptophan and Imiprimine with and without Attempted Potoniation by Liothyronine. *Archives of General Psychiatry, 26*, 234–241

Coppen, AJ (1974) Clinical Significance of Plasma Levels of Tricyclic Anti-Depressant Drugs in the Treatment of Depression. In: *Classification and Preduction of Outcome of Depression*. (Ed J Angst). Schattauer: Stuttgart

Corney, RH and Briscoe, ME (1977) Social Workers and their Clients: A comparison between primary health care and local authority settings. *Journal of Royal College of General Practitioners, 27*, 295–301

Covi, L, Lipman, RS, Derogatis, LR, Smith, JE and Pattison, JH (1974) Drugs and Group Psychotherapy in Neurotic Depression. *American Journal of Psychiatry, 131*, 191–198

Daneman, EA (1961) Imipramine in Office Management of Depressive Reactions (a double blind study). *Diseases of the Nervous System, 22*, 213–217

Davis, JM (1976) Maintenance Therapy in Psychiatry: II. Affective Disorders. *American Journal of Psychiatry, 133*, 1–13

Davis, JM and Janowsky, DS (1974) Recent Advances in the Treatment of Depression. *British Journal of Hospital Medicine, 2*, 219–227

Department of Health and Social Security (1977). *Health and Personal Social Service Statistics for England, 1977*. HMSO, London

Dunner, DL and Fieve, RR (1974) Clinical Factors in Lithium Carbonate Prophylaxis Failure. *Archives of General Psychiatry*

Electroconvulsive Therapy. Task Force Report 14. American Psychiatric Association. Sept. 1978. APA: Washington

Forman, JAS and Fairbairn, EM (1968) *Social Casework in General Practice*. London: Oxford University Press

Foulds, GA and Bedford, H (1975) Hierarchy of Classes of Personal Illness. *Psychological Medicine, 5*, 181–182

Freeman, CPL, Basson, JV and Crighton, A (1978) Double-Blind Controlled Trial of Electroconvulsive Therapy (ECT) and Simulated ECT in Depressive Illness. *Lancet, i*, 738–740

Friedman, AS (1975) Interaction of Drug Therapy and Marital Therapy in Depressive Patients. *Archives of General Psychiatry, 32,* 619–637

Fuchs, CZ and Rehm, LP (1977) A Self-Control Behaviour Therapy Program for Depression. *Journal of Consulting and Clinical Psychology, 45,* 206–215

Garfinkel, PE, Warsh, JL and Stancer, HC (1979) Depression: New Evidence in Support of Biological Differentiation. *American Journal of Psychiatry, 136,* 535–539

Glassman, AH, Kantor, SJ and Shostak, M (1975) Depression, Delusion and Drug Response. *American Journal of Psychiatry, 132,* 716–719

Goldberg, DP and Blackwell, B (1970) Psychiatric Illness in General Practice. *British Medical Journal, 2,* 439–443

Harvey-Smith, EA and Cooper, B (1970) Patterns of Neurotic Illness in the Community. *Journal of the Royal College of General Practitioners, 19,* 132–139

Helmchen, H (1979) Current Trends of Research on Antidepressive Treatment and Prophylaxis. *Community Psychiatry, 20,* 201–204

Henderson, AS (1977) The Social Network, Support and Heurosis. *British Journal of Psychiatry, 131,* 185–191

Hollon, S and Beck, AT (1978) Psychotherapy and Drug Therapy. In: *Handbook of Psychotherapy and Behaviour Change.* (Eds SL Garfield and AE Bergin). New York: Wiley

Imlah, NW, Ryan, E and Harrington, JA (1965) The Influence of Anti-Depressant Drugs on the Response to Electroconvulsive Therapy and on Subsequent Relapse Rates. *Journal of Neuropsychopharmacology, 4,* 438–442

Jenkins, CD and Hurst, MW (1979) Life Changes: Do People Remember? *Archives of General Psychiatry, 36,* 379–384

Kay, DWK, Fahy, T and Garside, RF (1970) A Seven-Month Double Blind Trial of Amitriptyline and Diazepam in ECT-treated Depressed Patients. *British Journal of Psychiatry, 117,* 667–671

Kedward, HB (1967) The Natural History of Minor Psychiatric Illness. MD Thesis: University of Manchester

Kendall, RE (1974) The Stability of Psychiatric Diagnosis. *British Journal of Psychiatry, 124,* 352–358

Kiloh, LG, Andrews, G, Nielson, M and Bianchi, GN (1972) The Relationship of Syndromes called Endogenous and Neurotic Depression. *British Journal of Psychiatry, 121,* 183–196

Klerman, GL, DiMascio, A, Weissman, M, Prusoff, B and Paykel, ES (1974) Treatment of Depression by Drugs and Psychotherapy. *American Journal of Psychiatry, 131,* 186–191

Kragh-Srensen, P, Asberg, M and Eggert-Hansen, C (1973) Plasma Nortriptyline Levels in Endogenous Depression. *Lancet, i,* 113–115

Kukopulos, A, Reginaldi, D, Tondo, L, Bernabei, A and Galiari, B (1977) Spontaneous Length of Depression and Response to ECT. *Psychological Medicine, 7,* 625–629

Kupfer, DJ, Foster, FG, Reich, L et al (1976) EEG-sleep Changes as Predictors in Depression. *American Journal of Psychiatry, 133,* 622–626

Kupfer, DJ, Picker, D, Himmelhoch, JM and Detre, TP (1976) Are there two types of unipolar depressions? *Archives of General Psychiatry, 32,* 716–719

Lambourn, J and Gill, D (1977) Is ECT Effective? The Preliminary Results of a Controlled Trial. *British Journal of Psychiatry, 1,* 317

Lazarus, AA (1968) Learning Theory and the Treatment of Depression. *Behaviour Therapy and Research, 6,* 83–89

Lewinsohn, PM (1974) A Behavioural Approach to Depression. In: *The Psychology of Depression: Contemporary Theory and Research.* (Eds RM Friedman and MM Katz). New York: Wiley

Lewinsohn, PM, Weinstein, MS and Alper, TA (1970) A Behaviorally Orientated Approach to the Group Treatment of Depressed Persons. *Journal of Clinical Psychology, 26,* 525–532

Lewis, A (1934) Melancholia: A Clinical Survey of Depressive States. *Journal of Mental Science, 80,* 277–378

Liberman, RP and Raskin, DE (1971) Depression: A Behavioral Formulation. *Archives of General Psychiatry, 24,* 525–532

Lipsedge, M (1976) Drug Treatment. In: *Recent Advances in Clinical Psychiatry,* No 2. Churchill Livingstone, London

Marks, IM (1974) Research in Neurosis: A Subjective Review. *Psychological Medicine, 4,* 1, 89–109

Marks, I (1978) Behavioral Psychotherapy of Adult Neurosis. In: *Handbook of Psychotherapy and Behavior Change.* (Eds SL Garfield and AE Bergin). New York: Wiley

McAuley, RR and Quinn, JT (1975) Behavioural Models of Depression. In: *Progress in Behaviour Therapy.* (Ed JC Breugelman). Berlin: Springer-Verlag

McLean, PD, Ogston, K and Graner, L (1973) A Behavioural Approach to the Treatment of Depression. *Journal of Behaviour Therapy and Experimental Psychiatry, 4,* 323–330

Medical Research Council. Report by Clinical Psychiatry Committee. *British Medical Journal, 1,* 881

Mendels, J (1976) Lithium in the Treatment of Depression. *American Journal of Psychiatry, 133,* 373–378

Mendlewicz, J, Fieve, RR and Stallone, F (1973) Relationship between the Effectiveness of Lithium Therapy and Family History. *American Journal of Psychiatry, 130,* 1011–1013

Mindham, RHS, Howland, C and Shepherd, M (1973) An Evaluation of Continuation Therapy with Tricyclic Antidepressants in Depressive Illness. *Psychological Medicine, 3,* 5–17

Montgomery, S (1975) The Relationship between Plasma Concentrations of Amitriptyline and Therapeutic Response. Paper read to the British Academy of Psycho-pharmacology, London

NIME Collaborative Program. The Psychobiology of Depression. *American Journal of Psychiatry, 136,* 1, 49–70

Nielsen, J, Juel-Nielsen, N and Stromgren, E (1965) A Five-year Survey of a Psychiatric Service in a Geographically De-limited Rural Population given Easy Access to this Service. *Comprehensive Psychiatry, 6,* 139–165

Noyes, R, Dempsey, M, Blum, A et al (1974) Lithium Treatment of Depression. *Comprehensive Psychiatry, 15,* 187–193

Odegard, O (1972) Epidemiology of the Psychoses. In: *Psychiatric der Gegenwart 11/1,* 2. Aufl. New York: Springer

Ottosson, JD (1960) Experimental Studies in the Mode of Action of Electroconvulsive Therapy. *Acta Psychiatrica Scandinavica, 35* (Suppl 145), 5–235

Pare, CBM and Mack, JW (1971) Differentiation of Two Genetically Specific Types of Depression by the Response to Antidepressant Drugs. *J. Med. Gen., 8,* 306–309

Parish, PA (1971) The Prescribing of Psychotropic Drugs in General Practice. *Journal of the Royal College of General Practitioners, 21,* Suppl 4

Parkes, CM (1972) Bereavement. *Studies of Grief in Adult Life.* London: Tavistock

Paykel, ES, Dimascio, A, Haskell, D and Prusoff, BA (1975) Effects of Maintenance Amitriptyline and Psychotherapy on Symptoms of Depression. *Psychological Medicine, 5,* 67–77

Paykel, ES (1979) Life Stresses and Attempted Suicide. In: *Suicide: A Comprehensive Handbook.* (Ed LD Hankoff). New York: Publishing Sciences Group Inc

Petursson, H (1979) Prediction of Lithium Response. *Comprehensive Psychiatry, 20,* 226–241

Prange, AJ and Wilson, JC (1972) Thyrotropic Releasing Hormones in Depression. *Psychopharmacologia (Berlin) 26,* 82

Rao, VA and Coppen, A (1979) Classification of Depression and Response to Amitriptyline Therapy. *Psychological Medicine, 9 :* 2, 321–326

Raskin, A, Schulterbrandt, JG, Reatig, N, Chase, C and McKeon, JJ (1970) Differential Responses to Chlorpromazine, Imiprimine and Placebo: A Study of Subgroups of Hospitalised Depressed Patients. *Archives of General Psychiatry, 23,* 164–173

Raskin, A (1974) Age-Sex Differences in Response to Antidepressant Drugs. *J. Ner. Ment. Dis., 159,* 120–130

Rush, AJ, Beck, AT, Kovacs, M and Hollon, SD (1977) Comparative Efficacy of Cognitive Therapy and Pharmacotherapy in the Treatment of Depressed Out-patients. *Cognitive Therapy and Research, 1,* 17–37

Seager, CP and Bird, RL (1962) Imipramine with Electrical Treatment in Depression – a Controlled Trial. *Journal of Mental Science, 108,* 704–707

Segal, SP (1972) Research on the Outcome of Social Work Therapeutic Interventiona: A Review of the Literature. *Journal of Health and Social Behaviour, 13*, 3

Seligman MEP (1975) *Helplessness.* San Francisco: WH Freeman

Sethna ER (1974) A Study of Refrectory Cases of Depressive Illnesses and their Response to Combined Antidepressant Treatment. *British Journal of Psychiatry, 124*, 265–272

Shepherd, M, Cooper, B, Brown, AC and Kalton, GW (1966) *Psychiatric Illness in General Practice.* Oxford University Press

Shepherd, M (1974) General Practice, Mental Illness, the British National Health Service. *American Journal of Public Health, 64*, 230–232

Simpson, GM, Lee, JH. Cuculic, Z et al (1976) Two dosages of Imipramine in Hospitalised Endogenous and Neurotic Depressives. *Archives of General Psychiatry, 33*, 1093–1102

Sloane RB. Staples, FR, Cristol, AH, Yorkston, NJ and Whipple, K (1975) Short Term Analytically Oriented Psychotherapy vs. Behaviour Therapy. Cambridge, Mass: Harvard University Press

Sylph, J Kedward, HB and Eastwood. MR (1969) Chronic Neurotic Patients in General Practice. A pilot study. *Journal of the Royal College of General Practitioners, 17*, 162–170

Taylor, Lord and Chave. S (1964) *Mental Health and Environment.* Longmans, London

Taylor, MA and Abrams, R (1975) Acute Mania: Clinical and genetic study of responders and non-responders to treatments. *Archives of General Psychiatry, 32*, 863–865

Tennant C and Bebbington. P (1978) The Social Causation of Depression – a critique of the work of Brown and his colleagues. *Psychological Medicine, 8*, 565–575

Thompson. KC and Hendrie, HC (1972) *Environmental Stress in Primary Depressive Illness*

Tyrer. P (1974) Indications for Combined Antidepressant Therapy. *British Journal of Psychiatry, 124*, 620

US National Commission for the Protection of Human Subjects of Biomedical and Behavioural Research (1977). *Report and Recommendations: Psychosurgery.* US DHEW Publ. No. (05) 77 0001

Valenstein, ES (1977) The Practice in Psychosurgery: A Survey of the Literature (1971–1976). In. *Psychosurgery, US National Commission for the Protection of Human Subjects of Biomedical and Behavioural Research*, Appendix 1-1-1-143. US DHEW Publ. No. (05) 77 0001

Weissman, MM, Prusoff, BA and Klerman, GL (1978) Application of Life Table. Method to Naturalistic Designs a Comparison of Efficacy of Tricyclic Antidepressants and Benzodiazepines in Ambulatory Depressives. *Comprehensive Psychiatry, 19*, 1, 27–36

Weissman, MM and Kasal, SV (1976) Help-seeing in Depressed Out-Patients Following Maintenance Therapy. *British Journal of Psychiatry, 129*, 252–260

Weissman MM, Prusoff, BA, Hanson, B and Paykel, ES (1974) Treatment Effects on the Social Adjustment of Depressed Patients. *Archives of General Psychiatry, 30*, 771–778

Weissman. MM. Prusoff, BA and Pincus, C (1977) Symptom Patterns in Primary and Secondary Depression. *Archives of General Psychiatry, 34*, 854–862

Weissman. MM. Prusoff, BA, Dimascio, A, Neu, C, Goklaney, M and Klerman, G (1979) The Efficacy of Drugs and Psychotherapy in the Treatment of Acute Depressive Episodes. *American Journal of Psychiatry, 135*, 555–558

Wheatley, D (1972) Potentiation of Amitriptyline by Thyroid Hormone. *Archives of General Psychiatry, 26*, 229 333

Wheatley, D (1972) Evaluation of Psychotropic Drugs in General Practice. *Proceedings of the Royal Society of Medicine, 65*, 317–320

Whyte. SF, Macdonald, AJ, Naylor, GJ and Moody, JP (1976) Plasma Concentrations of Protriptyline and Clinical Effects in Depressed Women. *British Journal of Psychiatry, 128*, 384 390

Willcox DRC, Gillan, R and Hare, EH (1965) Do Psychiatric Out-Patients take their Drugs? *British Medical Journal, 2*, 790–792

Williams P (1978) Physical Ill-Health and Psychotropic Drug Prescription – A Review. *Psychological Medicine, 8*, 683–693

Wing, JK (1976) A Technique for Studying Psychiatric Morbidity in In-Patient series and in General Population Samples. *Psychological Medicine, 6*, 665–71

Wirz-Justice, A, Puhringer, W and Hole, G (1976) Sleep Deprivation and Clomipramine in Engodenous Depression. *Lancet*

Wolpe, J (1971) Neurotic Depression: Experimental Analog, Clinical Syndromes and Treatment. *American Journal of Psychotherapy, 25,* 362—368

Woodruff, RA Murphy, GE, Herjanic, M (1967) The Natural History of Affective Disorders. *Journal of Psychological Research, 5,* 255—263

World Health Organisation (1973) *Psychiatry and Primary Medical Care* Copenhagen

CURRENT TRENDS IN SEX THERAPY

Keith Hawton

Introduction

With the publication of the work of Masters and Johnson (1970) there became available a rapid and successful method for treating sexual dysfunctions. Prior to this, sexual problems were viewed by many psychiatrists as having causes deeply-rooted in psychological development. They were only amenable to lengthy psychotherapy, and generally responded poorly to treatment.

Other workers, such as Helen Kaplan (1974), have added their own modifications to the basic Masters and Johnson approach. In this country it has proved possible to adapt the treatment to meet the needs of National Health Service patients (Bancroft, 1975).

As an introduction, the innovations of Masters and Johnson, and how they have been adapted for the N.H.S., will be summarised. Some of the more important developments that have occurred since sex therapy became established will be reviewed, and finally future needs in this field will be considered. (The treatment of sexual deviance will not be included in this review).

The Masters and Johnson Approach

One of the main developments in Masters and Johnson's work is the involvement throughout treatment of both partners, irrespective of whether one or other partner seems to pose the presenting problem. In addition, treatment is provided by two co-therapists, one male and one female. This is intended to ensure sensitivity to both male and female aspects of the problem, to act as a check against biased information, and to allow each of the partners to have a same-sex representative or spokesman.

After initial assessment the couple's problem is formulated with them in a 'round table' session. They are then guided through a carefully structured treatment programme. At first sexual intercourse and touching of genital and breast areas are banned. The partners are asked to take turns at pleasuring each other by general caressing. When this stage of 'sensate focus' is well established the couple proceed to involve the rest of the body areas in pleasuring ('genital sensate focus'). Sexual intercourse is introduced via an intermediate stage of 'vaginal containment' in which the penis is inserted into the vagina for a short while during which time the couple concentrate on pleasurable sensations without moving.

Where appropriate, specific measures are employed. For premature ejaculation, the couple will be instructed in the 'squeeze technique' (Semans, 1956), in which the female partner applies firm pressure to the ball of the glans penis in order to delay ejaculation. A couple where the female has vaginismus will be taught to use graded dilators. For the man with ejaculatory failure his partner will be instructed in the technique of 'super-stimulation' in which she provides vigorous penile stimulation in order to overcome the inhibitory block which is preventing ejaculation.

Masters and Johnson see their clients daily, seven days a week. Couples not living in St. Louis, where their treatment centre is based, are put up in a hotel. Each day the couple report back on how they have got on with their homework tasks. Resolution of the presenting problem is reported to occur after two to three weeks of treatment, sometimes earlier.

A common conception of this approach is that it is based purely on practical procedures. If progress is delayed, various psychotherapeutic techniques are used to resolve the difficulty. In addition, the partners are given detailed instructions on how to communicate, both verbally and non-verbally, about sex and their own sexual needs. Instruction in basic sexology, and education about what the couple might reasonably expect in their sexual relationship, form an integral part of treatment.

Outcome of treatment was reported by Masters and Johnson in terms of failure rates. The overall initial failure rate for 790 individuals was 18.9%. This represented an outstandingly high success rate and, understandably, led to widespread enthusiasm for their approach, both in the U.S.A. and elsewhere.

Sex Therapy in the National Health Service

Shortly after publication of Masters and Johnson's work in 1970, sex therapy began to develop in this country, with modifications to suit the needs of the N.H.S. The approach that has been developed in Oxford is fairly typical.

Instead of daily treatment, patients are seen on a weekly basis, treatment taking, on average, 12–14 sessions over the space of three to four months. Most couples are treated by single therapists, rather than co-therapists. Treatment is carried out by psychiatrists, psychologists, general practitioners, and occasionally by social workers or nurses. It includes many of the

217

components of the Masters and Johnson approach, but is somewhat more flexible. For example, where it seems appropriate, one of the partners might be seen on their own, possibly for several sessions.

The type of referrals are similar in distribution to those reported from elsewhere. However, the results, although reasonably satisfactory, bear little comparison with those obtained by Masters and Johnson. Thus, Bancroft and Coles (1976) found that 37% of couples treated in Oxford had a 'successful outcome' and a further 31% showed 'worthwhile improvement'. Other clinics in this country appear to have similar results (Duddle, 1975; Milne, 1976; Anderton et al, 1976).

Masters and Johnson's results have been the subject of considerable debate. Their patients appear to have been, by and large, intelligent, articulate, fee-paying, and highly motivated. In addition, outcome was classified only in terms of success or failure. Most therapists find that outcome frequently lies somewhere between the two.

Recent Developments

Since successful methods for treating sexual difficulties became established at the beginning of the 1970s there have been a number of further developments. One particularly notable trend has been the increasing attention that is paid to physical factors, both in the aetiology and treatment of sex problems. In addition the range of treatment techniques has expanded, firstly to meet the needs of a wider range of patients, including those without partners and secondly to make treatment more economical.

In considering recent developments, those of psychological and those of a physical nature will largely be considered separately. However it must be stressed that this is a somewhat artificial separation since there is often a closely interwoven relationship between the two.

Psychological Factors

Masters and Johnson (1970), and Kaplan (1974), have provided very thorough descriptions of the psychological factors which may cause and perpetuate sexual problems. Recent developments have largely concerned modifications of the original treatment method, and their evaluation.

Controlled Outcome Studies

The results described so far have not involved comparisons between one treatment and another, or between treatment and no treatment. To date there have been few well-controlled studies of outcome following sex therapy. One such study, reported by Ansari (1976), provided disappointing results. A total of 65 impotent males received one of three treatments:— a) modified Masters and

Johnson therapy, b) chemotherapy with oxazepam, or c) 'non-specific therapy'. No differences were found in outcome for the three groups. However, this study was unsatisfactory on several counts. Allocation of patients was not entirely random, the content of the modified Masters and Johnson technique is unclear, and the assessment procedures used were too non-specific.

Other studies have produced more encouraging results. Mathews et al (1976) in a carefully controlled trial treated 36 couples by one of three methods:— a) weekly Masters and Johnson treatment, b) an abbreviated form of treatment including postal instructions and occasional therapist contact, and c) systematic desensitisation. Although the differences at the end of treatment were modest they suggested that the modified Masters and Johnson treatment was the most beneficial. It is of interest that some of the subjects receiving treatment by postal instructions and occasional therapist contact did very well. Unfortunately, this study did not include a no-treatment control group.

In a study that included such a control group (Munjack et al, 1976) substantial evidence was obtained that treating women with orgasmic dysfunction by behavioural treatment, including homework assignments, was effective. In another study, Obler (1973) compared modified systematic desensitisation with group psychotherapy in the treatment of a range of sexual dysfunctions in a highly selected group of non-psychiatric patients. Eighty-two per cent of the systematic desensitisation group became 'sexually functional' compared with only 10 per cent of both the group therapy and no-treatment control patients.

With the exception of Ansari's trial, the results of controlled outcome studies strongly suggest that the new brief methods of treating sexual dysfunctions are more effective than less specific treatments, or no treatment at all.

Single Therapists

A male/female co-therapist team was said by Masters and Johnson to be necessary for the treatment of sexual problems. However, there is little evidence to support this contention. The controlled study of Mathews et al (1976) included both single and co-therapists. A trend favouring better outcome for those couples treated by dual therapists was found but this was not significant. In the National Marriage Guidance Council Marital Sexual Dysfunction Project (Barkla, 1977) no differences were found in outcome between patients treated by single and co-therapy procedures. On empirical grounds there appears to be no justification for using co-therapists for most couples. However, it is conceivable that a dual-therapist team might be advantageous for some, for example those with problems in their general relationship or where both partners experience dysfunctions.

Masturbation Training for Female Orgasmic Dysfunction

Masters and Johnson emphasised the notion of concentrating on erotic sensations while allowing sexual arousal to develop spontaneously. In the treatment of female dysfunction through masturbation training this philosophy has been challenged. This treatment was introduced by LoPiccolo and Lobitz (1972). Their nine-step masturbation programme includes visual examination of the genital region by the woman using a mirror, Kegel's (1952) exercises to improve tone in the pelvic musculature (particularly the muscles involved in orgasm), and tactile exploration of the genitals. The woman locates and stimulates sensitive areas in order to produce pleasure, this leading on to masturbation using a lubricant jelly. The woman is also encouraged to read erotic material and employ sexual fantasies to enhance arousal. Where difficulty in achieving orgasm is still experienced she is encouraged to use a vibrator. Some women are advised to role-play orgasm as a means of overcoming fear of loss of control.

When orgasm can be obtained through masturbation the woman is taught how to generalise this to a relationship if she has a partner. She teaches her partner how she masturbates so that he can take over. Finally, he is taught to stimulate her manually, or with a vibrator during intercourse. Lobitz and LoPiccolo (1972) reported 100 per cent success with their first thirteen women with primary orgasmic dysfunction, their criterion of success being attainment of orgasm on at least 50 per cent of occasions of intercourse.

Although masturbation therapy is particularly useful for the woman without a partner, it is also used as an adjunct to treatment of couples. Riley and Riley (1978), in this country, found that significantly greater success, in terms of orgasmic frequency, resulted from a directed masturbation programme combined with instruction in sensate focus and supportive psychotherapy, compared with sensate focus and supportive psychotherapy alone. Couples were randomly assigned to the two treatment conditions. Ninety per cent of women in the experimental group and 53 per cent of the control group were orgasmic by some means at the end of treatment. Eighty-five per cent and 47 per cent respectively were orgasmic during intercourse on three-quarters of occasions. Six out of eight women who had not been orgasmic in the control group became orgasmic during a subsequent directed masturbation programme. All the women who had become orgasmic during treatment continued to be so at the 12 month follow-up.

Group Treatment

Another notable diversion from Masters and Johnson's original programme has been treatment of patients in groups. This has economic advantages over couple therapy and may be particularly useful for patients without partners.

Group treatment has been used for women with orgasmic problems. Lonnie Barbach (1974) has described the approach used in her 'pre-orgasmic' groups.

Each group consists of six or seven women and two female co-therapists who meet twice weekly for 1½ hours at a time over a five week period. After discussion of the factors that have led to each of the group members' problems the women are instructed in homework exercises based on Lobitz and LoPiccolo's nine-step masturbation programme. Educational reading material is suggested. During the course of treatment, a film of female masturbation is shown to demystify the nature of orgasm. During the first few sessions, group members follow a standard programme; this is later individually tailored to each woman's needs.

Of the first 83 women treated, over 90 per cent had become orgasmic with masturbation by the end of ten sessions. Seventeen orgasmic women were followed up eight months after termination of their group treatment (Wallace and Barbach, 1974). All continued to be orgasmic. Sixteen of these women had partners and all but two of the women were orgasmic on at least some occasions with them. It should be emphasised that the women in these groups were largely self-selected.

In another report of the same approach (Leiblum and Ersner-Hershfield, 1977) rather poor generalisation of orgasm to partner stimulation or intercourse was found. The authors questioned whether orgasm through coitus alone was a reasonable goal. They also emphasised the need for involving the partner where there is evidence of his having a sexual problem.

Nevertheless, it does seem that group treatment for non-orgasmic women admirably meets the needs of some patients and is being tried in this country. In Oxford there have been two groups of women treated by similar methods to those described; 60 per cent have become orgasmic by the end of treatment. Patients with psychiatric disorders appeared to have a poor outcome.

Groups have also been used successfully in the treatment of premature ejaculation, both for couples, (Kaplan et al, 1974) and for men without partners (Zilbergeld, 1975). Zeiss et al (1978) reported treatment of two small groups each consisting of three males with premature ejaculation. Two male therapists conducted the groups. All the participants had partners and were expected to relay instructions to them. Although the outcome was reasonable, these authors also warned of the dangers of offering this type of treatment to all such patients.

Economically, group treatments are a major advance, but there should be cautious assessment of individual patients to determine those who might benefit most from this approach. Many patients will be unwilling to discuss their personal lives with others. In addition, group treatment is unlikely to be successful for an individual who is involved in a difficult relationship or where the partner has a sexual problem.

Biofeedback

Some interest has been shown in biofeedback as a possible treatment for sexually dysfunctional individuals who lack partners. Rosen (1977) demonstrated that normal male volunteers were able to suppress erections effectively with biofeedback while listening to tape recorded erotic material. Biofeedback also appeared to be effective in facilitating erection, although there was no control for increased comfort in the experimental situation.

Csillag (1976) gave six impotent patients and six volunteer controls 'treatment' in which erectile response to erotic fantasy and erotic pictures, both with and without feedback, were recorded. There were sixteen sessions over the space of eight days. The control subjects responded well at first but their responses gradually decreased over the sixteen sessions, perhaps due to boredom. However, the impotent subjects' responses, which at first were poor, gradually increased. There was some evidence for generalisation of these gains to real life situations. However this study did not distinguish a specific effect of biofeedback from other possible factors.

As Rosen (1977) has suggested, since impotence is often associated with strong interpersonal conflicts, it is unlikely that biofeedback will play a major role in the treatment of sexually dysfunctional men. There is considerable doubt whether treatment gains in the laboratory will transfer to the real life situation, and biofeedback may itself actually increase performance anxiety. So far, there have been no reports of the use of biofeedback for sexual problems in females, presumably because methods of measuring their physiological arousal were unavailable until very recently.

Predictive Factors

Finally, in the consideration of psychological aspects of treatment, there remains the important question of how we can predict who is likely to do well with sex therapy and who will do badly. There is a paucity of such information, although gradually some factors predictive of outcome are being clarified.

It seems that when patients have major psychiatric problems in additon to their sexual disorders, prognosis is likely to be poor, at least when treated by brief sex therapy methods (Myer et al, 1972; Lansky and Davenport, 1975; O'Connor, 1976).

Another important factor is the extent to which couples are experiencing marital discord. Some therapists (McGovern et al, 1975; Fordney-Settlage, 1975) have emphasised the need to resolve matital conflicts if successful outcome of the sexual problem is to occur. Whitehead and Mathews (1977) showed that outcome is also related to the extent to which the partners find each other 'sexually attractive'.

We have little information regarding other predictive factors. O'Connor (1976), in a review of possible factors, made some suggestions that warrant further examination. One was that once over the age of 40, males are likely to do worse the older they get. Another was that the longer the symptoms have persisted the worse the outcome is likely to be, particularly for females. He also suggested that males generally either do well or badly with treatment, whereas females show a greater tendency for partial improvement. Presumably the most likely explanation, if this is true, would be that a female with a partially resolved problem would be able to engage in intercourse, whereas a male with a similar degree of dysfunction might not, because of mechanical factors.

Physical Factors

Over the past few years greater attention has been paid to physical factors in both the aetiology and treatment of sexual problems. This has probably been related to growing awareness of the diversity of individuals with sexual problems, including those not amenable to primarily psychological methods of treatment. Particular attention has been paid to hormonal factors. In addition, we have learned more about the role drug treatments may have in causing sexual difficulties, and about the sexual problems of the physically disabled.

Hormones

The technical difficulties involved in hormonal assays and their conflicting results have meant that our understanding of the role of hormones in the causation of sexual problems remains both confused and somewhat rudimentary. As a result the effects of hormonal treatments are even less well understood. Nearly all studies of hormonal causes of sexual dysfunction and their treatment have involved males.

a) *Testosterone*. Consideration of the relationship between testosterone and male sexual disorders illustrates the current state of confusion. Plasma testosterone levels in impotent men have been found to be either normal (Lawrence and Swyer, 1974) or low (Raboch et al, 1975). Testosterone response to administration of human chorionic gonadotrophin in impotent males was found to be low in one study (Ismail et al, 1970), and normal in another (Delitala et al, 1977). One reason for the contradictory results may be that impotence has been treated as a homogenous phenomenon in these studies. Hormonal factors are likely to be more important in impotence of gradual onset, particularly where this is associated with decline in sexual interest. There has been some experimental support for this notion (Ismail et al, 1970; Cooper et al, 1970) but also some contradictory results (Racey et al, 1970).

Studies of the effects of treating male sexual dysfunctions with androgens have also produced conflicting findings. As long ago as 1944, Heller and Myers reported that older impotent men with low testosterone and raised gonadotrophin levels improved with androgen treatment. The results of other studies of testosterone therapy for impotence have been more equivocal. Positive effects were claimed by Bruhl and Leslie (1963) and by Jacobvits (1970), but both on the basis of poorly designed studies. Cooper et al (1973) found only a small transient effect of testosterone. In all three studies relatively low doses of hormone were used.

Clearly much work is required in this area, firstly to delineate appropriate sub-groups of impotent males, including those with androgen insufficiency, and secondly to assess which of these sub-groups are likely to respond to androgen replacement. In addition we need to know the effects of androgen therapy combined with counselling because, even if impotence were due to lowered androgen concentrations, there are likely to be secondary psychological effects that may persist even when androgen levels return to normal.

b) *Gonadotrophins*. Where testicular failure has caused impotence, gonadotrophin levels, especially LH, are likely to be high. However, low testosterone levels are often accompanied by low gonadotrophin levels which then suggests a central cause such as a deficiency of luteinizing hormone releasing-hormone (LH-RH) production. Mortimer et al (1974) found that LH-RH treatment of hypogonadal males with hypothalamic or pituitary lesions resulted in improved sexual responsiveness, even before circulating androgens increased.

Two other studies of LH-RH treatment of impotence have been reported (Benkert et al, 1975; Davis et al, 1976) both having unimpressive results. However, neither controlled for pre-treatment hormonal levels. It is likely that LH-RH will be effective in some cases.

c) *Prolactin*. Recently there has been much interest in the possible role of prolactin in male sexual dysfunctions. Hyperprolactinaemia can result from a number of causes including pituitary tumours and phenothiazine medication. Franks et al (1978) investigated 29 males with raised serum prolactin levels and pituitary tumours and found a complete lack of libido and impotence in 17, impaired libido and potency in six, and normal sexual functioning in the remaining six. In nearly all of those with impotence serum testosterone was low, but this was only found in one of those with normal potency. Where prolactin levels returned to normal as a result of treatment serum testosterone rose and potency returned. Failure of potency to return was associated with persisting hyperprolactinaemia.

The role of prolactin in the aetiology of impotence is obscure. It may have a central effect on gonadotrophin release. However, in spite of our lack of understanding of the possible relationship between hyperprolactinaemia and impotence, there has been a small spate of studies of bromocriptine treatment for this condition. Bromocriptine is an ergot alkaloid that inhibits prolactin release from the pituitary.

Bromocriptine treatment of impotence has so far had a doubtful and brief career. It has been reported in two poorly designed studies as having no useful action. In the study reported by Cooper (1977), increasingly large doses of bromocriptine, eventually combined with an androgen, were given to a series of males with 'non-pscychogenic' impotence. However, prolactin levels were not evaluated at the outset so it is uncertain whether any patients suffered from hyperprolactinaemia. Ambrosi et al (1977) found no significant difference between patients treated with the active drug or those receiving placebo. However, although serum testosterone and prolactin levels were measured, nearly all subjects had normal prolactin levels at the outset. In an uncontrolled study reported by Thorner and Besser (1977) bromocriptine treatment resulted in restoration of potency in 19 out of 23 impotent males with hyperprolactinaemia.

A well controlled study of bromocriptine therapy in appropriate patients is now needed. Ideally this should include comparison of patients with markedly high prolactin and lowered testosterone levels and those with mildly elevated levels of prolactin and normal testosterone. It is likely that bromocriptine may only be of use in the former.

At present we have very little information about the role hormones might play in either the aetiology and/or treatment of sexual dysfunctions in females.

The possible effects of the contraceptive pill on female sexual functioning are very uncertain. In the report of the Royal College of General Practitioners' Study (1974) a four-fold frequency of impaired sexual functioning was found in pill users compared with controls. However, the difficulty in unravelling physiological from psychological effects was made clear. It has been suggested, for example, that sexual side effects of the pill may be secondary to mood changes (Cullburg, 1973).

There have been several reports indicating that increased sexual interest in the female may result from androgen treatments for medical conditions (Shorr et al, 1938; Greenblatt et al, 1942; Solomon and Geist, 1943).

Although there have been no systematic trials of testosterone therapy alone for impaired female libido, a recent study in Oxford (Carney et al, 1978) suggested that testosterone treatment, when combined with psychosexual counselling, was more effective than diazepam plus counselling. An unlikely explanation of this result might have been that diazepam actually impaired sexual interest. Further research of the effects of testosterone therapy in female unresponsiveness is required before this can be justifiably incorporated into clinical practice.

Now that hormone replacement therapy for post-menopausal women is so much in vogue, one awaits systematic evaluation of its effects where there is impaired sexual functioning. It would be surprising if beneficial effects were not found if only because of the well-established effects of oestrogen therapy on the post-menopausal vaginal mucosa (Campbell and Whitehead, 1977).

Two final comments must be made concerning the possible relationships between hormones and sexual dysfunctions. Firstly, in future studies a careful distinction needs to be made between effects of hormones on sexual interest and on sexual performance as these are likely to differ. Secondly, although most of the work in this field has been based on the assumption that changes in sexual attitudes and behaviour can result from changes in hormone levels, there may well be a strong two-way relationship between them. That is, sexual attitudes and behaviour may also influence hormone levels.

Physical Handicap and Side-Effects of Medication

A vast group of patients whose sexual problems have been neglected until recently are the physically disabled. In a study carried out by the Committee on Sexual Problems of the Disabled it was found that over 50 per cent of disabled people experienced sexual problems (Stewart, 1975). Unfortunately there was no control group of non-disabled persons for comparison.

There is growing awareness of the types of problems that disabled people face and an increasing amount of literature giving guidance on their management, Heslinga's 'Not Made of Stone' (1974) being an excellent example. It has been pointed out (Stewart, 1978) that although the solutions to these problems are often extremely simple, the main difficulties lie in the lack of awareness amongst staff caring for the disabled and the inhibitions of staff and patients preventing their introduction. Fortunately it seems that the situation is undergoing radical change at present.

Sexual aids may have a place in the treatment of sexual problems of both the disabled and the non-disabled but are in need of careful evaluation. The use of vibrators in treatment of female orgasmic dysfunction has already been mentioned. A penile ring of electro-galvanic plates has been advocated in the treatment of impotence but has not proved any more effective than a 'placebo' penile ring (Cooper, 1974).

However, penile prostheses have undergone some promising evaluation (Mallor and Von Eschenbach, 1977; Furlow, 1978). Inflatable penile prostheses can be surgically implanted in patients with irreversible impotence. It appears that 90 per cent of such patients are pleased with the appearance and performance of the prosthesis. However, approximately a quarter develop complications requiring further operations.

It often proves difficult to distinguish whether impotence is due to a psychological or an organic cause. Observations of the pattern of nocturnal erections has been recently suggested as one reliable method (Fisher et al, 1975; Karacan et al, 1977). Nocturnal erections are closely associated with REM sleep in normal males (Fisher et al, 1965). Karacan and colleagues (1977) claimed that in a sample of over 2,000 males with normal sexual function all exhibited normal nocturnal erections. In a high proportion of males with impotence, they found impaired nocturnal erections and in most were able to identify an organic cause (Karacan et al, 1975). A series of diabetics with impotence had abnormal nocturnal erectile patterns compared with both impotent subjects without

226

medical disorders and normal controls (Karacan et al, 1977). Evaluation of the pattern of erections during sleep seems a rather cumbersome assessment procedure but might prove of use in impotent patients where, after using more traditional methods of assessment, there remain doubts as to whether the problem is of psychogenic or organic origin.

We are becoming increasingly aware of the extent to which medication, prescribed for both physical and psychological disorders, may influence sexual functioning, and the need for taking a careful history of drug usage when assessing patients with sexual problems. Drugs may affect both libido and sexual performance. Libido may be impaired by tranquillisers, some anti-hypertensives, and anti-convulsants. Their effects may be due to sedation, a central inhibitory effect, or both (Kaplan, 1974; Turner, 1978).

Anti-convulsants, particularly phenytoin, may also reduce the levels of free circulating testosterone by induction of sex hormone binding globulin (Victor et al, 1977; Baragry et al, 1978). A high incidence of impotence has been reported in male epileptic patients on anti-convulsants (Christiansen et al, 1975), such patients showing decreased excretion of androgens (Luhdorf et al, 1977).

It has been known for some time that major tranquillisers may impair ejaculatory function due to anti-adrenergic effects. Thioridazine may cause dry ejaculation through paralysis of the internal sphincters of the bladder with resultant retrograde emission into the bladder. Both MAOI and tricyclic antidepressants may have mild effects on erectile and ejaculatory functions as a result of anti-cholinergic and anti-adrenergic activity respectively. Finally, there is some evidence that Lithium may occasionally impair potency (Vinarova et al, 1972).

The wide range of medication which can affect sexual function highlights the importance of ruling out such a cause before starting sex therapy proper. If practical, the medication can be changed or stopped, the patient reassured, and the re-assessment carried out after a suitable time period to check that normal sexual functioning has been restored.

Conclusions

Although our current methods of treating sexual difficulties only generally became available at the beginning of the 1970s there have clearly been considerable developments in sex therapy since then. There is now no doubt that the brief behavioural methods of treatment are relatively effective. Recent work has mostly been concerned with finding more economical ways of providing treatment and with the development of a wider range of approaches in order to meet the diverse needs of patients.

Treatment in groups has obvious economic advantages but it is unlikely to suit more than a minority of patients in this country, at least for the present. For most couples with sex problems treatment by a therapist working on his or her own is probably as effective as two therapists working together. We are now in a better position to help patients, particularly females, who do not have partners.

What are likely future developments? The current interest in physical factors in both the causation and treatment of sexual problems will certainly continue in parallel with improvements in hormone assay techniques and the development of greater understanding of the hormonal basis of sexual interest and response.

The pattern of sex problems referred is likely to change. Already some sex therapists, including Masters and Johnson (1977), have noted that the proportion of relatively simple problems being referred has declined. There may be more than one explanation, for example changes in sexual attitudes and education, or improved treatment of sexual problems by general practitioners. In addition, a number of self-help books have recently appeared based on the new treatment methods (e.g. Barbach, 1975; Heiman et al, 1976; Brown and Faulder, 1977). It is difficult to know how effective these are, or whether they are used, but presumably individuals with less difficult problems would be the most likely to benefit from them.

There are several areas that should prove fruitful for future research. The interaction of drug treatment with counselling is one. We need to know more about the factors which predict treatment outcome. Finally, we are relatively ignorant as to the long-term durability of changes resulting from sex therapy.

COMMENTARY ON CURRENT TRENDS IN SEX THERAPY

Maurice Yaffe

Introduction

Dr. Hawton's paper is an excellent account of the state of the art of sex therapy today and, as he points out, to a large extent *art* it still is. In a recent comprehensive review of the literature on the treatment of sexual dysfunction Wright et al (1977) at McGill could only find eighteen outcome studies which made a criterion sample size of ten or more, and only three of these, using directive sex therapies (Ansari, 1976; Wincze and Caird, 1976; and Obler, 1973) qualified as controlled studies. For some reason the British Oxford Group Study (Mathews et al., 1976) and the one Paul Brown conducted for the National Marriage Guidance Council (Barkla, 1977) were not cited.

I want to discuss what I believe are eleven central issues concerning sex therapy that arise out of Dr. Hawton's paper, but before doing so I wish to dispel the misconception some may have that treatment for sexual problems is rather at the luxury end of the market, that those presenting with such problems are really not ill, and that perhaps the therapy should not be available on the NHS. Firstly, those presenting with problems in the psychosexual domain are usually suffering and/or causing concern to their partner (if they have one), just as are those with other kinds of difficulties. Secondly, good sexual relationships generally provide stabilising influences on a marriage; and thirdly, parents who have a good sex life generally transmit this to their children, implicitly or otherwise and indicate to them that they (both parents and children) need time for themselves. This has the general effect of reducing the communication and potential learning of conservative and rigid sexual attitudes, and even the likelihood of incestuous practices. Furthermore, offering psycho-sexual help enables some groups, for example the physically disabled, to have sexual activity and thereby to some extent overcome their disability. It is also very cheap compared with some other therapies. Though

Dr. Hawton chose not to include the treatment of sexual deviation in his review, it is necessary to mention that the sex therapist from time to time is called upon to help individuals to cope with expressions of a deviant sexual interest, usually of a transvestite or homosexual nature (for example, Latham and White, 1978), within a heterosexual marriage. My own experience indicates that given a relationship where there is basic caring for each other and motivation for change on the part of the person with the deviant interest, the preferred therapeutic approach is that of improving heterosexual function within the relationship, followed if necessary, by self-control of unwanted sexual behaviour; however, incorporation of the paraphiliac interest within the shared sexual activity of the couple, i.e. positive adaptation to the deviant role, may be a feasible alternative (e.g. Bancroft, 1979), especially so in fetishistic transvestitism.

As Trimmer (1979) points out, the treatment of sexual dysfunction 'presents a persistent difficulty for we do not really know what "normal", "healthy", "adequate", or "inadequate" sexual behaviour really is, and we have therefore, adopted a patient-centred definition of the problem'. He states that 'a sex problem exists when an individual expresses a complaint about one or more cognitive, affective, or behaviour elements of sexual functioning or sexual relations'. But what are these and how extensive are they? Dr. Hawton assumes that we all know.

Incidence/Prevalence

Levin and Levin (1975) studied workers in the US and discovered that 12–18% wives married for less than a year were dissatisfied with their sex life. In this country similar figures were obtained by Thorns and Collard (1979) i.e. 12–21% of wives were initially sexually dissatisfied, but sexual difficulties rarely precipitate marital disruption (Dominian, 1979) though continuing absence of orgasm or pleasure is likely gradually to erode the relationship. Frank et al (1978) in Pittsburg examined the frequency of sexual problems experienced of 100 predominantly white, well educated, and happily married couples who responded to a self-report questionnaire, and related them to sexual satisfaction. They found that although over 40% of the men reported erectile or ejaculatory dysfunction, and 63% of the women reported arousal or orgasmic dysfunction, 50% of the men and 77% of the women reported difficulty that was not dysfunctional in nature (for example, lack of interest or inability to relax); interestingly, the number of 'difficulties' reported was more strongly and consistently related to overall sexual dissatisfaction than the number of 'dysfunctions'. In a study of the marital sexual enjoyment and frustration of 59 professional men in the Eastern United States, Heath (1978) found an association between increasing sexual frustration, i.e. dissatisfaction, and what he calls 'psychological unhealthiness', interpersonal immaturity, inadequate marital communication, and marital unhappiness.

A very recent study of Swan and Wilson (1979) was designed to identify those patients referred to a psychiatric out-patient clinic in north-east England who had sexual or marital difficulties and who could be offered help with their problems; none of the patients had been referred primarily for sexual or marital therapy, but 12% had such difficulties and were offered treatment.

The pattern of presenting problems is apparently changing. Ginsberg et al (1972) suggests there is an increase in the number of complaints of erectile problems among younger men in the US and puts this down to demands made upon men for sexual satisfaction by members of the Women's Liberation movement. On the other hand US women's complaints seem to have changed from 'frigidity', problems of finding husbands, and difficulties in raising children (in the 1950s) to conflict about professional versus personal identity, divorce, and extra-marital affairs (in the 1970s) according to Moulton (1977).

Assessment and Classification

Classification

Dr. Hawton does not spell out the range of specific dysfunctions in his paper, but these can be divided usefully into *disorders of performance* that prevent or significantly alter functioning during the sexual cycle, and *disorders of satisfaction* that decrease enjoyment during the sexual cycle. In men disorders of performance include erectile and ejaculatory (premature, retarded, *and retrograde) problems;* both can be *primary* i.e. dysfunction always present, or *secondary,* i.e. disturbed function was once intact, and can be *partial* or *complete.*

In women disorders of performance include *dyspareunia* (pelvic or vaginal discomfort/pain associated with penetration and intercourse, and *vaginismus* (a spasm of the perivaginal musculature making penetration difficult if not impossible).

Disorders of satisfaction in men include *split orgasm* (emission without ejaculation — semen leaks from the urethera) and *orgasm without pleasure* (emission and ejaculation but no concomitant pleasurable sensation). In women these dysfunctions include *general sexual dysfunction* (no vasocongestive genital response or subjective erotic feeling); *sexual anaesthesia* (lubrication without the feeling of arousal or enjoyment); and *anorgasmia* (the inability to reach orgasm though sexual arousal is present).

Money (1977) classifies problems of human sexuality into too little (hypophilia); too much (hyperphilia) and too peculiar (paraphilia); he explains that these difficulties develop at specific stages of the three phases of sexual or erotic pair-bonding the *proceptive* (when solicitation and attraction occurs), *acceptive* (physical receptiveness and activity between partners) and *conceptive* (the non-invariable sequel to the previous phases).

Hypophilias and paraphilias have been studied extensively but hyperphilias

231

appear to have been neglected despite the fact that quite a number of husbands and probably some wives put excessive demands on their partners.

There are also some common interpersonal problems that generate dysphoric feelings and interfere with sexual functioning (Redmond, 1978).

1. *Ambivalent commitment to relationship.* Occurs commonly when one partner wants greater intimacy and the other withdraws.
2. *Incongruency between fantasy and reality.* Concern, protection, and care-taking; when dissonant needs between partners can lead to resentment.
3. *Competition.* Competitiveness, for example, who should reach orgasm first, can lead to deterioration of the physical relationship.

Assessment

Dr. Hawton indicates that "evaluation of the pattern of erections during sleep seems a rather cumbersome assessment procedure" but Rosen and Keefe (1978), Fisher et al (1979), and Karacan et al (1978) indicate nocturnal penile tumescence recording is an important and straightforward procedure for the differential diagnosis of erectile problems, especially for the diabetic.

In addition to improved psychophysiological assessment procedures for the male, Hatch (1979) reviews the contribution of vaginal photoplethysmographic procedures for measuring physiological sexual arousal in the female; these recent developments represent an important source of information previously unavailable.

A full review of assessment procedures for measuring both sexual behaviour and arousal patterns (Barlow, 1977) indicates the complexity of this rapidly growing field. Derogatis and Meyer (1979) assessed the psychological characteristics of 47 male and 40 female dysfunctional patients cf. 200 heterosexual normals, using the authors' Sexual Functioning Inventory. They found significant differences between dysfunctionals and normals: both male and female patients showed higher levels of psychological distress and dysphoric affect than normals and also revealed decrements on sexual information.

Particularly noteworthy among male dysfunctionals were lowered sex drive levels and a constricted repertoire of sexual experiences. Male dysfunctionals also revealed gender role definitions less polarised in the masculine direction. Compared to their male counterparts female patients were assessed to be more creative and less constrained in their sexual activities. The authors conclude that sexually dysfunctional patients do maintain a characteristic psychological profile, but one distinct for males and females. Interestingly, in the Maudsley Study (Stoll — personal communication) of their series of over 190 couples 63% of the male presenters had a partner with a dysfunctional problem and so did 59.2% of the female presenters, and the suggestion is that a proportion of these select dysfunctional partners in the first place, and they sometimes attempt to sabotage treatment.

Physical Factors

Dr. Hawton has covered this section very thoroughly and I would endorse his recommendation to conduct controlled trials on androgen effects in dysfunctional males and females both with and without counselling in order to tease out the contribution of each, as well as to provide support to patients who are left with residual psychological sequelae after hormone levels are adjusted in those where they were found to be deficient.

As far as psychotropic drug effects on sexual functioning are concerned recent reviews by Barnes et al (1979) and in the BMT (Editorial 1979) make a plea for their careful use especially in hypertension, epilepsy, depression, and psychosis, particularly phenothiazines.

The contraceptive pill has been shown to lead to a reduction of female-initiated sexual activity at ovulation (Adams et al, 1978) and must be taken into account when prescribing and assessing dysfunctions. Moreover, recent information from Denmark (Wagner – personal communication) indicates that primary complete erectile dysfunction may be due to the presence of an arteriovenous fistula communicating with the corpora cavernosa and spongiosum. Regarding the physically disabled a new social group has started in London called the Outsiders Club which teaches sex education and offers therapeutic advice to those without partners.

Sexual Dysfunction and Psychopathology

Crisp (1979) presents a formulation of sexual pathology as it presents in the psychiatric clinic of a general hospital and gives illustrations of how biological, social, and experimental aspects of sex come to be disturbed either primarily or secondarily. He lists four categories of mechanisms involving diet, affect, personality, fantasy, and human relationships. In the first, body image considerations in the obese and anorexic affect subjective estimations of attractiveness and availability of partners; in the second, amenorrhea in a woman who had experienced incest at age 9; in the third, patients who presented with pre-menstrual tension, agoraphobia, and a sleep disturbance – all with underlying inter-personal and sexual conflicts; in the fourth, he describes disturbance of sexual experience and behaviour as consequences of, or part of, psychiatric illness – especially when those with high levels of anxiety or with severe depressive illness are judged, compared to other diagnostic categories, to be less sexually active than before their illness.

McFalls (1979) documents the relationship between psychological stress and coital inability with respect to erectile problems, vaginismus, and dyspareunia. According to McFalls psychological stress is the single most important cause of coital inability; this tends to have a much greater impact on an individual's fecundity than do many conceptive-failure and pregnancy-less factors, which as he indicates, may simply lower the probability of conception and successful pregnancy. In a study cited by McFalls (Stallworthy) of 1000 infecund married couples 5% of the women were virgins.

Controlled Trials of Treatment

In addition to those cited by Dr. Hawton there are several other studies that throw some light on effectiveness of various therapeutic approaches on the treatment of the dysfunctions. Kockott (1973) found Masters and Johnson therapy superior to desensitisation in cases of erectile insufficiency but Everaerd (1976) for the same complaint, found the two procedures equal in effectiveness. McMullen and Rosen (1976) found explicit sexual films no better than explanatory handouts for anargasmia; and Kilmann (1979) in a review suggests useful hypotheses for future orgasmic dysfunction research.

For general dysfunction Crowe (1978) found Masters and Johnson treatment with behavioural marital therapy superior to supportive marital therapy, and for these problems Crowe et al (1979) and Arentewicz (1978) found two therapists better than one. Whereas Crowe et al showed that Masters and Johnson therapy is no better than behaviour marital therapy with relaxation, Arentewicz (1978) obtained no differences between long-term and short-term therapy.

Munjack and Kanno (1979) indicate that to date no controlled trials have been conducted on evaluating appropriate treatment procedure for retarded ejaculation and their impression is that it is either more common than previously assumed or is increasing in frequency.

Kilmann and Auerbach (1979) in a critical review of the literature on treatment of premature ejaculation and psychogenic impotence indicate that the studies which used systematic desensitisation and those which assessed the extensive retraining programmes reported the most consistently positive results. Dr. Hawton dismisses the usefulness of co-therapy over using a single therapist.

The value in using two therapists rather than one is twofold: in order to train a junior therapist, and to exchange views enabling continuous active review of cases.

Group Treatment

Group procedures have been shown to be effective for couples with mixed sexual dysfunctions without severe marital discord (Leiblum et al, 1976); individuals without available partners, for women (e.g. Sotice and Kilmann, 1978) and for men with single and mixed dysfunctions i.e. erectile and ejaculatory problems in different individuals (Zilbergeld, 1975, 1978; Lobitz and Baker, 1979); and by Gillan and Yaffe (1979) for both single and mixed dysfunctions i.e. erectile and ejaculatory problems together in the same patients *and* in different members of the same group. However, primary problems may be better directed to a social skills group initially, particularly if the individual has severe heterosexual social skills deficits and/or anxiety. Our experience is *not* that men are unwilling to disclose and discuss their sexual difficulties in a group, as Dr. Hawton suggests might be the case. Furthermore Becker and Watson (personal communications) have successfully conducted a group treatment programme for the treatment of vaginismus: seven weekly sessions, each of an hour's duration — included general sex education and visual aids, relaxation, and homework assignments. By the end of treatment all patients had achieved either full or partial penetration by their partners.

The Use of Sexually Explicit Materials

One interesting therapeutic development that Dr. Hawton does not discuss is the role of sexually explicit materials as an adjunct to other procedures. They usually comprise photographic illustrations, drawings and, most commonly, films, and have a place both in the treatment of sexual dysfunctions (for education, desensitisation, and stimulation therapy) (Reisinger, 1978) and in the treatment of sexual deviations (psycho-physiological assessment of tumescence, aversion therapy — commonly in tranvestitism (Rosen and Kopel, 1977) and in re-conditioning therapy, where there is a paucity of, or weak appropriate, fantasies (Keller and Goldstein, 1978) as, for example, in most paedophiles.

Basically two different modes of presentation have been used: massed and spaced (Bjorksten, 1976); the former utilises a 'workshop' format and the latter divides exposure to materials into stages that are separated by a longer period of time. The rationale for using massed presentations is to bombard individuals over a short period of time with explicit sexual imagery with a view to producing desensitisation to material so that participants are more comfortable with their own sexual thoughts and with discussion of sexual topics. This is the method of the Sexual Attitude Re-Structuring programme of the National Sex Forum, San Francisco (Glide Foundation, 1971). On the other hand, spaced presentations tend to be used as part of on-going therapy (individual or group) as a demonstration rather than as a way of changing anxiety levels or attitudes. Examples of this approach include: illustration of sex education lectures to medical students (Stanley, 1977); demonstration of anatomical models to patients in order to teach them accurately about the structure of genitalia; teaching therapists and patients specific techniques, e.g. massage exercises, the squeeze technique, and about various coital positions; and showing scenes to individuals who have a paucity of fantasies.

Indications for the therapeutic use of sexually explicit materials include: inability to discuss sexual matters using specific terms due to inhibition; anxiety about sexual behaviour and about having sexual fantasies; paucity of sexual fantasies; excessively restrictive conservative attitudes about ones own sexual behaviour; sexual naivety and ignorance; unrealistic expectations of sexual performance in self or partner; sexual identity confusion; sexual enrichment of couples with no specific dysfunction, e.g. the 'humdrum' marriage; and for couples with communication difficulties.

Sexually explicit materials are poorly tolerated by psychotics, especially where paranoid features are in evidence, in severe depression accompanied by feelings of performance inadequacy, and in those with a strong, non-defensive, moral indignation, and are therefore contra-indicated in therapy. Sexually explicit materials have a definite place as an adjunct to other procedures in sex education and therapy, and Wilson (1978) suggests that this kind of material also has a positive role to play in the prevention of sexual problems.

Cross-Cultural Aspects/Ethnic Factors

There is a wide range of special populations where sexual dysfunction is presented as a problem and Dr. Hawton has dealt with the physically handicapped, who most commonly present with spinal cord injuries, and diabetics with erectile failure. Other groups who are starting to be offered help with their sexual difficulties include the elderly, the pregnant, the post-coronary male, and those in chronic renal failure (Green, 1975; Meyer, 1976). But probably one of the most interesting groups are the ethnic minorities; increasingly we are now seeing West Indians, Africans, Indians, and Pakistanis in our Psycho-Sexual Problems Clinic but relatively few Asians. A literature on how to deal with these patients in an inter-racial treatment situation has now started to appear (e.g. Chipman, 1978) — issues include symbolic meanings of the symptom in the patient's schema, feelings about racial self-image, and the options that allow for individual identity.

Prognostic Factors for Positive Outcome

Dr. Hawton recommends research emphasis should be placed on outcome factors and Stoll (personal communication) on the basis of his Maudsley Study, suggests that positive outcome in sex therapy is directly related to the following: higher socio-economic class, higher education, good non-sexual relationship and commitment to marriage, perceived physical attractiveness of presenter to partner, and good homework ratings. Negative outcome was significantly associated with poor living conditions.

Prevention

Dr. Hawton does not deal with this issue. Qualls et al (1978), in their book which deals solely with prevention of sexual disorders, suggest that "given that there are strong cultural influences on sexual functioning and that these influences affect the prevalence of the dysfunctions (they conservatively estimate that at least 5% of the adult population are sexually dysfunctional at any given time), prevention may be a more appropriate way to promote effective sexual functioning than our present treatment, a remedial effort at best. 'Clearly there are insufficient resources to treat everyone if we so desire.'

Contentious issues here include the accusation of invasion of individual privacy as a result of preventive interventions, the re-distribution of precious medical and para-medical resources, and an implication of re-ordering of social values — even at the level of individual behaviour (viz fitness, smoking and diet). The question of which sexual disorders should be prevented is also of central concern, for example where does homosexuality fit into the picture? Qualls et al (1978) provide some of the answers on how to deal with preventive issues once the political disputes have been resolved.

Ethics

The rights of clients and the responsibilities of therapists is of fundamental importance (Hare-Mustin et al, 1979) especially in the sensitive field of sex therapy (Masters et al, 1977), to which Dr. Hawton does not allude. In a survey of 460 U.S. physicians' attitudes and practices regarding erotic and non-erotic contact with patients, 5–7.2 per cent indicated they engaged specifically in sexual intercourse (Kardener et al, 1973). In a follow-up paper Kardener et al (1976) suggest that the freer a physician is with non-erotic contact with patients, the more statistically likely he is to engage in erotic contact. Holroyd and Brodsky (1977) in their nationwide survey with a 70% return rate found 5.5% male and 0.6% of female licensed PhD psychologists reported having had sexual intercourse with patients and of these 80% repeated it. An additional 2.6% of the males and 0.3% of the females reported having had sexual intercourse with patients within three months after the termination of therapy. Taylor and Wagner (1976) conclude that the majority of therapist-client sexual liaisons have negative effects but they suggest specific ways in which this kind of involvement develops, as well as therapeutic aspects of sexual feelings and fantasies. Perhaps closer to home is the recent U.S. report that 25% of the recent female graduates had had some sexual contact (i.e. genital stimulation or intercourse) with their educators (Pope et al, 1979).

Other ethical issues concern confidentiality of sex clinic files and correspondence, and the question of informal consent regarding research and treatment practices in the sexual area. (Masters et al, 1977), e.g. showing a sexually explicit film.

Future Research and Therapy

I am not so pessimistic as Dr. Hawton regarding the suitability of individuals to join a sex dysfunction group; our experience at Guy's is extremely positive for both men and women (e.g. Gillan & Yaffe, 1979).

I agree with Dr. Hawton that the role of physical factors should become

237

clearer with 'improvements in hormone assay techniques and a greater understanding of the hormonal basis of sexual interest and response'. I also agree with his assessment that the pattern of responses presented is likely to change, but with the advent of sex education procedures for both the health professional (Rosenzweig & Pearsall 1978) and the individual (Wilson, 1978), the next generation should be in a better position to have a balanced view with respect to their sexuality.

Recommendations

1. In future studies it will be necessary to match or balance treatment groups on subject variables: *type*, i.e. primary or secondary, and *extent* of the disorder must be specified; and larger and more homogeneous samples need to be used. Given developments in diagnostic criteria, it is not valid any more to talk of 'frigidity' or 'impotence'. It will be necessary in future to specify the problem as fully as possible on several dimensions (e.g. erectile insufficiency, primary/secondary, difficulty in obtaining/maintaining erections, percentage of full erection obtained during sexual activity, whether it is specific to one partner/all partners, whether it occurs during masturbation, before/during intercourse. Full assessment is critical for different people with the same global classification, e.g. premature ejaculation; they may exhibit subtle differences in the dysfunction and may require different treatments accordingly, i.e. re-education, supportive, or re-training procedures.

2. Lower socio-economic groups are under-represented, and components of therapeutic effectiveness need to be evaluated using component analysis methods.

3. Studies using homosexually-oriented persons with dysfunctions are needed, as are systematic treatment trials of the married bisexual where one partner presents with dysfunctional difficulties.

4. Data needs to be reported on duration of disorder, age of patient, socio-economic status, and cooperativeness of his/her most frequent partner, as well as assessment of the motivation for treatment.

5. Specificity of treatment procedures as to constituent parts is necessary to enable replication attempts, and it is important to use one treatment at a time in order to make useful measurement possible.

6. No-treatment control or control waiting list procedures need to be used to enable comparison with the experimental treatment.

7. Systematic evaluation of different treatments for the same dysfunction need to be determined, and effective therapeutic ingredients of programmes require isolation as some treatment components can have variable importance for different patient types and/or problems. Self-report ratings by patients of

the relative effectiveness of different components of treatment would provide valuable information in this respect.

8. The influence of the therapist-variable on treatment outcome needs to be evaluated; therapist experience and training are often not reported. As a result, more than one therapist should be used for the same treatment format.

9. Method of conducting follow-up assessment of outcome is seldom reported if this takes place at all. It will be necessary to seek verification from *both* sexual partners regarding treatment effects, the partner's validation of the presenters self-reports (and vice versa), and specification of criteria adopted for evaluation of outcome. It would be preferable for each person's treatment goals to be used as outcome criteria.

10. The contribution of treatment to other dimensions of personal adjustment should be assessed both pre and post-treatment using multiple dependent measures, including the standardised interview, sexual knowledge questionnaires, and sexual anxiety questionnaires.

11. It would be useful to know to what extent partner participation is crucial for optimal results, and under what circumstances.

12. Since verbal report, approach behaviour, and physiological responses are often not highly correlated after therapy, physiological measures obtained in response to sexual slides or videotapes can provide important information.

13. It will be necessary to match a specific therapeutic programme to a particular patient (rather than apply the same format to a wide variety of patients) and any future studies of mixed populations will need to identify both the level of non-sexual psychopathology and non-marital sexual functioning.

14. Evaluation of the effectiveness of sex therapies used singly, e.g. in combination with a non-sexual treatment 'package' regardless of theoretical orientation, is necessary for patients who have both sexual and non-sexual psychopathology.

15. It would be useful to conduct a study on the effectiveness of sex therapy alone, as against this procedure in combination with marital therapy, e.g. an operant-interpersonal approach on couples who present with non-sexual marital problems.

16. There is a paucity of long-term follow-up data and a need to assess the durability of treatment procedure outcomes.

17. I would also like to recommend an alternative to conventional massage exercises: Japanese finger acupressure is easy to learn, pleasurable, relaxing, and arousing (Ohashi, 1977).

18. It would be beneficial in order to reduce the drop-out rate to offer patients an immediate assessment interview at the time the referral agent makes his request for the patients to be seen.

19. Alcohol is probably the most commonly used drug affecting sexual function and its role in the aetiology and maintenance of dysfunction needs to be assessed.

20. Perhaps it would be useful to promote non-consummation as a distinct and separate diagnostic entity for it usually brings with it a unique constellation of factors.

21. Most authors consider orgasm as the unit of sex and one necessary criterion for successful therapeutic outcome. This needs to be re-evaluated as it promotes standard setting.

22. I would wholeheartedly recommend increase in the use of Health Centres and G.P. practices for running psycho-sexual problem clinic sessions, rather than the large hospitals — especially Departments of Psychiatry, which are still somewhat stigmatised.

In conclusion I can do no better than quote from Wright et al (1979):

"Tremendous advances have been achieved in the treatment of sexual dysfunction in the last 15 years. There is, however, a clear danger that some of these promising treatment procedures are being applied indiscriminately with inadequately selected populations. The result is that the directive sex-therapies as they are practised on the population at large are probably achieving much lower success rates than is often assumed. And finally, the risk of treatment-provoked deterioration is ever present."

I hope that Dr. Hawton's paper and these comments will help us to move in the right direction in the sensitive area of psycho-sexual problems and their resolution.

COMMENTARY ON CURRENT TRENDS IN SEX THERAPY

Colin Wilson

Keith Hawton's Paper is extremely comprehensive and I'm afraid doesn't leave much unsaid. There is, however, one area of increasing importance in the field of sex therapy which he does not mention; that of the role of the media, which by its very nature, is able to be more effective or more damaging than all the efforts of the medical profession. I have some experience of the media from working both on radio and in magazines, and perhaps my experiences will be of interest.

As a clincian I am primarily concerned with the attitudes of people coming to see me, their expectations as well as their problems and of course, the attitudes of society which change all the time and which mould their thoughts. At times we may all be forgiven for our fears that we are inadequate therapists and that there are new treatment methods that we have never heard of and which our patients assure us other doctors on our doorsteps are practising with amazing results! Sex therapy more than many branches of clinical psychiatry reflects peoples' expectations rather than their actual needs. The media play a vital part in this phenomenon. They never actually cause trends in behaviour to happen but may magnify or speed up a process that is already established. There are many examples of this; one good one being the numerous scares about the contraceptive pill.

Many women are clearly unhappy about altering their bodily functions with chemicals that they see as unnatural. All medical evidence to the contrary does not convince them, neither can they logically accept that it is worth taking the minimal risk of the pill in order to achieve the goal of a trouble-free and pregnancy-free sex life. Because 'the pill' is such an emotive subject the media, especially popular newspapers, exploit each item of obvious news value. Journalese remarks in the press about little publicised preliminary pieces of research may spark off a massive public response. This year's sharp rise in birth rate can largely be blamed on the media accelerating a move away from the pill to less efficient methods of contraception or none at all. If used responsibly,

241

however, the media can promote a sensible attitude to sex and help ordinary people resist extremes.

The involvement of the media in sexual matters has a very long history. The loosening of the stranglehold of the medieval Church on literacy coupled with the rise of the secular universities and the introduction of printing by Caxton into England in 1497 began the process. The use of the broadsheet as a vehicle for public information, however, did not become widespread until the Civil War of 1642 and the problem page first made its appearance as part of the tremendous upsurge in the cultural life of England that occurred in the forty years that followed Cromwell's rule.

On 10th March 1691, John Dunton, a 32 year old Bookseller, 'who spoke of morality, but knew more about sin', launched the Athenian Gazette in London. This was the first device for audience participation in the history of publishing. The range of Dunton's problem pages was far broader than that of a 20th Century agony column with less than half the letters dealing with sex. Alas, even this earliest venture had its critics. Dr. Johnson himself was of the opinion that the letters were not genuine. In fact, Dunton was so overloaded with letters that his Gazette soon became a twice weekly paper. Dunton noticed some phenomena which are still familiar; his correspondents came from widely different social backgrounds and all were interested in obtaining medical advice for two pence that would cost a guinea to obtain from a visit to the doctor!

The first womens' magazine quickly followed; the Ladies Mercury was launched in 1693. This offered more sexual advice to women in the strict moral tone of the time. One is forced to ponder the question of whether these early 'agony columnists' were really fitted to the task. Dunton became insane — possibly as a result of a public whipping he received for 'profanely cursing Queen Anne' — in April 1708. Nevertheless, he continued to pour out his correspondence, even more avidly received than ever, between 1708 and 1711.

The first female agony aunt was Mrs. Eliza Haywood who took over the Female Spectator in 1744 and since that time advice columnists, mainly female, have reflected their times and have been a consistent element in the world of magazines and newspapers, often providing the only source of information and comfort in personal and sexual problems for a large section of the population.

World War II gave the agony column a new lease of life. For 250 years advice columns had counselled people who had nowhere else to turn and 1939 to 1945 was their greatest test. The popularity of the agony column today is a direct legacy of the war years. With the rise of the National Health Service and the advent of free medicine for all the agony column added a new role to its functions, that of a referral agency to the increasing range of voluntary organisations which plugged the gaps in the state system.

The first media response to the change in sexual attitudes started by the Second World War appeared in the soft pornographic press of the late 1950s. The appearance of Penthouse Magazine in 1965 made its predecessors, Titbits,

Esquire, Reveille, and Men Only look very tame. For the first time a specifically sexual advice column was included but once again, like Dr. Johnson, people assumed that the letters were fictitious. 'Surely people didn't actually write about their sexual problems!'

It is true that the early editions of Penthouse laid particular emphasis on subjects like Flagellation, Transvestism, and pubic shaving but this reflected the attitude of the editorial staff rather than that of the readers. Eventually, such interest was shown that the first magazine to deal specifically with sexual attitudes and problems — Forum — was launched in April, 1968, as an offshoot from Penthouse. It has remained popular but controversial ever since. After Forum had led the way the agony columns in leading womens' magazines became far more open in their handling of sexual matters. The modern agony aunts typified by people like Clare Rayner and Anna Raeburn give sensible, sympathetic advice, backed up by a body of expert medical knowledge to prevent too many mistakes; a very effective formula.

'If you think you've got problems' was launched on the radio in the late sixties and was the first counselling programme dealing with actual relationships often, but not primarily, sexual. This was followed in 1975 by Capital Radio's Open Line on which I still work as the doctor with Anna Raeburn. This programme is extremely successful and carries the technique of the agony column onto the air. Advice on sexual problems that helps to promote a sane attitude to sex, not only in the enquirer but in all the listeners, can usually be given. The enormous popularity of this sort of programme is evidence of the continuing need of people for this form of counselling.

It is organs like these rather than the efforts of doctors and a medical environment which have changed society's attitude and in turn forced doctors to recognise new problems which we have now to become competent to solve.

In the last five years the therapeutic role of the media has also changed. One of the most obvious factors is that whilst medical sex therapists used only to see highly motivated patients who were brave enough to come out into the open with their problems the agony columns, problem magazines, radio and TV programmes reach a far wider population. The experiences of the Forum Clinic emphasise this. In 1971 a clinic for sexual problems was started by Forum Magazine and when I started to work there in 1972, whilst a Registrar at UCH, to gain experience in psychosexual problems the first thing to strike me was that the clientele were universally afraid of doctors and the clinical approach but readily responded to the non-medical atmosphere of the Clinic which was held in the Magazine's offices. What started as a simple one-off counselling service rapidly expanded; it's main task being to introduce potential patients who needed help to the idea of therapy and send them on to places where longer term treatment was available. It was the pioneering work of the Clinic that made Forum Magazine respectable and safe for doctors to identify with.

Forum went through several crises when its medical staff threatened to dissociate themselves from it when moves were made to guide it in a more pornographic direction but these were countered successfully. This sensible approach prepared potentially interested doctors for working more closely with the media.

My experiences in this field are not atypical. I have found editors and programme producers very sympathetic to the treatment role of doctors and in practice it is not difficult to satisfy both the needs of the therapist to treat and the media to entertain. Indeed, serious advice that enables the audience to identify strongly with both the doctor and the patient is one of the best forms of entertainment there is!

The standard of medical and sexual advice has risen steadily and the public response is slowly becoming more sophisticated. I second Keith Hawton's observation that the nature of the problems referred has changed. The number of people possessing insight is slowly increasing and sexual problems are no longer treated in total isolation from the enquirer's lifestyle. I have worked on Capital Radio's Open Line for five years now; it has increased its audience to an estimated 750,000 in London and South East England most of whom are regular listeners. Because of the lasting interest shown the education potential here is vast. Although people joke about it, there is no doubt that the callers are genuine and many receive help that would otherwise be unavailable; even if it is only a plea for them to visit their own doctors. Of course there is the odd 'telephone wanker' but handling these can be a useful lesson as well. I am aware of the power of the media and try always to steer a middle course as well as to work from first principles and to educate people to modify their sexual expectations of themselves and their partners.

With the regular listeners this is much easier. Week after week the same sort of problems crop up and I am able to work at conveying the same basic principles to them so that when it comes to solving their own problems they are able to take a more sensible attitude. Unfortunately, people still expect magic cures without effort from themselves and now there are actually proper 'sex therapists' who 'cure you with pills' their expectations are higher than ever. Callers to a radio programme like Open Line, like those attending the Forum Clinic, want the intimacy of a one to one relationship without the risk of an interview with the doctor. Surprisingly, even though 750,000 people may be listening it is still possible to create the atmosphere of a one to one relationship over the radio. I simply forget about the listeners and talk exclusively to the caller and it does not take long to build up a rapport. One also learns to read between the lines and make quite reasonable appraisals of their personalities. Because they are on the air, the listeners feel important and because they are talking to the Open Line team, Anna Raeburn, Adrian Love and myself, the contact is personal.

We often argue over what they are saying. They are, therefore, far more likely to remember what is said and be able to use that in future. It is important for me

244

to be able to convey the image of a doctor as approachable and sympathetic and this in turn may prepare the listener for more advanced therapy with a doctor in a real life situation later on. It also helps, of course, the process of education which is so vital in changing sexual bigotry. Alas, the image of doctors as clinical and unapproachable robs us of a great deal of our effectiveness in sex therapy.

There is no doubt that the media are going to play an increasingly important part in sex therapy by sex education programmes, agony columns, advice magazines, TV presentations and phone-in programmes so it is really up to us, the medical profession, who have both the knowledge and the common sense to learn to use this therapeutic tool more effectively. I sympathise with my colleagues who shy naturally away from any contact with the media on the grounds that they do not consider themselves to be experts and that by broadcasting they would risk the jealousy of their colleagues. You do not have to be an expert to be a good broadcaster. The technique to learn is simply to make sure of your basic facts, never to venture into fields that you know nothing about except when talking from first principles and rely on your natural sympathy for the patient to carry you through.

In Britain at the moment there are fewer than twenty doctors who broadcast regularly or who are associated with the popular press. There should be many more.

It is not surprising that the sort of problems seen for treatment have changed since Masters & Johnson started their centre in the late 1960s. The increasing sophistication of the patients and their higher expectations of themselves, in which process as I have explained the media played a vital part, are responsible. There is now a strong emphasis on taking sex therapy away from the realm of doctors, white coats, and illness into the realm of self-help organisations. This brings me to the second topic I would like to raise, briefly mentioned by Keith — that of the role of the self-help group. This offers a range of behavioural treatment and practical experience to women or couples and also a smattering of psychotherapy. In some of the womens' groups, where problems end and politics and philosophy start is often unclear. Self-help groups for inorgasmic women are often led by feminists who are primarily motivated by the ideal of freeing women from the age-old slavery; a potent and effective message. The treatment of men with similar problems seems a less attractive proposition but perhaps Maurice Yaffe can comment on this?

Traditionally, prostitutes were entrusted with the practical side of the treatment of impotent men, but alas, that is not how the prostitute sees her role. Prostitutes make a purely commercial contract with their clients which is cold and unyielding and, in my experience, usually makes men worse rather than better if they had little confidence to start with. Male prostitutes for women are a very rare commodity indeed and no substitute for the self-help group. I doubt if prostitutes as they operate at present can ever be a therapeutic proposition.

245

Indeed, a letter from the leader of the prostitutes union to me recently made this very clear. I had made the mistake of asking her to help a young Greek Cypriot whose wife was refusing him sex. She said that any emotional involvement, however superficial, was out of the question, so as a current trend in sex therapy prostitutes are out. Women on the whole are less sexually competitive than men and under greater pressure from society to conform to moral standards. Perhaps this is why the self-help group or pre-orgasmic group workshop for women is so effective. Many therapists are ardent entrepreneurs with high ideals, much practical experience, and plenty of charisma, but no medical training. Ann Hooper and Sylvia Fairbrother, who both run womens' workshops in London, are good examples. Neither have any medical training; they use brief, simple, behavioural methods. Over five or six sessions the group members discuss their sexual attitudes and experiences; many women have never done this. They go on to self-examination, learning the use of the speculum to remove their fears about their bodies and then progress to mutual massage and instruction on masturbation techniques. I have referred four women to Ann Hooper's group and have followed them up afterwards. They were all helped by her down to earth woman to woman approach and have learned to adapt towards their own femininity. Three out of four became orgasmic; a good example of what Keith Hawton describes as brief behavioural techniques in action. I have no doubt that for this sort of problem the behavioural group is far more effective than psychotherapy by itself rather like the difference between learning to swim by talking about it on the couch or getting in the water and actually doing it. Similar groups for couples aimed at removing inhibitions and increasing communication are equally helpful and use similar techniques. These, like the pre-orgasmic workshop for women, originated in America and have found a valuable place in the British scene.

In its present perilous state, the National Health Service is unlikely to expand, and its role in sex therapy is bound to remain very limited. The inevitable expansion of the field in order to meet ever-increasing demand will have to come from the very limited number of doctors practising in the private sector, from charity organisations like the Marriage Guidance Council and the Brook Advisory Centres, or from self-help groups like the ones I have mentioned right outside medical control.

So far, all the lay workers that I have met in this field have been dedicated to their task, sensitive to their patients' needs, honest, and amenable to medical advice. I am afraid it will only be a question of time, however, before people with no such scruples appear on the scene as they already have in the United States. There will be no means of checking them and they will bring the whole concept of sex therapy, with all that it means, into disrepute. In order to prevent this there will have to be far more involvement with us, the medical profession, in an advisory capacity so that by helping with the inevitable psychiatric problems as they occur we can influence the way the self-help groups develop and play a more dominant role in shaping them.

246

RESPONSE TO COMMENTARIES BY MR YAFFE AND DR WILSON

Keith Hawton

Compared with the other topics we have been discussing during this conference, sex therapy in its current form has had a very brief career. It has really only blossomed since Masters and Johnson published their treatment work in 1970. However, there is a considerable need for sex therapy in this country. Most sex therapy clinics have long waiting lists. Maurice Yaffe has referred to the frequency of sexual problems in various populations. I would like to comment on just one of those studies, that of Franks and colleagues from New York, carried out last year and published in the New England Journal of Medicine. They studied a hundred 'normal' couples and took their samples from various Rotary Clubs, so it is doubtful whether this sample can be described as normal! Nevertheless, their's and other studies have demonstrated that there are large numbers of people who require help for sexual problems.

Colin Wilson has remarked that current enthusiasm for sex therapy reflects peoples' expectations rather than their needs. I would agree that the media has had a tremendous effect on peoples' expectations, particularly the womens' magazines, many of which have set unreasonable standards. I remember one article some years ago in a glossy magazine, describing the multi-multi orgasmic female capable of having fifty orgasms in quick succession. A patient referred to me about that time complained that she could only have about eight successive orgasms and that the quality was not quite right!

While I cannot deny that sex therapy explicitly presents a value system, and I think there are dangers in this, we are seeing some elderly patients who come along only too glad to receive help for problems which they have been unhappy with for many years, who have been helped and this makes me feel that we are also meeting needs rather than just setting up expectations. I agree with Maurice Yaffe that sex therapy should not be a luxury, in view of the obvious effect of sexual problems on marriages and on the children of those marriages.

I would now like to summarise some of the developments in sex therapy as I

247

see them, and at the same time comment on the other papers. Finally I would like to summarise where we go from here.

Firstly, there have been advances in the interests of economy, so that one can meet the needs of the greatest number of patients most efficiently. Secondly, new treatment methods have been developed in the last decade. Thirdly, there have been important developments concerning the role of physical factors, especially hormones, in sexual problems.

Among developments in the interests of economy has been the increasing use of single therapists in treatment, as opposed to co-therapists as originally used by Masters and Johnson in their work. There is no conclusive evidence that work with co-therapists is superior to that with single therapists, at least not in the field of sex therapy.

In Oxford we have been treating most couples with single therapists for several years now and by doing this we have been able to treat twice the number of patients that would have been possible had we used co-therapists. However, there may be exceptions to this. There are certain situations where co-therapy may, in fact, be more useful, for example, where general marital problems, as well as specific sexual problems, exist. Michael Crowe's findings would support this. Where both partners are experiencing specific sexual dysfunctions, co-therapists may also be useful. Co-therapy also has a very useful training role. I found that I had many blind spots about female sexuality, which were revealed to me quite forcefully by a female co-therapist.

A second advance of economic relevance in sex therapy, which Maurice specifically referred to, has been the use of groups — the pre-orgasmic groups for women, started by Lonnie Barbach in California, and the treatment of couples in groups, which again Maurice has referred to. Nevertheless, I do feel that many of our clients are going to be unwilling to share their sexual problems in a group. I am referring particularly to experience in Oxford, but what is acceptable in London now may, of course, eventually be acceptable in Oxford.

The third development in the field of economy is in the use of instructional material, particularly self-help books. David Delvin's 'Book of Love' is an excellent book which we ask all our clients to read. Paul Brown and Christine Faulder's book 'Treat yourself to Sex' is also good. The use of manuals and of written postal instructions has been found to be successful for a limited number of couples.

I agree with Colin Wilson that the media have an important role to play in education, in the prevention of sexual problems and in providing advice. However, we must be cautious about this. I would like some reassurance or some evidence that advice given over the Radio or through magazines is effective. John and Judy Bancroft, as many people know, chaired a television programme called 'Man and Woman', following which they had 9000 requests for the manual which they produced in conjunction with the programme. Unfortunately, they were never able to find out how effective the manual actually was in helping viewers with their sexual problems.

Now I would like to turn to the special needs of patients and how they are being met. One aspect which Colin Wilson specifically referred to was masturbation training for women who have failed to achieve orgasm, based on the Lobitz and LoPiccolo programme which I have described briefly in my paper. In Oxford we have run two groups like this, both of which have used sexually explicit material. A film of a woman masturbating was felt to have been crucial in the achievement of orgasm by women within the group. Other than this, I have had little experience in the use of sexually explicit material in therapy, apart from my experiences in educating medical students.

Another development in the treatment of patients with special needs concerns those without partners. Until a few years ago we were all very depressed when we were faced with people who did not have partners available to help them in treatment, but now a great deal can be done to help this group. Masturbation training for women is an example of this, and treatment of premature ejaculation too can also be done on an individual basis. I feel it is important to follow up these individuals, so that in the event of them meeting a partner and making a relationship we can help with any subsequent problems that develop and make sure that the gains they made during individual treatment are not wasted. The same applies to the use of surrogate therapy, referred to earlier. Masters and Johnson actually gave up using surrogates because of the legal problems involved, particularly when they were treating an individual whose real life partner took objection to the surrogate.

A third group of patients with special needs referred to by Maurice Yaffe were medical patients. We are becoming increasingly aware of the many sexual problems that patients in medical and surgical wards face as a result of their illnesses or their operations. A particularly important group are coronary patients. I think it is our duty to educate physicians to be aware of the particular problems that these people face after their illnesses, and some of the anxieties that they have about what they can or cannot do after a coronary. Good counselling, in my experience, can do a great deal to alleviate these difficulties and to dispel the many myths which abound about sexual abilities after such episodes.

Now I would like to turn briefly to some developments in physical methods of treatment, particularly the role of hormones in treatment, and in the causation of sexual problems. As I pointed out in my paper earlier, and as Maurice Yaffe has also said, we are at a very early stage in understanding the complex interaction between hormones and sexual functioning. I would particularly like to mention testosterone and its role in the treatment of impotent males which has recently been extensively studied. In the majority of these studies, however, the hormone levels in the patients prior to treatment with testosterone were not measured. It seems probable to me that testosterone would only be useful in males who had previously low testosterone levels. I say this in spite of the enormous sale of attractively packed products containing testosterone by certain drug companies, claiming to put a tiger in their patient's tank so to speak, which are on the whole totally ineffective! In any case, we know that oral testosterone is very poorly absorbed in the gut. So, if you are intending to use hormone treatment, please get your patient's hormone levels measured at the outset, otherwise it is like giving someone a blood transfusion for supposed anaemia without ever having measured the haemoglobin beforehand!

Similar objections apply to the interest at present being paid to prolactin. There is some evidence that hyperprolactinaemia may be associated with sexual difficulties. It is, however, unlikely to be a cause of impotence, except in very few cases. Evidence so far indicates that prolactin levels have to be very high and testosterone levels lower than normal for treatment with bromocryptine to be effective. We clearly need to know a great deal more about this.

I would also like to comment briefly on the use of androgens in women with impaired libido. Although the study in Oxford mentioned on Wednesday morning indicated that women with low libido benefited from androgens in conjunction with sexual counselling, this has not been supported in clinical practice, either in Oxford, Edinburgh or London, and I think this needs further evaluation. The same objections apply to that study as applied to the previous one I mentioned; that hormone levels were neither measured before or during the study. I am glad to say Andrew Mathews is now carrying out a study in which hormone levels will be measured. Again, it seems likely to me that if androgens are going to be effective, it will only be so in the women who have low androgen levels at the outset.

The second problem I would like to mention here relates to the physically handicapped. Contrary to popular opinion, their problems are no more difficult to treat than those of people presenting normally at sexual dysfunction clinics, provided a little imagination and common sense are used. The major problem is frequently the attitude of the staff, who are too embarrassed to discuss sexual difficulties with their patients. I would also like to mention here the recent literature on the use of penile prostheses: I refer to the inflatable prosthesis, which is surgically implanted and which can be pumped up when it is required. The results from the U.S.A. indicate that this is a useful device and satisfactory for many patients who have tried it, but I wonder whether it is likely to become available here in view of the financial straits of the National Health Service. This would seem to be a particularly useful way of helping, for example, the young diabetic who has developed peripheral neuropathy and is impotent.

I would also like to comment on the use of rapid eye movement sleep in the differential diagnosis of psychogenic and organic impotence. An individual's sleep and erectile patterns are monitored to check whether erections occur at times of rapid eye movement sleep. In organically caused impotence this relationship is disturbed. There are many other assessment methods which are far simpler, do not take eight hours in the laboratory, and which are quite

effective for distinguishing between psychogenic and organic impotence. I am
thinking of procedures like testicular sensation in diabetic neuropathy:
sensation to firm squeeze on the testicles is generally impaired. Simpler
procedures such as these are more readily employed by the clinician. The paper
by Fisher, in the Archives of General Psychiatry, which Maurice Yaffe quoted
in his address, noted a mis-diagnosis rate of psychogenic and organic cases of
impotence of 15% so the method is not perfectly reliable.

Before finishing with the physical aspects of sexual disorders, I would like to
comment on the very serious side-effects of many drugs, which have been
reviewed in a number of articles recently. We are becoming increasingly aware
that many drugs used to treat important medical conditions can have a profound
effect on sexual functioning. For instance, many anticonvulsants decrease the
availability of free testosterone in the blood: blood samples of patients who
have been on Epanutin for a long time often show high testosterone levels. This
is due to an overall increase in testosterone, but the amount of free testosterone
is reduced due to induction of hormone-binding globulin. I remember seeing a
patient recently who had been on high levels of Probanthine several years
before for a short period, and had become impotent and had then remained
impotent. It was clear that his impotence had initially been caused by the
Probanthine, but that subsequently psychological factors had perpetuated the
situation.

I would like to make a few further comments on Maurice Yaffe's paper at
this stage. I agree with him that there has been a change in the approach to
treating people with deviancy problems. The focus of therapy has moved from
the deviant behaviour to a consideration of the person's sexual relationships,
and this has been far more successful.

Maurice raised a very important point in stressing that it has become
increasingly important to try to understand different cultural attitudes towards
sex. We often get referrals of people from other cultural groups, and find these
referrals particularly difficult because the cultural and language problems may
be formidable. The same problems apply to lower social class patients of our
own culture, but in a more subtle way. Sex therapy, as I said earlier, involves an
implicit value system which may not be acceptable to such patients, so I would
urge people working in this field to exercise caution. Therapists must try to
meet the needs of individual patients by setting reasonable goals even if this
means modifying their own concepts of satisfactory sex.

I was very interested to hear Maurice Yaffe's comment on the Keith Stoll
study and his findings that lower social class was often associated with poor
outcome in sex therapy. Prevention of sexual problems has been touched upon
by the other two papers. Educationalists are in a very powerful position to
implement this, although, as we all know, currently they are politically
vulnerable. Much can be done through education to dispel sexual myths. Young
people engaging in sexual encounters for the first time may be enabled to have

greater confidence and less anxiety, and this may lead to fewer sexual problems in the future.

Although I have not commented on the ethical problems of sex therapy, this matter does concern me greatly. My personal view is that sexual contact between therapist and patient is indefensible. I hope very much that this is at least one American trend which will not be followed here in Britain.

So, where do we go from here in regard to sex therapy? I agree with the first 16 of Maurice Yaffe's 17 points about research and clinical needs, although I have reservations about Japanese finger acupressure. We need to know more about what predicts a good outcome for treatment, so that therapists do not become involved in lengthy treatment with patients who are not likely to respond, and so that couples who will not respond can be offered alternative treatment methods. An extremely productive research area may concern the interaction between counselling and hormone therapy. We also need to know about the long-term durability of treatment effects. Masters and Johnson's original findings, which included a five year follow-up on their patients, were taken to indicate that the effects of sex therapy were very durable, but this was based on unsatisfactory reporting of their results. Their recent book on homosexuality indicates that their original reporting of an 18% failure rate did not necessarily imply that the remaining 82% were successes. This means that the implications of their original results are not clear. Therapists who have felt depressed in the past at not being able to reach Masters and Johnson's original high success rate can take comfort from this.

Finally, I must touch on the area of training people in sex therapy. There is an obvious need for many more people to work in this field. I am particularly interested in what constitutes the psychotherapeutic component of sex therapy. The sex therapy model provides one with a very useful behavioural framework, which a couple can follow through various stages and which is likely to lead to rewards and is, therefore, to some extent self-maintaining. However, there are blocks in treatment with every couple and psychotherapeutic skills must be used to overcome these blocks. We are currently trying to define the psychotherapeutic techniques used to overcome these difficulties in treatment. This will enable us to train people far more effectively.

I envisage that sex therapy may move out of the area of psychiatry and psychology and do not consider this to be a bad thing. In the United States, for instance, many gynaecologists practise sex therapy, although I find it difficult to imagine British gynaecologists doing the same thing. The training of general practitioners, particularly for future work in Health Centres, for instance, is a promising development. Perhaps in group practices at least one general practitioner could specialise in sexual problems. I am also glad to see that the Marriage Guidance Council trains many of its counsellors in sex therapy. I would like to see an increasing movement of sex therapy into the hands of General Practice and Marriage Guidance, and I see the future roles of psychiatrists lying in the training of other therapists, in dealing with particularly difficult cases, in the development of new treatment methods, and in research.

References

Adams, DB, Gold, AR and Burt, AD (1978) Rise in Female-Initiated Sexual Activity at Ovulation and its Suppression by Oral Contraceptives. *The New England Journal of Medicine, 229,* 1145–1150

Ambrosi, B, Bara, R, Travaglini, P, Weber, G, Peccoz, PB, Rondena, M, Elli, R and Faglia, G (1977) Studey of the Effects of Bromocriptine on Sexual Impotence. *Clinical Endocrinology, 7,* 417–21

Anderton, KJ, Copper, FS, Holdsworth, AV and Tonge, WL (1976) The Team Approach to the Outpatient Treatment of Sexual Dysfunction. *Journal of Family Planning, 1,* 6–9

Ansari, JMA (1976) Impotence: A Controlled Study. *British Journal of Psychiatry, 178,* 194–198

Arentewicz, G (1978) Partner Therapy with Sexual Dysfunctions: Final Report of a Controlled Study with 202 Couples. Paper Presented at *Third International Congress of Medical Sexology,* Rome, Oct

Bancroft, JHJ (1975) The Masters and Johnson Approach in a National Health Service Setting. *British Journal of Sexual Medicine, 1,* 6–10

Bancroft, J and Coles, L (1976) Three Years' Experience in a Sexual Problems Clinic. *British Medical Journal, 1,* 1575–7

Bancroft, JHJ (1979) Treatment of Deviant Sexual Behaviour. Ch. 18 in Gaind RR and Hudson, BL (Eds) *Current Themes in Psychiatry 2.* London: Macmillan

Barbach, LG (1974) Group Treatment of Preorgasmic Women. *Journal of Sex and Marital Therapy, 1,* 139–45

Barbach, LG (1975) *For Yourself: The Fulfilment of Female Sexuality.* Signet

Barkla, D (1977) *An Account of the NMGC Marital Sexual Dysfunction Project.* National Marriage Guidance Council

Barlow, DH (1977) Assessment of Sexual Behaviour. In: *Handbook of behavioral Assessment,* Ciminero, A; Calhoun, KJ and Adams, HE (Eds) New York: Wiley

Barragry, JM, Makin, MLJ, Trafford, DJH and Scott, DF (1978) Effects of Anticonvulsants on Testosterone and Sex Hormone Binding Globulin Levels. *Journal of Neurology, Neurosurgery and Psychiatry, 41,* 913–4

Benkert, O, Jordon, R, Danlen, IIG, Schneider, HPG and Gammel, G (1975) Sexual Impotence: A Double-Blind Study of LMRh Nasal Spray versus Placebo. *Neuropsychobiology, 1,* 203–10

Bjorksten, OJW (1976) Sexually Graphic Material in the Treatment of Sexual Disorders. Ch. 8 in Meyer, JK (Ed) *Clinical Management of Sexual Disorders.* Baltimore: Williams & Wilkins

Brown, P and Faulder, C (1977) *Treat Yourself to Sex.* Dent and Sons: London

Bruhl, DE and Leslie, CH (1963) Afrodex: Double-Blind Test in Impotence. *Medical Records and Annals, 56,* 22

Campbell, S and Whitehead, M (1977) Oestrogen Therapy and the Menopausal Syndrome. *Clinics in Obstetrics and Gynaecology, 4,* 31–47

Carney, A, Bancroft, J and Mathews, A (1978) Combination of Hormonal and Psychological Treatment for Female Sexual Unresponsiveness: A Comparative Study. *British Journal of Psychiatry, 133,* 339–46

Chipman, A (1978) Psychogenic Impotence and the Blackman's Burden. *American Journal of Psychotherapy, 32,* 603–612

Christiansen, P, Deigaard, J and Lund, M (1975) Potency, Fertility and Sexual Hormones in Young Male Epileptics. *Ugeskr. Laeg., 137,* 2402–5. (Quoted in *British Journal of Sexual Medicine, 5,* No. 34, 14–6)

Cooper, AJ, Smith, CG, Ismail, AAA and Loraine, JA (1973) A Controlled Trial of Potensan Forte in Impotence. *British Journal of Medical Science, 142,* 155–61

Copper, AJ (1974) A Blind Evaluation of a Penile Ring – A Sex Aid for Impotent Males. *British Journal of Psychiatry, 124,* 402–6

Cooper, AJ (1977) Bromocriptine in Impotence. *Lancet, ii,* 567

Crisp, AH (1979) Sexual Psychopathology in the Psychiatric Clinic. *British Journal of Clinical Practice, Supplement, 4,* 4–11

Crowe, MJ (1978) Conjoint Marital Therapy: A Controlled Outcome Study. *Psychological Medicine, 8,* 623–36

Crowe, MJ, Gillan, P and Golombok, S (1979) Form and Content in the Conjoint Treatment of Sexual Dysfunction. (In preparation)

Csillag, ER (1976) Modification of Penile Erectile Response. *Journal of Behaviour Therapy and Experimental Psychiatry, 7,* 27–9

Cullberg, J (1973) Mood Changes and Menstrual Symptoms with Different Gestrogen/Oestrogen Combinations. *Acta Psychiatrica Scandinavia,* Supplement 236

Davies, TF, Mountjoy, CQ, Gomez-Pan, A, Watson, MJ, Hankes, JP, Besser, GM and Hall, R (1976) A Double-Blind Crossover Trial of Gonadotrophin Releasing Hormone (LH–RH) in Sexually Impotent Men. *Clinical Endocrinology, 5,* 601–8

Delitala, G, Masala, A, Alagna, S and Lotti, G (1977) Luteinizing Hormone, Follicle Stimulating Hormone and Testosterone in Normal and Impotent Men Following LH–RH and HCG Stimulation. *Clinical Endocrinology, 6,* 11–15

Derogatis, LR and Meyer, JK (1979) A Psychological Profile of the Sexual Dysfunctions. *Archives of Sexual Behaviour, 8,* 201–223

Dominian, J (1979) Choice of Partner. *British Medical Journal,* 8th Sept. 594–6

Duddle, CM (1975) The Treatment of Marital Psycho-Sexual Problems. *British Journal of Psychiatry, 127,* 169–70

Everaerd, W (1976) Comparative Studies of Short-Term Treatment Methods for Sexual Inadequacies. In: Gemme, R and Wheeler, CC (Eds) *Progress in Sexology.* New York: Plenum, pp. 153–65. Selected papers from the proceedings of the 1976 International Congress of Sexology

Fisher, C, Gross, J and Zuch, J (1965) Cycle of Penile Erection Synchronous with Dreaming (REM) Sleep. *Archives of General Psychiatry, 12,* 29–45

Fisher, C, Schiavi, R, Leah, H, Edwards, A and Witkin, RL (1975) The Assessment of Nocturnal REM Erection in the Differential Diagnosis of Sexual Impotency. *Journal of Sex and Marital Therapy, 1,* 277–89

Fisher, C, Schiavi, RC, Edwards, A and Others (1979) Evaluation of Nocturnal Penile Tumescence in the Differential Diagnosis of Sexual Impotence. *Archives of General Psychiatry, 36,* 431–7

Fordney-Settlage, DS (1975) Heterosexual Dysfunction: Evaluation of Treatment Procedures. *Archives of Sexual Behaviour, 4,* 367–87

Frame, E, Anderson, C and Rubinstein, D (1978) Frequency of Sexual Dysfunction in 'Normal' Couples. *New England Journal of Medicine, 299,* 111–115

Franks, S, Jacobs, HS, Martin, N and Nabarro, JDN (1978) Hyperprolactinaemia and Impotence. *Clinical Endocrinology, 8,* 277–87

Furlow, WL (1978) The Current Status of the Inflatable Penile Prosthesis in the Management of Impotence. Mayo Clinic Experience Updated. *Journal of Urology, 119,* 363–4

Garrard, J, Vaikus, A and Chilgren, RA (1976) Follow-up Effects of a Medical School Course in Human Sexuality. *Archives of Sexual Behaviour, 5,* 331–340

Gillan, P (1978) Therapeutic Use of Obscenity. Ch. in Dhavan, R and Davies, C (Eds) *Censorship and Obscenity,* pp. 127–147. London: Martin Robertson

Gillan, P and Yaffe, M (1979) *Men's Sex Therapy Groups: The British Experience.* Paper to be presented at the Fourth World Congress in Medical Sexology. Mexico City, December

Gillan, P, Golombok, S and Becker, T (1979) The Future of Women's Sex Therapy Groups. Paper to be presented at the *Fourth World Congress of Medical Sexology,* Mexico City, December

Ginsberg, GL, Frosch, WA and Shapiro, T (1972) The New Impotence. *Archives of General Psychiatry, 26,* 218–222

Glide Foundation (1971) Effect of Erotic stimuli used – National Sex Forum Training Courses in Human Sexuality. In: *Tech. Rep. of Com. Obsc. and Porn. 5*, Societal Control Mechanism, Government Printing Office, Washington D.C.

Green, R (Ed) (1975) *Human Sexuality: A Health Practitioner's Text.* Baltimore: Williams and Wilkins

Greenblatt, RB, Mortara, F and Torpin, R (1942) Sexual Libido in the Female. *American Journal of Obstetrics and Gynaecology, 44*, 658–63

Hare-Mustin, RJ, Marecek, J, Kaplan, AG and Liss-Levinson, N (1979) Rights of Clients: Responsibilities of Therapists. *American Psychologist, 34*, 3–16

Hatch, JP (1979) Virginal Photoplethysmography: Methodal Considerations. *Archives of Sexual Behaviour, 8*, 357–74

Heath, DH (1978) Marital Sexual Enjoyment and Frustration of Professional Men. *Archives of Sexual Behaviour, 7*, 463–76

Heiman, J, Lopiccolo, L and Lopiccolo, J (1976) Becoming Orgasmic: A Sexual Growth Programme for Women. Prentice-Hall: New Jersey

Heller, CG and Myers, GB (1944) The Male Climacteric: Its Symptomatology, Diagnosis and Treatment. *Journal of the American Medical Association, 126*, 472–7

Heslinga, K (1974) *Not Made of Stone.* Charles L Thomas: Illinois

Holyroyd, JC and Brodsky, AM (1977) Psychologists' Attitudes and Practices Regarding Erotic and Non-Erotic Physical Contact with Patients. *American Psychologist, 32*, 843–9

Ismail, AAA, Davidson, DW, Loraine, JA, Cullen, DR, Irvine, WJ, Cooper, AJ and Smith, CG (1970) Assessment of Gonadal Function in Impotent Men. In: Reproductive Endocrinology (Ed) Irvine, WJ. Livingstone: Edinburgh

Kaplan, HS (1974) The New Sex Therapy. Bailliere Dindall: London

Kaplan, H, Kohl, RN, Pomeroy, WB, Offit, AK and Hogan, B (1974) Group Treatment of Premature Ejaculation. *Archives of Sexual Behaviour, 3*, 443–52

Karacan, I, Williams, RL, Thornby, JI and Salis, PJ (1975) Sleep-Related Penile Tumescence as a Function of Age. *American Journal of Psychiatry, 132*, 932–7

Karacan, I, Brantley-Scott, F, Salis, PJ, Attia, SL, Ware, JC, Altinel, A and Williams, RL (1977) Nocturnal Erections, Differential Diagnosis of Impotence and Diabetes. *Biological Psychiatry, 12*, 373–80

Karacan, Salis, Ware, Dervent, Williams, Scott, Attia and Beutler (1978) Nocturnal Penile Tumescence and Diagnosis in Diabetic Impotence. *American Journal of Psychiatry, 135*, 191–7

Kardener, S, Fuller, N and Mensh, I (1973) A Survey of Physicians' Attitudes and Practices Regarding Erotic and Non-Erotic Contact with Patients. *American Journal of Psychiatry, 130*, 1077–81

Kardener, S, Fuller, M and Mensh, I (1976) Characteristics of 'Erotic' Practitioners. *American Journal of Psychiatry, 133*, 1324–5

Kegel, AH (1952) Sexual Function of the Pubococcygeus Muscle. *Western Journal of Obstetrics and Gynaecology, 60*, 521

Keller, DJ and Goldstein, A (1978) Orgasmic Reconditioning Reconsidered. *Behaviour Research and Therapy, 16*, 299–301

Kilmann, PR and Auerbach, R (1979) Treatments of Premature Ejaculation and Psychogenic Impotence: A Critical Review of the Literature. *Archives of Sexual Behaviour, 8*, 81–100

Kockott, MD, Dittmar, F and Musseett, L (1979) Systematic Desensitization of Erectile Impotence: A Controlled Study. *Archives of Sexual Behaviour, 4*, (5)

Lansky, MR and Davenport, AE (1975) Difficulties in Brief Conjoint Treatment of Sexual Dysfunction. *American Journal of Psychiatry, 132*, 177–9

Latham, JD and White, GD (1978) Coping with Homosexual Expressions within Heterosexual Marriages: Five Case Studies. *Journal of Sex Marital Therapy, 4*, 198–212

Lawrence, DM and Swyer, GIM (1974) Plasma Testosterone and Testosterone Binding Affinities in Men with Impotence, Oligospernia, Asoospernia and Hypogonadism. *British Medical Journal 1*, 349–51

Leiblum, SR and Ersner-Hershfield, R (1977) Sexual Enhancement Groups for Dysfunctional Women: An Evaluation. *Journal of Sex and Marital Therapy, 3*, 139–52

Levin, RJ and Levin, A (1975) *Sexual Pleasure: The Surprising Preference of 100,000 Women.* New York Red Books

Lobitz, WC and Baker, EL (1979) Group Treatment of Single Males with Erectile Dysfunctions. *Archives of Sexual Behaviour, 8,* 127–38

Lobitz, WC and Lopiccolo, J (1972) New Methods in the Treatment of Sexual Dysfunction. *Journal of Behaviour Therapy and Experimental Psychiatry, 3,* 265

Lopiccolo, J and Lobitz, WC (1972) The Role of Masturbation in the Treatment of Orgasmic Dysfunction. *Archives of Sexual Behaviour, 2,* 163–71

Luhdorf, K, Christiansen, P, Hansen, JM and Lund, M (1977) The Influence of Phenytoin and Carbamazepine on Endocrine Function: Preliminary Results. In: *Epilepsy: Proceedings of the 8th International Symposium.* Ed Penry, JK. New York: Raven Press

McGovern, K, Stervart, R and Lopiccolo, J (1975) Secondary Orgasmic Dysfunction: I. Analysis and Strategies for Treatment. *Archives of Sexual Behaviour, 4,* 265–75

McMullen, SJ and Rosen, RC Self-Administered Masturbation Training in the Treatment of Primary Orgasmic Dysfunctions. (I Press)

Malloy, TR and Voneschenbach, AC (1977) Surgical Treatment of Erectile Impotence with Inflatable Penile Prosthesis. *Journal of Urology, 118,* 49–51

Masters, WH and Johnson, VE (1970) *Human Sexual Inadequacy.* Churchill: London

Masters, WH and Johnson, VE (1976) In: *Ethical Issues in Sex Therapy and Research* Ed Masters, WH and Johnson, VE and Kolodny, RC. Little, Brown & Co., Boston

Masters, WH, Johnson, VE and Kolodny, RC (Eds) (1977) *Ethical Issues in Sex Therapy and Research.* Boston: Little Brown

Mathews, A, Bancroft, J, Whitehead, A, Hackman, A, Julier, D, Bancroft, J, Gath, D and Shaw, P (1976) The Behavioural Treatment of Sexual Inadequacy: A Comparative Study. *Behaviour Research and Therapy, 14,* 427–36

Meyer, JK, Schmidt, CW, Lucas, MJ and Smith, ES (1975) Short-Term Treatment of Sexual Problems: Interim Report. *American Journal of Psychiatry, 132,* 172–6

Meyer, JK (Ed) (1976) *Clinical Management of Sexual Disorders.* Baltimore: Williams & Wilkins

Milne, HB (1976) The Role of The Psychiatrist. In: *Psycho-Sexual Problems* (Ed Milne, H and Hardy, SJ). Bradford University Press

Money, J (1977) Paraphilias. In: Handbook of Sexology. (Eds) Money, J and Mustaph, H. Amsterdam: Elsevier/N-Holland

Mortimer CH, McNeilly, AS, Fisher, RA, Murray, MAF and Besser, GM (1974) Gonadotrophin-releasing Hormone Therapy in Hypogonadal Males with Hypothalamic or Pituitary Dysfunction. *British Medical Journal, 4,* 617–21

Moulton, R (1977) Some Effects of the New Feminism. *American Journal of Psychiatry, 134,* 1–6

Munjack, D, Cristol, A, Goldstein, A, Phillips, D, Goldberg, A, Whille, K. Staples, F and Kanno, P (1976) Behavioural Treatment of Orgasmic Dysfunction: A Controlled Study. *British Journal of Psychiatry, 129,* 497–502

Munjack, DJ and Kanno, PH (1979) Retarded Ejaculation: A Review. *Archives of Sexual Behaviour, 8,* 139–150

Obler, M (1973) Systematic Desensitisation in Sexual Disorders. *Journal of Behaviour Therapy and Experimental Psychiatry. 4,* 93–101

O'Connor, JF (1976) Sexual Problems, Therapy and Prognostic Factors. In: Clinical Management of Sexual Disorders (Ed) Mayer, JK. Baltimore: Wilkins & Wilkins

Ohashi, W (1977) Do-It-Yourself SHIATSU. New York: Mandala

Pope, KS, Levenson, H and Schover, LR (1979) Sexual Intimacy in Psychology Training: Results and Implications of a National Survey. *American Psychologist, 34,* 682–9

Qualls, CB, Wincze, J and Barlow, DH (1978) The Prevention of Sexual Disorders: Issues and Approaches. New York: Plenum

Raboch, J, Mellan, J and Starka, L (1975) Plasma Testosterone in Male Patients with Sexual Dysfunction. *Archives of Sexual Behaviour, 4,* 541–5

Racey, PA, Ansari, MA, Rowe, PH and Glover, TD (1973) Testosterone in Impotent Men. Journal of Endocrinology, 59, xxiii

Redmond, AC (1978) Common Sexual Dysfunctions. In: *Clinical Psychopathology*, (Eds) Baylis, GU, Wurmser, L, McDaniel, E and Grenele, RG. *The Psychiatric Foundation of Medicine, 4*, Boston: Butterworth

Reisinger, JJ (1978) Effects of Erotic Stimulation and Masturbatory Training Upon Situational Orgasmic Dysfunction. *Journal of Marital Sex Therapy, 4*, 177–185

Riley, AJ and Riley, EJ (1978) A Controlled Study to Evaluate Directed Masturbation in the Management of Primary Orgasmic Failure in Women. *British Journal of Psychiatry, 133*, 404–9

Rosen, RC (1977) Operant Control of Sexual Responses in Man. In: *Biofeedback: Theory and Research* (Ed) Schwartz and Beatty, J. Academic Press: London

Rosen, RC and Keefe, FJ (1978) The Measurement of Human Penile Tumescence. *Psychophysiology, 15*, (4): 366–76

Rosen, RC and Kopel, SA (1977) Penile Plethysmography and Biofeedback in the Treatment of a Transvestite–Exhibitionist. *Journal of Cons. Clinical Psychology, 45*, 908–16

Rosenzweig, N, Pearsall, FP (1978) *Sex Education for the Health Professional: A Curriculum Guide*. New York: Grune & Stratton

Royal College of General Practitioners (1974) *Oral Contraceptives and Health*. Pitman, London

Salmon, UJ and Geist, SH (1943) The Effects of Androgens upon the Libido in Women. *Journal of Clinical Endocrinology, 3*, 235–8

Semans, JH (1956) Premature Ejaculation: A New Approach. *Southern Medical Journal, 49*, 353–7

Shorr, E, Papanicolaou, GN and Stimmel, BJ (1938) Neutralisation of Ovarian Follicular Hormone in Women by Simultaneous Administration of Male Sex Hormone. *Proceedings of the Society of Experimental Biology and Medicine, 38*, 759–62

Stanley, E (1977) *A Course in Human Sexuality for Medical Students* at St George's Hospital. *British Journal of Family Planning, 3*, 16–17

Stewart, WFR (1975) *Sex and the Physically Handicapped*. National Fund for Research into Crippling Diseases, Horsham Sussex

Stewart, WFR (1978) Sexual Fulfilment for the Handicapped. *British Journal of Hospital Medicine*, 676–80

Taylor, BJ and Wagner, NN (1976) Sex Between Therapists and Clients: A Review and Analysis. *Professional Psychology, 7*, 593–601

Thorner, MO and Besser, GM (1977) Hyperprolactinaemia and Gonadal Function. In: *Prolactin and Human Reproduction*, (Ed) Grosignami, PG and Robyn, C. Academic Press, London

Thorn, B and Collard, J (1979) *Who Divorces*. London: Routledge & Keegan Paul

Trimmer, E (1979) Sexual Dysfunctions. *British Medical Journal*, 7th July: 28–30

Turner, P (1978) Effects of Drugs on Sex and Bladder Function. *Prescriber's Journal, 18*, 94–8

Victor, A, Lundberg, PO and Johansson, EDB (1977) Induction of Sex Hormone Binding Globulin by Phenytoin. *British Medical Journal, 2*, 934–5

Vinarova, E and Uhlir, O, Stika, L and Vinar, O (1972) Side Effects of Lithium Administration. *Activitas Nervosa Superior, 14*, 105–7

Wallace, DH and Barbach, LG (1974) Preorgasmic Group Treatment. *Journal of Sex and Marital Therapy, 1*, 146–54

Whitehead, A and Mathews, A (1977) Attitude Change During Behavioural Treatment of Sexual Inadequacy. *British Journal of Social and Clinical Psychology, 16*, 275–81

Wilson, WC (1978) Can Pornography Contribute to the Prevention of Sexual Problems? Ch. 7 in: The Prevention of Sexual Disorders: Issues and Approaches. (Eds) Brandon Qualls, Wincze and Barlow. New York: Plenum

Wincze, JP and Caird, WK (1976) The Effects of Systematic Desensitisation and in the Treatment of Essential Sexual Dysfunction in Women. *Behaviour Therapy, 7*, 335–342

Wishnoff, R (1978) Modelling Effects of Explicit and Non-Explicit Sexual Stimuli on the Sexual Anxiety and Behaviour of Women. *Archives of Sexual Behaviour, 7*, (5), 455–61

Wright, J, Perreault, R and Matthieu, M (1979) The Treatment of Sexual Dysfunctions: A Review. *Archives of General Psychiatry, 34,* 881–90

Yaffe, M (1979) The Therapeutic Uses of Sexually Explicit Materials. Paper Presented at: Symposium on Aspects of Psychosexual Problems. Liverpool: April 1979

Zeiss, RA, Christensen, A and Levine, AG (1978) Treatment for Premature Ejaculation Through Male Only Groups. *Journal of Sex and Marital Therapy, 4,* 139–43

Zilbergeld, B (1975) Group Treatment of Sexual Dysfunctions in Men Without Partners. *Journal of Sex and Marital Therapy, 1,* 204–214

Zilbergeld, B (1978) *Men and Sex: A Guide to Sexual Fulfilment.* London: Souvenir

258